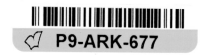

Wolf-Heidegger's

Atlas of
Human Anatomy
Volume 1

Petra Köpf-Maier, Berlin

Wolf-Heidegger's

Atlas of Human Anatomy

Volume 1
**Systemic Anatomy, Body Wall,
Upper and Lower Limbs**

5th, completely revised
and supplemented edition, 2000

586 figures of which 452 are in color

KARGER

Editor
Univ.-Prof. Dr. med. Petra Köpf-Maier
Professor of Anatomy
Freie Universität Berlin
Königin-Luise-Strasse 15
D–14195 Berlin (Germany)

This Atlas is published in two volumes:
Volume 1: Systemic Anatomy, Body Wall, Upper and Lower Limbs
Volume 2: Head and Neck, Thorax, Abdomen, Pelvis, CNS, Eye, Ear

Until 1989 the Atlas was published as
'Atlas of Systematic Human Anatomy', vol. I–III
1st edition 1954
2nd edition 1960
3rd edition 1972
Spanish translation: Salvat Editores S.A., Barcelona
Portuguese translation: Editors Guanabara Koogan S.A., Rio de Janeiro

4th edition 1990
Published as 'Wolf-Heidegger's Atlas of Human Anatomy'
Japanese translation: Nishimura Co., Ltd., Tokyo
Indonesian translation: Penerbit Widya Indonesia, Jakarta

The original Latin nomenclature version with German and English captions is also available under the titles: "Wolf-Heideggers Atlas der Anatomie des Menschen"/ "Wolf-Heidegger's Atlas of Human Anatomy"
Bd./Vol. 1: Allgemeine Anatomie, Rumpfwand, obere und untere Extremität/Systemic Anatomy, Body Wall, Upper and Lower Limbs: ISBN 3–8055–6754–5
Bd./Vol. 2: Kopf und Hals, Brust, Bauch, Becken, ZNS, Auge, Ohr/Head and Neck, Thorax, Abdomen, Pelvis, CNS, Eye, Ear: ISBN 3–8055–6755–3
Complete set: ISBN 3–8055–5442–7

Library of Congress Cataloging-in-Publication Data

Wolf-Heidegger's atlas of human anatomy. — 5th, completely rev. and supplemented [English] ed. / [editor] Petra Köpf-Maier.
p.   cm.
"The original Latin nomenclature version with German and English captions is available under the titles: 'Wolf-Heideggers Atlas der Anatomie des Menschen'/ 'Wolf-Heidegger's Atlas of Human Anatomy'" — T.p. verso.
Includes bibliographical references and index.
Contents: v. 1. Systemic anatomy, body wall, upper and lower limbs —
           v. 2. Head and neck, thorax, abdomen, pelvis, CNS, eye, ear.
ISBN 3–8055–6852–5 (v. 1: hardcover). – ISBN 3–8055–6853–3 (v. 2: hardcover) –
ISBN 3–8055–6854–1 (complete set: hardcover)
1. Human anatomy Atlases.   I. Wolf-Heidegger, G. (Gerhard)
II. Köpf-Maier, P. (Petra)   III. Title: Atlas of human anatomy.
[DNLM: 1. Anatomy atlases.   QS 17 W859 1999]
QM25.W633   1999b
611'.022'2—dc21
DNLM/DLC
for Library of Congress   99-33383
                                                                  CIP

KARGER

Basel · Freiburg · Paris · London · New York · New Delhi · Bangkok · Singapore · Tokyo · Sydney

© Copyright 2001 by S. Karger AG,
P.O. Box, CH–4009 Basel (Switzerland)
Printed in Switzerland on acid-free paper by Reinhardt Druck, Basel
ISBN 3–8055–6852–5

The editor dedicates
this book to her grandson

Leander Leonin

Homage to Those Who Bequeathed Their Bodies to Science

'Hic locus est ubi mors gaudet succurrere vitae'

'This is the place where death delights in helping life'
(Inscription above the Anatomical Theatre of Bologna)

The present atlas of human anatomy shall not begin without paying due homage and returning thanks to those who freely bequeath their bodies to anatomy. Such donations testify to an admirable, unselfish, and idealistic sense of sacrifice and nothing can compensate for the invaluable service rendered to science and society. Anatomy and medicine owe these individuals a tremendous debt of gratitude. By bequeathing their bodies, they enable medical students to learn through real observation and direct 'grasping', and even now, at the end of the twentieth century, there is no alternative to this. Thus, even beyond death, these altruistic people help the living – medical students, physicians, and their patients alike. This is how the above inscription should be interpreted. Students should make every endeavour to be worthy of these voluntary and generous body donations by respecting and honoring the dead as well as by working hard and learning eagerly.

Contents

VIII Preface to the 5th Edition
IX Preface to the 1st Edition
X Concept of the New Version of the Atlas and
Illustration Credits
XII Information for Users

1–26 Systemic Anatomy

2–5 Skeleton, parts, regions, and axes of the body
6 Body types
7–10 Motor system
11 Skin
12–14 Cardiovascular system
15–17 Lymphoid and organ systems
18–21 Surface projections of thoracic and abdominal viscera
22–25 Central and peripheral nervous systems

27–80 Body Wall

28–39 Vertebral column and vertebrae
40–45 Thorax, ribs, and sternum
46–51 Joints and ligaments of the vertebral column
52 Surface anatomy of the back
53–59 Muscles of the back
60–61 Blood vessels and nerves of the back
62 Surface anatomy of the thorax and abdomen
63–68 Muscles of the ventral body wall and inguinal region
69 Diaphragm
70–74 Breast and axilla
75–79 Blood vessels and nerves of the ventral body wall

81–168 Upper Limb

82–94 Bones of the pectoral girdle and upper limb
95–104 Joints of the pectoral girdle and upper limb
105 Surface anatomy of the upper limb
106–113 Muscles of the shoulder and arm
114–119 Muscles of the forearm
120–129 Muscles of the hand
130–131 Tendinous sheaths of the hand
132–134 Cutaneous innervation of the upper limb and
brachial plexus
135–143 Blood vessels and nerves of the shoulder and arm
144–149 Sections and tomograms of the arm
150–155 Blood vessels and nerves of the forearm
156–159 Sections and tomograms of the forearm
160–165 Blood vessels and nerves of the hand
166–167 Sections and tomograms of the hand

169–282 Lower Limb

170–189 Bones of the pelvis and lower limb
190–215 Joints of the pelvis and lower limb
216–217 Surface anatomy of the lower limb
218–229 Muscles of the hip and thigh
230–235 Muscles of the leg
236–241 Muscles of the foot
242–244 Cutaneous innervation of the lower limb and
lumbosacral plexus
245–247 Lymphatic vessels and veins of the lower limb
248–257 Blood vessels and nerves of the gluteal region
and thigh
258–265 Sections and tomograms of the thigh
266–271 Blood vessels and nerves of the leg
272–277 Sections and tomograms of the leg
278–281 Blood vessels and nerves of the foot

283 Subject Index

Contents of Volume 2:
Head and Neck, Thorax, Abdomen, Pelvis, CNS, Eye, Ear

Preface to the 5th Edition

Macroscopic anatomy is a fundamental branch of medicine without which clinical facts cannot be understood.

Throughout history, the importance of anatomy for medicine – and thus for medical studies – has fluctuated considerably. Five hundred years ago, at the end of the Renaissance, Leonardo da Vinci and Andreas Vesal laid the foundation stones of modern anatomy and modern medicine. In those days, anatomy – then exclusively macroscopic – was the only fundamental speciality medical students were confronted with during their studies, along with the clinical subjects internal medicine, surgery and botany (in the meaning of use of herbal drugs).

The first half of the twentieth century saw the development of microscopic anatomy besides macroscopic anatomy; physiology became an independent speciality and physiological chemistry and biochemistry made huge progress. Research in these fields provided new knowledge on functional and molecular interactions in the mammalian organism which fundamentally altered our understanding of diseases and opened new perspectives in clinical diagnosis and therapy. As a consequence of these developments, macroscopic anatomy was somehow relegated to the background during the 1960s and 1970s, and seemed to have retained its essential importance only for surgical specialities.

Apart from these developments, new diagnostic imaging technologies have become clinically established in the second half of the twentieth century: computed tomography, magnetic resonance imaging, and ultrasonography. These imaging techniques opened up new visions of the morphology of the living organism, enabled a very detailed identification of structures and thus laid the foundation stone of rapid and unexpected progress in clinical diagnosis. However, the interpretation of normal and pathologically altered structures in two-dimensional images of the human body with all these techniques demands extremely precise anatomical knowledge. In recent years, this has led to the revival and to a considerable increase in the significance of macroscopic anatomy both for clinical medicine and the education of medical students.

Successful clinical work without well-founded knowledge in topographical and sectional anatomy is thus no longer possible. This is the reason why the editor urges present and future medical students to study macroscopic anatomy intensively.

As a matter of fact, it is the establishment of the new imaging techniques in clinical medicine that prompted this new revised version of Professor Wolf-Heidegger's Atlas of Human Anatomy, which had been continued by H. Frick, B. Kummer, and R. Putz in its 4th edition, and the supplementation of its 5th edition with numerous anatomical sections, computed and magnetic resonance imaging tomograms and ultrasonograms. Such a new design of an atlas of the anatomy of the whole human body is only possible with the collaboration of many enthusiastic forces. Thus I am deeply indebted to Dr.

R. Andresen and Priv.-Doz. Dr. D. Banzer (Berlin) for most of the new radiographs as well as the computed and magnetic resonance tomograms included in this atlas. Prof. Dr. G. Bogusch (Berlin), Prof. Dr. E. Fleck (Berlin), Dr. M. Jäckel (Göttingen), Dr. H. Kellner (Munich), Priv.-Doz. Dr. T. Riebel (Berlin), Priv.-Doz. Dr. C. Sohn (Heidelberg), Dr. D. Zeidler (Berlin) and Prof. Dr. W.G. Zoller (Munich) contributed some further radiographs, tomograms and ultrasonograms for which I would like to thank them.

I am moreover deeply indebted to Prof. Dr. M. Herrmann (Ulm) who provided the anatomical sections for most of the computed and magnetic resonance tomograms of the present atlas and thus considerably enriched it. The sections on which these illustrations are based were prepared and photographed by Mr. E. Voigt (Ulm), whom I would like to thank as well.

Valuable help in translating the Latin terms of the original Latin nomenclature version into English equivalents was contributed by Prof. A.W. English, Ph.D. (Atlanta, Georgia, USA). I thank him very much for his engagement.

I also express my thanks to Mrs. G. Heymann-Monhof, Mr. H. Jonas, Mrs. H. Heinen, Mrs. I. Tripke, Mrs. C. Naujok and Mr. F. Geisler who prepared about 230 new anatomical drawings for the present edition.

My special thanks go to Dr. h.c. Th. Karger for his constructive collaboration during the past years. Dr. Karger always lent an understanding ear to my concepts, which were often difficult and expensive to realize, and was a partner whose expert advice and understanding always helped me in my work with the atlas. Many thanks in particular to Mr. B. Pfäffli as well as to all the personnel of S. Karger Publishers and Neue Schwitter AG who helped in the production of Wolf-Heidegger's atlas.

Mrs. M. Risch, my secretary, has been a great and dependable help over the past years, which has eased my work in many respects. I would like to thank her as well.

This new edition of Wolf-Heidegger's Atlas of Systematic Human Anatomy has been supplemented by numerous new anatomical drawings, radiographs, tomograms, ultrasonograms and anatomical sections. As the editor, I am confident that this new edition will indeed 'help one to see' – one of the most difficult things, according to the quote from Goethe, which Wolf-Heidegger chose as the motto for the first edition of his atlas – and that it will give medical students better access to anatomy and clinical medicine:

'What is the hardest of aught? What seemeth the simplest to you: With your eyes to see that which is in front of your eyes.'

Johann Wolfgang von Goethe,
Distichon 155 of the 'Xenien' (translated by M. Pfister, Berlin)

Berlin, Spring 1999   Petra Köpf-Maier

Preface to the 1st Edition

«Was ist das Schwerste von allem? Was dir das Leichteste dünket:
Mit den Augen zu sehn, was vor den Augen dir liegt.»*

Accustomed during his school years to place greater trust in the written word than in his own senses, the young medical student in his first pre-clinical term is faced with a problem which Goethe aptly describes as 'hardest of all': He has to learn how to see. To teach him to do so, by the aid of anatomical preparations and plates as the most effective means at his disposal, is the foremost task of the pre-clinical instructor. The aim of the present Atlas is to give to the medical student and to the physician wishing to revise his anatomical knowledge a picture, as true and exact as possible, of the organs of our human body. The drawings were made partly from specimens preserved in the large collection of the Basle Anatomical Institute, partly from special preparations. Nearly all the plates in the section on muscles were drawn from fresh preparations in order to exclude the deformities caused by preservation. Our aim was always to avoid individual peculiarities and, by using a larger number of similar preparations, to produce as general and universal a picture as possible. With a few exceptions, noted in the legends, the right side of the body was always chosen in all bilaterally symmetrical organs or parts.

We were for a long while undecided whether or not the illustrative material should be accompanied by a short written text. As stated above, we are of the opinion that the Atlas is the primary aid in anatomical instruction, but it neither can nor should be a substitute for the detailed textbook and the spoken word; these are indispensable in preparing the student for what he is to see and in fixing what he has seen firmly in his mind. Students tend to regard a short Atlas text as a source of information sufficient for their needs, but it can never deal exhaustively with all noteworthy and necessary aspects of the subject; we therefore decided finally to publish the present volume without text, but to pay great attention to the labelling of the separate illustrations. The Atlas can thus be used in combination with any textbook of anatomy. On the other hand, for the sake of clarity, care was taken not to overload the separate plates with too many pointers; thus, parts and details which have already been shown are not re-labelled in plates in which they are not important for purposes of instruction. Sketches of the body surface, copied partly from well-known sculptures, have been inserted beside the plates showing the superficial muscular layers; it is hoped that these will help the student and qualified doctor to fit the muscle relief into the body of the patient. X-ray photographs of all important skeletal parts and junctures have been included with the intention of preparing the student for a form of examination which is of vital importance in clinical medicine and only possible on the basis of a sound knowledge of the normal anatomical picture. We had also planned, and partly completed, some treatment of general morphology, constitutional types, evolution, and the mechanics of joints, also a summarising survey in tabular form of the musculature; but all this had to be omitted in order to keep the volume of handy size and accessible price for the student.

Pending the establishment – we hope at a not too distant date – of a standard anatomical nomenclature, internationally recognised and scientifically and linguistically acceptable, we have made use in the present work of the Jena nomina anatomica; this is the terminology most widely used in the German-speaking countries. The Basle nomenclature has, however, been substituted for a few linguistically incorrect or in our opinion inappropriate terms.

I wish to take this oppportunity of expressing once again may sincere thanks to the publisher, Dr Heinz Karger, who by his energy and expert knowledge, his optimism and kindly, confident encouragement has made possible the wearisome and costly realisation of this work. I wish to thank further my faithful artistic collaborators: Mr Adolph Dressler (junctures), Mr Rolf Muspach (osteology), and above all Mr Robert Schlumpf (myology), who as sculptor with many years' dissecting room experience has in the course of our prolonged collaboration far surpassed his original function as artist and become a knowledgeable and indispensable scientific colleague, invaluable at every stage of the work from the preparation of muscle specimens to the typographical composition of the plates and the correction of proofs. For untiring and invaluable help I owe sincere thanks to my former Viennese assistant, Dr Arthur von Hochstetter (now Fribourg, Switzerland). Nearly all the X-ray photographs I owe to the kindness of Dr Emil A. Zimmer (Basle/Berne). For important suggestions and active help I wish to thank in particular my kind and highly esteemed anatomy instructor, Professor Eugen Ludwig, M.D. (Basle), and also Dr Walter Bejdl (Vienna/Basle), Dr Leopold Drexler (Vienna), Mr Willy Jäggi of S. Karger Ltd., Dr Walter Krause (Vienna), Dr Kurt S. Ludwig (Basle), Dr Carl Rudolf Pfaltz (Basle), Professsor Joseph Tomasch, M.D. (Kingston, Canada; formerly Vienna/Basle), Mr Armin Wolf, dissector (Basle), and Dr Wolfgang Zürcher (Basle).

In deep gratitude I wish finally to pay tribute to the memory of my mother who by her devoted and untiring energy made it possible for me, after the early death of my father, to follow the profession of my choice and thus to bring this Atlas into being.

Basle, Autumn 1953   Gerhard Wolf-Heidegger

* J.W. Goethe: 'Xenien.' From the posthumous papers.
   Weimar Edition, Vol. 5, part 1, p. 275, No. 45, 1893.

Concept of the New Version of the Atlas and Illustration Credits

The present 5th edition of the *Atlas of Human Anatomy,* published in 1954, 1960, and 1972 by Professor Dr. Gerhard Wolf-Heidegger and edited in 1990 by Prof. Dr. H. Frick, Prof. Dr. B. Kummer, and Prof. Dr. R. Putz, has been thoroughly revised in several aspects and supplemented in comparison to the previous four editions.

1. Retained Anatomical Drawings

The classical drawings of the three previous editions prepared by Wolf-Heidegger and his illustrators have been retained, recolored and – in the case of black-and-white drawings – colored didactically in order to make them clear also for beginners. Moreover, most of the figures prepared by Frick, Kummer, and Putz for the 4th edition, were revised and incorporated into the current 5th edition.

2. New Anatomical Pictures

The original illustrations of the previous four editions have been supplemented with about 230 new, mostly topographical drawings. These drawings were realized by six illustrators from Berlin, whom I would like to thank here for their enthusiasm. First of all, Mrs. Gertrud Heymann-Monhof, who possesses the talent to represent anatomical situations both true to detail and in an aesthetically convincing fashion. Mr. Hendrik Jonas drew most of the new illustrations of the locomotor apparatus and the head and succeeded very well in maintaining them in the style of the earlier editions. Mrs. Hildegard Heinen prepared numerous schematized drawings in a didactically clear manner. Other, mostly smaller drawings were done by Mrs. Ilona Tripke; three illustrations whose originals had been lost where painted in water colors by Mrs. Corinna Naujok. Mr. Frank Geisler prepared some new pictures and revised several others of the last edition.

Mrs. Gertrud Heymann-Monhof
Volume 1: Cover picture; Figs. 18, 19, 20, 21, 48b,c, 54b, 59, 60c, 75, 77a,b, 79a, 82, 83, 87a, 134a, 170, 171, 244a, 246a–c, 253, 254
Volume 2: Cover picture; Figs. 79, 95a, 107a, 113, 115b, 118a, 160c, 166, 172, 209a–c, 211b, 227, 243a, 250a,b, 251a,b, 256a–c, 285a, 336a, 342, 352, 382a, 395c

Mr. Hendrik Jonas
Volume 1: Figs. 90a,b, 99a, 103a, 123b, 125a–c, 127a–c, 131a–d, 137b,c, 138a,b, 155a, 163a, 167c–e, 175b, 176c, 177b, 181e, 189a–c, 191a,b, 193c, 196a,b, 200b–e, 201b–e, 209b, 213b, 220b, 221a,b, 225a,b, 226b, 249b,c, 250a,b, 257a–c, 280b
Volume 2: Figs. 264a,b, 265a, 276b, 277b, 281a,b, 290a,b, 292a, 321a,b, 324b, 325b, 329a,b, 332a,b, 368a, 369a,b, 394a,b, 395a, 399a

Mrs. Hildegard Heinen
Volume 1: Figs. 40b,c, 41b,c, 67a,b, 69b,c, 71c, 73a
Volume 2: Figs. 95b,c, 106b, 114c, 122b, 123b, 137a–c, 144a–c, 145a–c, 146a,c, 147a,c, 178b, 212a, 235b,c, 237b, 246b,c, 247a,b, 272a–e, 273a,b, 392a,b,d

Mrs. Ilona Tripke
Volume 1: Figs. 5c, 23b, 24, 63b, 79, 134b, 244b, 248b, 249a
Volume 2: Figs. 45b, 49b, 60a,b, 80a, 81a, 84a,b, 86b, 87b, 88b, 89b, 90b,c, 183c, 184a,b, 199b, 214b–e, 231b, 249, 293a–c, 371d, 379a, 382b, 383b

Mrs. Corinna Naujok
Volume 1: Fig. 252
Volume 2: Figs. 320a,b

Mr. Frank Geisler
Volume 1: Figs. 6a–c, 18, 19, 20, 21
Volume 2: Figs. 27b, 53a,b, 405a

Other anatomical illustrations, that is 3D reconstructions of the coronary arteries (Vol. 2, Figs. 148a–d), were contributed by Prof. Dr. Eckart Fleck and Dr. Helmut Oswald, Deutsches Herzzentrum Berlin. I acknowledge Dr. Martin Jäckel, Universitätsklinik Göttingen, for the laryngoscopic pictures in Volume 2 (Figs. 69a–d) of the present atlas, and Prof. Dr. Dieter Sasse, Universität Basel, for giving us access to the Anatomical Collection of the University of Basel and allowing Hansjörg Stöcklin to photograph the corrosion casts of the pulmonary, hepatic and renal vessels for the present atlas (Vol. 2, Figs. 115a, 119a, 183a, 213c, 214a).

3. Presentation of Imaging Techniques

The present atlas also aimed at giving imaging techniques due attention. Most radiographs, CT[1] and MRI[2] images published in the previous edition were technically superseded and, thus, replaced by new pictures. Besides conventional radiographs, the editor was anxious to incorporate computed and MRI tomograms of the whole human body and to represent ultrasonography by some selected images. For an anatomist, this could only be achieved by the close collaboration with enthusiastic radiologists: two radiologists from Berlin, Dr. Reimer Andresen and Priv.-Doz. Dr. Dietrich Banzer, Krankenhaus Zehlendorf, Behring-Krankenhaus Berlin. They have both untiringly searched for 'normal' anatomical images, which proved much more difficult and time-consuming than expected. Most MRI tomograms were done by use of a Philips Gyroscan ACS-NT MRI tomograph which had fortunately been installed a few years ago in the Zehlendorf Hospital.

[1] CT = Computed tomography, computed tomogram
[2] MRI = Magnetic resonance imaging, magnetic resonance image

Nearly 200 radiographs, CT and MRI tomograms as well as ultrasonograms were taken from Dr. Reimer Andresen's and Priv.-Doz. Dr. Dietrich Banzer's 'treasury':

Volume 1: Figs. 3a,b, 7b, 8d, 33b, 36a,b, 37b, 38a,b, 39b, 43, 45d, 51a,b, 55c, 71a,b, 73b, 85b, 87b, 91a,b, 93a,b, 97a,b, 100a,b, 101a,c, 103c, 106b, 120, 121, 123a, 129b, 137a, 139, 144b, 145b, 146b, 147b, 149a–c, 151b, 155b, 156b, 157b, 158b, 159b, 163b, 164b, 166a, 167a, 173a,b, 181f, 185, 188c, 194a,b, 195a–c, 197a,b, 202a–c, 203a–c, 204a,c,e, 205, 208b, 209a, 210a,b, 247a,b, 251, 258c,d, 259b, 260b, 261b, 262b, 263b, 264b, 265b, 269, 272b, 273b, 274b, 275b, 276a–c, 281a,b

Volume 2: Figs. 5, 7, 12b, 26c,d, 41b, 43c, 53c,d, 59a, 61a,b, 71a–c, 72a, 75a, 78, 110a, 118b, 119b, 126, 127, 128a, 129a, 130a, 131a, 156a, 157a, 159a,b, 175a–c, 182a,b, 186b,d, 188b, 189c,d, 194b, 197a,b, 198b, 201a,b, 203b, 208c, 215a–e, 217a,b, 218c, 219, 221, 223b, 224b, 229, 244b, 253a,b, 255a,b, 257a–c, 259a–c, 261a,b, 271b, 278a,b, 287a–c, 305, 336b, 339, 341, 343, 347, 349, 367b, 378b, 385a,b, 387a,b

Moreover, I gratefully acknowledge the following colleagues for other radiographs and ultrasonograms:

Prof. Dr. Eckart Fleck and Dr. Helmut Oswald, Deutsches Herzzentrum Berlin:
Volume 2: Figs. 136a–c, 138a–h, 146b,d, 147b,d

Dr. Martin Jäckel, HNO-Klinik, Universität Göttingen:
Volume 2: Figs. 9, 11, 395b, 406a–c, 407a–c

Dr. Herbert Kellner, Medizinische Poliklinik, Klinikum Innenstadt, Universität München:
Volume 1: Fig. 173c

Priv.-Doz. Dr. Thomas Riebel, Strahlenklinik, Virchow-Klinikum, Humboldt-Universität Berlin:
Volume 1: Fig. 177a

Priv.-Doz. Dr. Christof Sohn, Frauenklinik, Universität Heidelberg:
Volume 2: Figs. 74a, 238b, 242a–d, 245b,c

Dr. Diethmar Zeidler, dentist, Berlin:
Volume 2: Figs. 40e,f

Prof. Dr. Wolfram Zoller, Medizinische Poliklinik, Klinikum Innenstadt, Universität München:
Volume 2: Figs. 185a, 186c, 199c, 210e, 218b, 236b,c

I thank Prof. Dr. Gottfried Bogusch, formerly Institut für Anatomie der Freien Universität Berlin, now Humboldt-Universität Berlin, for giving me the permission to inspect the collection of radiographs and tomograms set up by him and to use the following pictures for the atlas:
Volume 1: Figs. 194a, 199a,b, 214b, 222b
Volume 2: Figs. 23c, 59b, 73a, 74a, 107a, 158a,b, 160a,b 161a,b, 176b, 213a, 222b, 225b, 278c,d, 301b, 302a,b

4. Anatomical Sections

In order to facilitate the understanding of the radiological sections (CTs and MRIs), the present atlas was designed to enable direct comparison with anatomical sections. While many institutes of anatomy pay attention to sectional anatomy, only few institutes possess complete series of sections of the whole human body. I would like to thank very much Prof. Dr. Martin Herrmann and Mr. Ernst Voigt, Abteilung Anatomie der Universität Ulm, for these illustrations; Mr. Voigt prepared and photographed all the sections.

A total of 90 anatomical sections contributed by Prof. Dr. M. Herrmann, Universität Ulm, have been included in the present new edition of Wolf-Heidegger's atlas:

Volume 1: Figs. 37a, 39a, 60b, 101b,d, 103b, 129a, 144a, 145a, 146a, 147a, 148a,b, 156a, 157a, 158a, 159a, 166b, 167b, 204b,d,f, 208a, 211, 258a,b, 259a, 260a, 261a, 262a, 263a, 264a, 265a, 272a, 273a, 274a, 275a, 277a–c

Volume 2: Figs. 62a,b, 63a,b, 68c, 72b, 73b, 74b, 75b, 128b, 129b, 130b, 131b, 156b, 157b, 158c, 159c, 164, 165, 213b, 220, 222a, 223a, 224a, 225a, 252a,b, 254a,b, 258a–c, 260a,b, 355a,b, 356a,b, 357a,b, 358a,b, 359a,b, 360a,b, 361a,b, 362a,b, 386a,b, 400b,c, 408a,b

5. Organization

The first three editions of Wolf-Heidegger's *Atlas of Systematic Human Anatomy* were published in three volumes organized in a somewhat modified manner according to the classical division into three parts:
Volume 1: Bones, joints, muscles
Volume 2: Viscera, skin, sensory organs
Volume 3: Nervous system, vascular system

In the 4th edition, prepared by H. Frick, B. Kummer, and R. Putz, the main contents of the previous three volumes were concentrated into one volume and reorganized according to topographical aspects.

The present 5th edition is divided into two volumes; the topographical arrangement of the illustrations has been taken over from the 4th edition, but the chapters have been arranged as follows:
Volume 1: Systemic anatomy, body wall, upper and lower limbs
Volume 2: Head and neck, thorax, abdomen, pelvis, central nervous system, eye, and ear.

This arrangement is based on the organization of the dissection courses into two main parts in many institutes of anatomy:
Part 1 – dissection of the locomotor apparatus: Ventral and dorsal body wall, upper and lower limbs
Part 2 – dissection of the viscera: Thorax, abdomen, pelvis, neck, head, brain

This division of the atlas into two volumes should make it easier for students to carry the atlas around during the dissection course and should moreover facilitate future supplementations.

Information for Users

1. Anatomical Nomenclature

In the present atlas, the designation of anatomical structures follows the most current international anatomical nomenclature, the *Terminologia Anatomica* (TA), in its latest edition of 1998. In this edition of the TA, a list of English terms in common usage was taken up for the first time. The American English variants of these terms (e.g., cecum instead of caecum, esophagus instead of oesophagus, fiber instead of fibre, gray instead of grey, tenia instead of taenia) were used throughout in the present atlas. Many of the synonyms that appear in the TA are listed in the subject index, an arrow referring to the main term given by the TA.

2. Abbreviations

In some cases, the following abbreviations were used:

Singular			Plural		
a.	=	artery	aa.	=	arteries
br.	=	branch	brr.	=	branches
cut.	=	cutaneous			
eth.	=	ethmoidal			
fem.	=	femoral			
inf.	=	inferior			
lig.	=	ligament	ligg.	=	ligaments
m.	=	muscle	mm.	=	muscles
n.	=	nerve	nn.	=	nerves
post.	=	posterior			
r.	=	ramus	rr.	=	rami
rad.	=	radiation			
rt.	=	right			
sup.	=	superior			
v.	=	vene	vv.	=	venes

3. Brackets

Parentheses ( ) are used to note terms also shown in parentheses in the TA, and for designating varieties, additional information, and explanations. Moreover, in the legends, the relative size of images referred to the originals is given as percentage in parentheses.

Commonly used, but not official TA terms are noted in pointed parentheses ⟨ ⟩.

Numbers of vertebrae and cranial nerves are placed in square brackets [ ], as in the TA.

4. Dashes

A dash *following* (left column) or *preceding* (right column) an entry indicates that one or several specific entries for the same body part will follow. The generic term is shown above it – usually without a pointer:

Examples	*Body of fibula*	or	*Infraclavicular part*
	Lateral surface –		*of brachial plexus*
	Anterior border –		*– Lateral cord*
	Medial surface –		*– Medial cord*
	Interosseous border –		*– Posterior cord*

5. Pointers and Dots

If dots on a pointer identify two or more anatomical structures or if several dots appear on a pointer, the various designations are separated by a comma; their order follows that of the arrangement of the anatomical structures in the figure. In both columns, the labelings are arranged according to the following principle: left first, then right; in the case of branched pointers, above first, then below.

6. Notation of Sizes

Unless otherwise indicated in the legends, the anatomical drawings in the present atlas always represent the situation in adults; the percentages given in parentheses in the legends denote the relative size of the image referred to the original. With a view to the considerable biological variations in body size, the percentages have been rounded off and should only be considered as indicative.

7. MRI Tomograms

Enhancement of the tissue-specific relaxation parameters T_1 and T_2 in MRI tomograms is noted in the legends as T_1 or T_2 weighting. T_1- and T_2-weighted tomograms represent the various structures of the human body in different brightnesses and different contrasts. Thus, in T_1-weighted tomograms, liquid-filled spaces are shown black, muscles dark, and the bone marrow white. In T_2-weighted tomograms, liquid-filled spaces appear white, bones dark, and muscles light gray.

8. Tomograms and Anatomical Sections

In current clinical practice, transverse computed and magnetic resonance imaging tomograms of the human body are always viewed from caudal, that is from below and looking up. This is the reason why, in the present atlas, the anatomical sections – with the few exceptions noted in the legends – are also viewed from caudal, that is from the feet of the patient. While this view of the tomograms and sections is doubtless difficult for beginners, it does correspond to the physician's perspective when he approaches the supine patient from the foot end of the patient's bed. The accompanying figure illustrates this view from caudal (bottom) to cranial (top) and makes clear that in this perspective the organs located on the patient's right (R) side appear on the left in the figure and the organs located on the left (L) side appear on the right side of the figure.

R 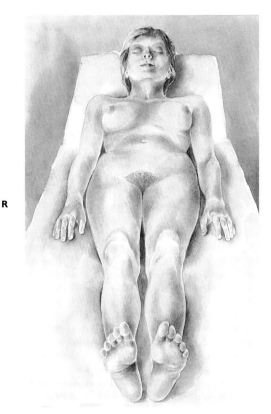 L

(Painted by G. Heymann-Monhof, Berlin)

Systemic Anatomy

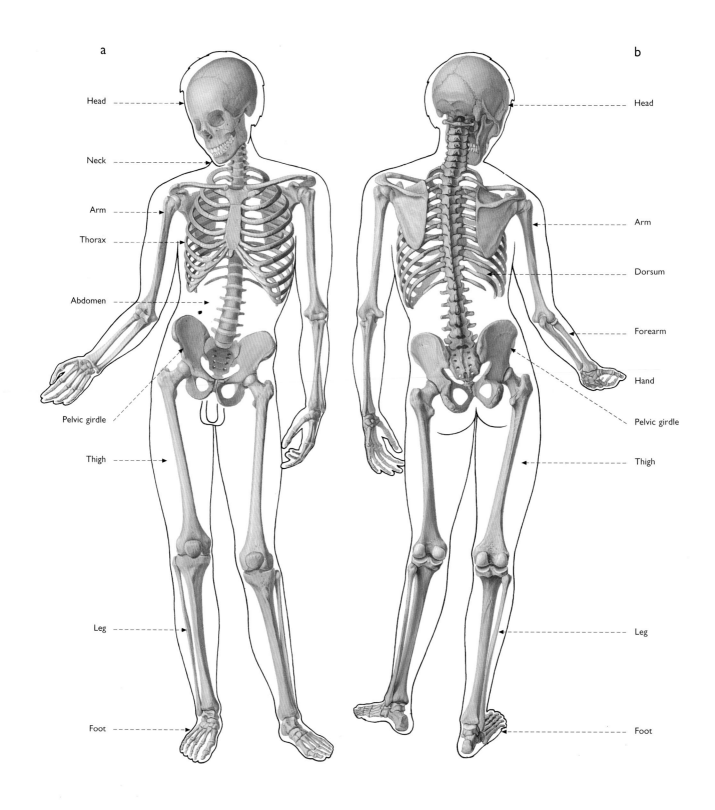

a   b

Head   Head

Neck

Arm   Arm

Thorax

                                                  Dorsum

Abdomen

                                                  Forearm

                                                  Hand

Pelvic girdle   Pelvic girdle

Thigh   Thigh

Leg   Leg

Foot   Foot

2 Skeleton and parts of the human body (10%)

    Male skeleton
a Ventral aspect
b Dorsal aspect

3 Skeleton of the human body (10%)

Male skeleton, scan of bones using ^{99m}Tc

a Ventral aspect
b Dorsal aspect

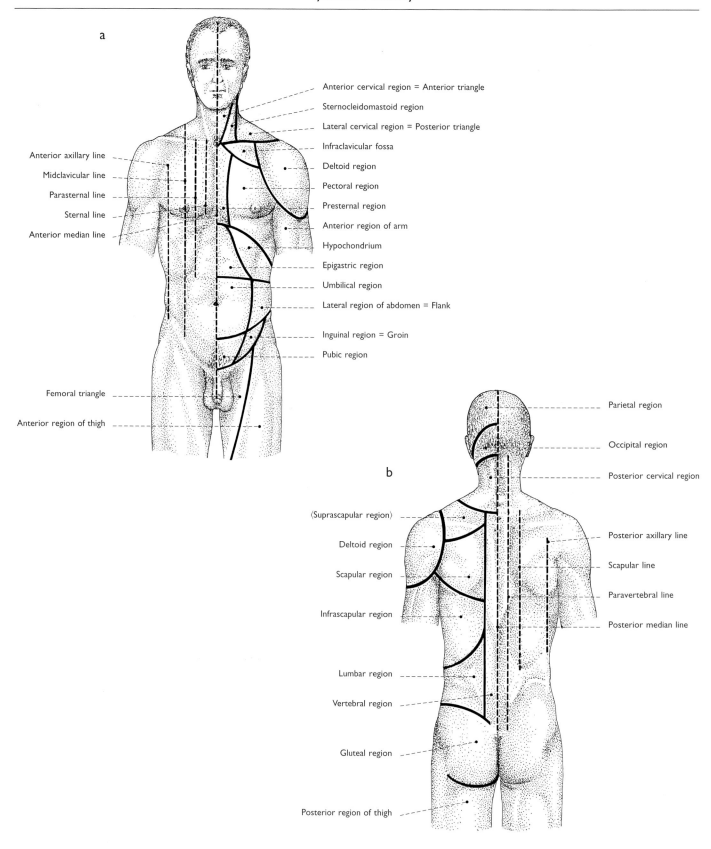

a

Anterior cervical region = Anterior triangle
Sternocleidomastoid region
Lateral cervical region = Posterior triangle
Infraclavicular fossa
Deltoid region
Pectoral region
Presternal region
Anterior region of arm
Hypochondrium
Epigastric region
Umbilical region
Lateral region of abdomen = Flank
Inguinal region = Groin
Pubic region

Anterior axillary line
Midclavicular line
Parasternal line
Sternal line
Anterior median line

Femoral triangle
Anterior region of thigh

b

Parietal region
Occipital region
Posterior cervical region

⟨Suprascapular region⟩
Deltoid region
Scapular region
Infrascapular region

Posterior axillary line
Scapular line
Paravertebral line
Posterior median line

Lumbar region
Vertebral region

Gluteal region

Posterior region of thigh

4 Regions and lines of the human body
a   Ventral aspect
b   Dorsal aspect

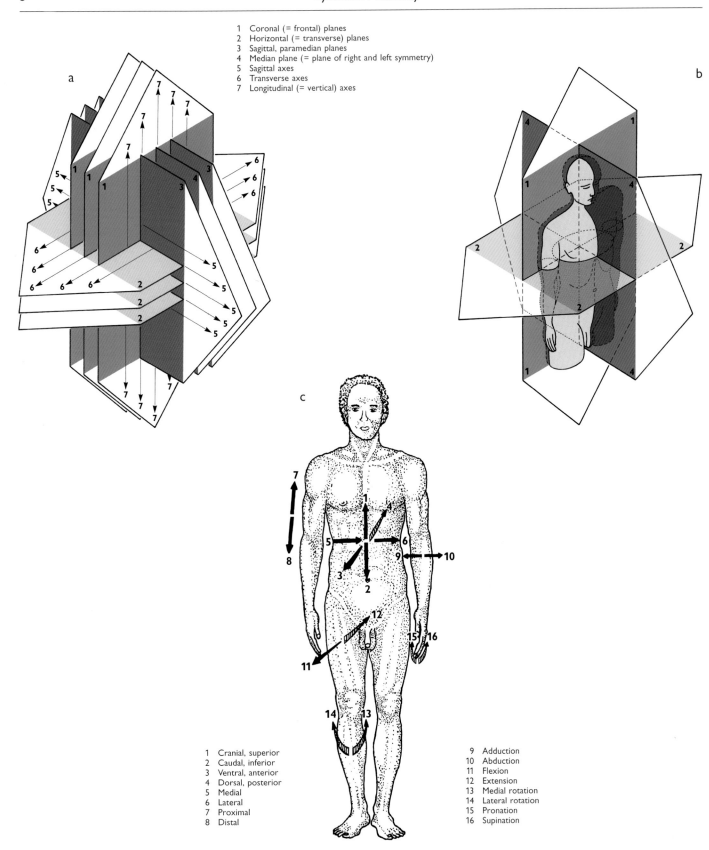

1 Coronal (= frontal) planes
2 Horizontal (= transverse) planes
3 Sagittal, paramedian planes
4 Median plane (= plane of right and left symmetry)
5 Sagittal axes
6 Transverse axes
7 Longitudinal (= vertical) axes

1 Cranial, superior	9 Adduction
2 Caudal, inferior	10 Abduction
3 Ventral, anterior	11 Flexion
4 Dorsal, posterior	12 Extension
5 Medial	13 Medial rotation
6 Lateral	14 Lateral rotation
7 Proximal	15 Pronation
8 Distal	16 Supination

5 Planes and axes

a Planes and axes
b Planes
c Spatial orientations and directions of motion

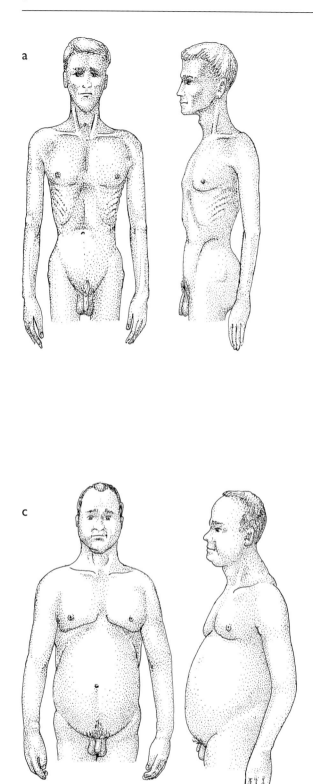

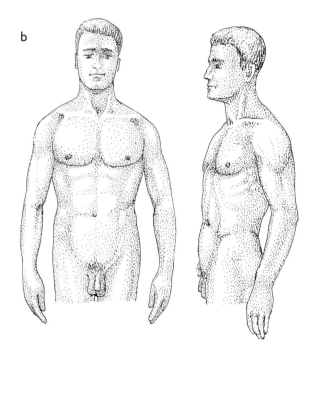

a

b

c

6 Body types

Ventral and lateral aspects
a Leptosomatic person
b Athletic person
c Eurysomatic, pyknic person

a

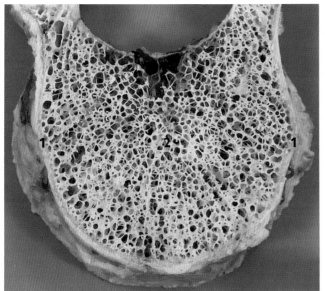

b

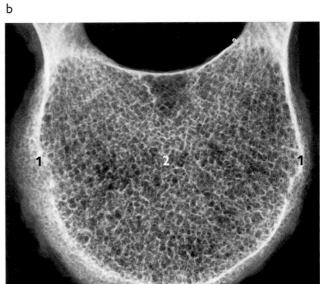

1   Compact bone
2   Spongy bone

c

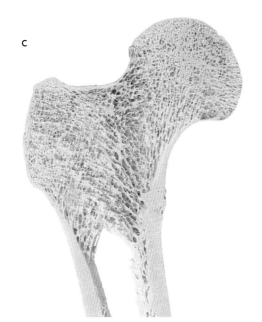

d

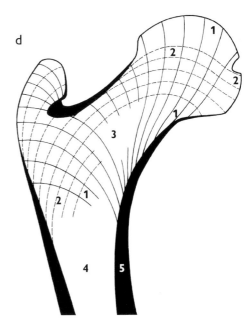

1   Compressive stress trajectories (solid lines)
2   Tensile stress trajectories (dashed lines)
3   WARD's triangle
4   Medullary cavity
5   Compact bone of shaft

7   Compact and spongy bone

a, b   Vertebral body (200%) (R. Andresen, Berlin)
   a   Anatomical cross-section
   b   Corresponding radiograph
c, d   Trabecular architecture, proximal end of the femur (80%)
   c   Coronal section
   d   Stress trajectories

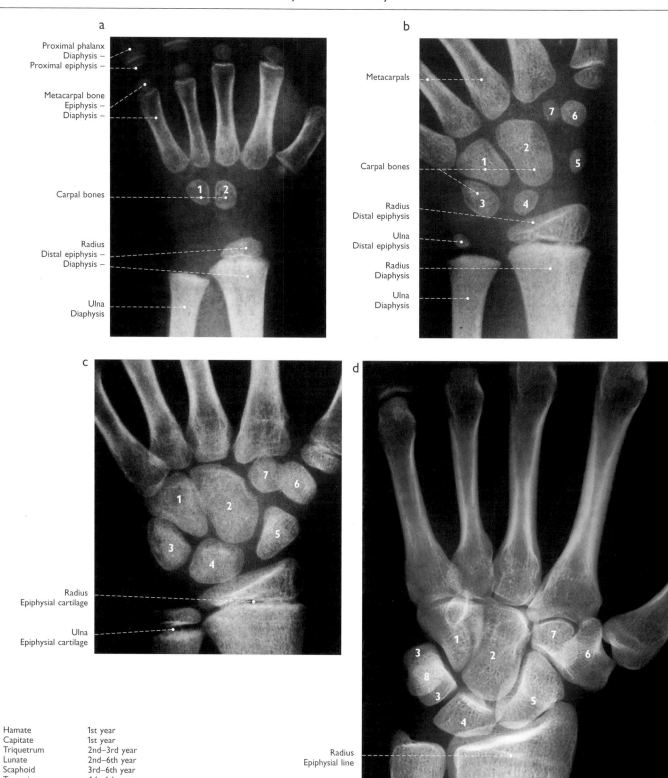

a
Proximal phalanx
Diaphysis –
Proximal epiphysis –
Metacarpal bone
Epiphysis –
Diaphysis –
Carpal bones
Radius
Distal epiphysis –
Diaphysis –
Ulna
Diaphysis

b
Metacarpals
Carpal bones
Radius
Distal epiphysis
Ulna
Distal epiphysis
Radius
Diaphysis
Ulna
Diaphysis

c
Radius
Epiphysial cartilage
Ulna
Epiphysial cartilage

d
Radius
Epiphysial line

1	Hamate	1st year
2	Capitate	1st year
3	Triquetrum	2nd–3rd year
4	Lunate	2nd–6th year
5	Scaphoid	3rd–6th year
6	Trapezium	4th–6th year
7	Trapezoid	4th–6th year
8	Pisiform	8th–12th year

8 Development of bones

Dorsopalmar radiographs of the hand (100%)
a 1st year of life
b 2nd year of life
c 12th year of life
d 26th year of life

a

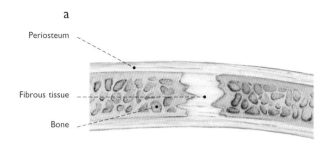

Periosteum

Fibrous tissue

Bone

b

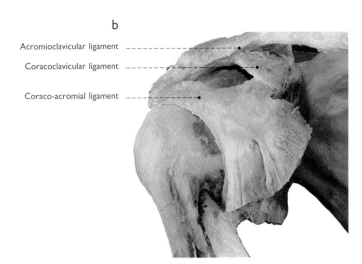

Acromioclavicular ligament

Coracoclavicular ligament

Coraco-acromial ligament

c

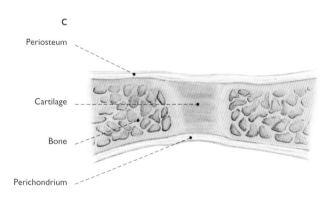

Periosteum

Cartilage

Bone

Perichondrium

d

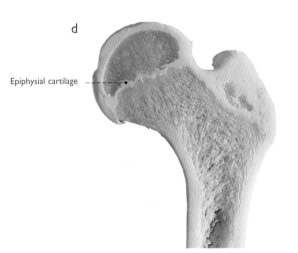

Epiphysial cartilage

e

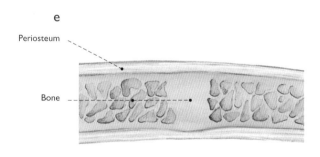

Periosteum

Bone

f

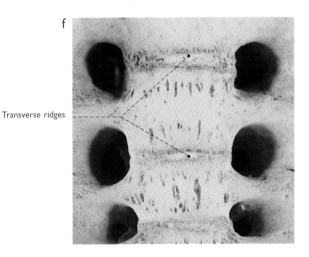

Transverse ridges

9 Joints

a Fibrous joint (syndesmosis)
b Example, ligaments of the glenohumeral girdle (75%), ventral aspect
c Cartilaginous joint (synchondrosis)
d Example, epiphysial cartilage in the proximal part of the femur
    of a 12-year-old child (75%), coronal section
e Bony union (osseous joint, synostosis)
f Example, sacrum (200%), ventral aspect

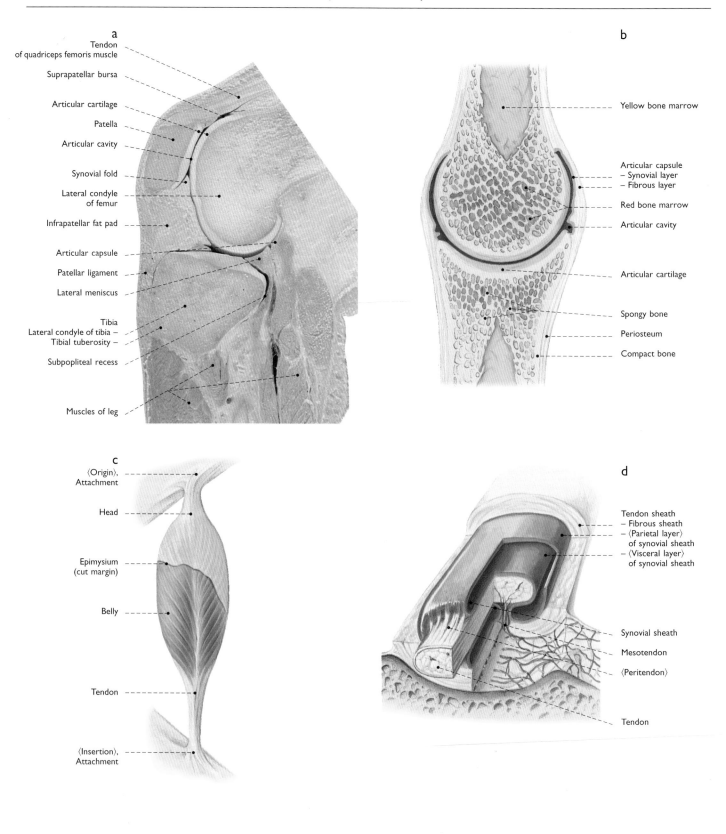

a
Tendon
of quadriceps femoris muscle
Suprapatellar bursa
Articular cartilage
Patella
Articular cavity
Synovial fold
Lateral condyle
of femur
Infrapatellar fat pad
Articular capsule
Patellar ligament
Lateral meniscus
Tibia
Lateral condyle of tibia –
Tibial tuberosity –
Subpopliteal recess
Muscles of leg

b
Yellow bone marrow
Articular capsule
– Synovial layer
– Fibrous layer
Red bone marrow
Articular cavity
Articular cartilage
Spongy bone
Periosteum
Compact bone

c
⟨Origin⟩,
Attachment
Head
Epimysium
(cut margin)
Belly
Tendon
⟨Insertion⟩,
Attachment

d
Tendon sheath
– Fibrous sheath
– ⟨Parietal layer⟩
of synovial sheath
– ⟨Visceral layer⟩
of synovial sheath
Synovial sheath
Mesotendon
⟨Peritendon⟩
Tendon

10 Synovial joint (diarthrosis), muscle and tendon
a Flexed right knee joint, sagittal section (60%),
   medial aspect of the lateral part
b Schematized section through a spheroidal joint
c Parts of a muscle
d Tendon sheath, schematic representation

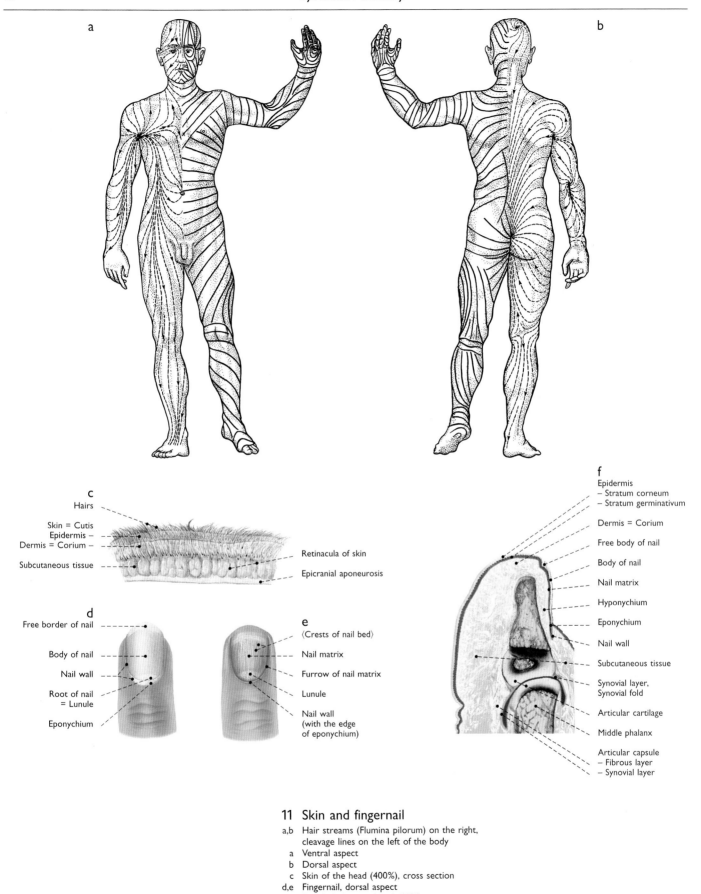

a

b

c

Hairs

Skin = Cutis
Epidermis –
Dermis = Corium –

Subcutaneous tissue

Retinacula of skin

Epicranial aponeurosis

d

Free border of nail

Body of nail

Nail wall

Root of nail
= Lunule

Eponychium

e

⟨Crests of nail bed⟩

Nail matrix

Furrow of nail matrix

Lunule

Nail wall
(with the edge
of eponychium)

f

Epidermis
– Stratum corneum
– Stratum germinativum

Dermis = Corium

Free body of nail

Body of nail

Nail matrix

Hyponychium

Eponychium

Nail wall

Subcutaneous tissue

Synovial layer,
Synovial fold

Articular cartilage

Middle phalanx

Articular capsule
– Fibrous layer
– Synovial layer

11　Skin and fingernail

a,b　Hair streams (Flumina pilorum) on the right,
　　　cleavage lines on the left of the body
　a　Ventral aspect
　b　Dorsal aspect
　c　Skin of the head (400%), cross section
d,e　Fingernail, dorsal aspect
　d　Distal phalanx with nail (80%)
　e　Distal phalanx without body of nail (80%)
　f　Distal phalanx (200%), longitudinal section

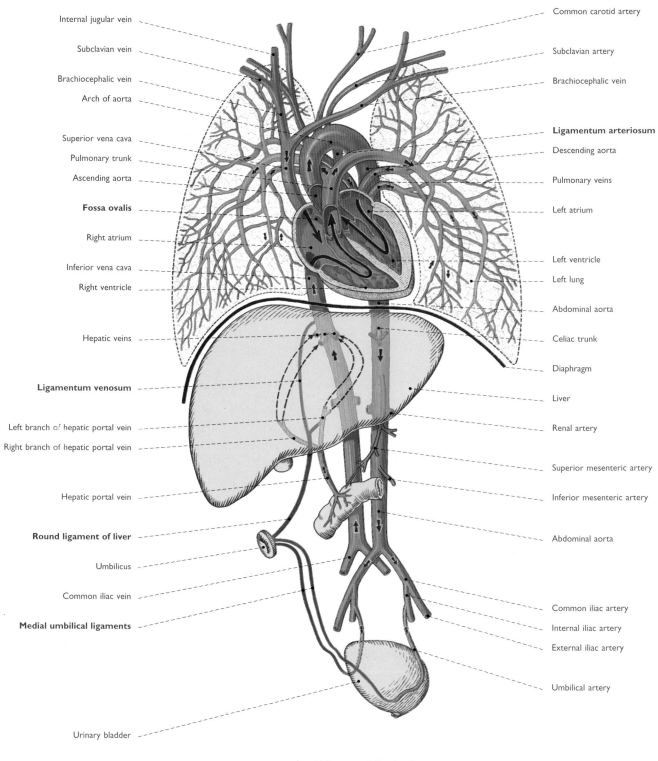

Internal jugular vein

Subclavian vein

Brachiocephalic vein

Arch of aorta

Superior vena cava

Pulmonary trunk

Ascending aorta

Fossa ovalis

Right atrium

Inferior vena cava

Right ventricle

Hepatic veins

Ligamentum venosum

Left branch of hepatic portal vein

Right branch of hepatic portal vein

Hepatic portal vein

Round ligament of liver

Umbilicus

Common iliac vein

Medial umbilical ligaments

Urinary bladder

Common carotid artery

Subclavian artery

Brachiocephalic vein

Ligamentum arteriosum

Descending aorta

Pulmonary veins

Left atrium

Left ventricle

Left lung

Abdominal aorta

Celiac trunk

Diaphragm

Liver

Renal artery

Superior mesenteric artery

Inferior mesenteric artery

Abdominal aorta

Common iliac artery

Internal iliac artery

External iliac artery

Umbilical artery

Arterial (oxygenated) blood **red**,
venous (deoxygenated) blood **blue**,
obliterated embryonic vessels **brown**

12 Adult cardiovascular system
Ventral aspect

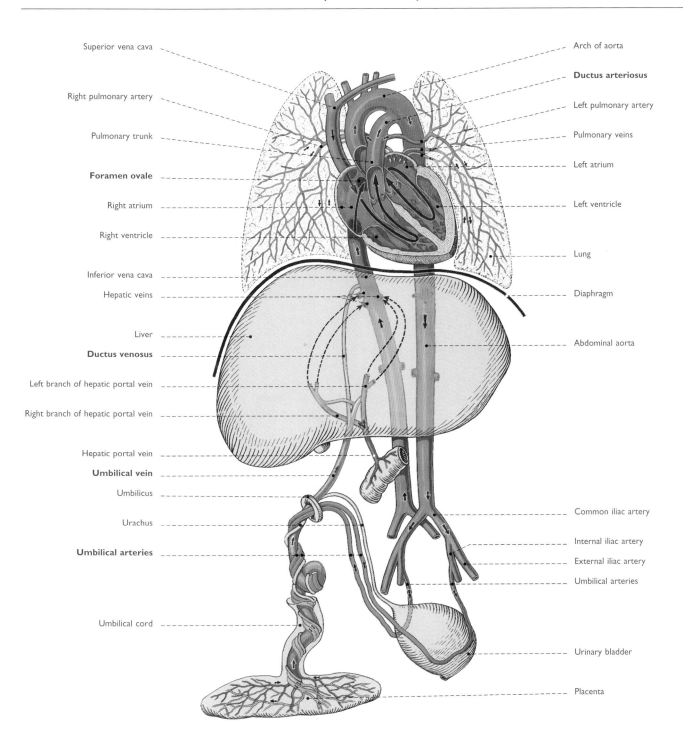

Superior vena cava

Right pulmonary artery

Pulmonary trunk

Foramen ovale

Right atrium

Right ventricle

Inferior vena cava

Hepatic veins

Liver

Ductus venosus

Left branch of hepatic portal vein

Right branch of hepatic portal vein

Hepatic portal vein

Umbilical vein

Umbilicus

Urachus

Umbilical arteries

Umbilical cord

Arch of aorta

Ductus arteriosus

Left pulmonary artery

Pulmonary veins

Left atrium

Left ventricle

Lung

Diaphragm

Abdominal aorta

Common iliac artery

Internal iliac artery

External iliac artery

Umbilical arteries

Urinary bladder

Placenta

Arterial (oxygenated) blood **red**,
venous (deoxygenated) blood **blue**,
mixed blood **violet**

13 Fetal cardiovascular system
Ventral aspect

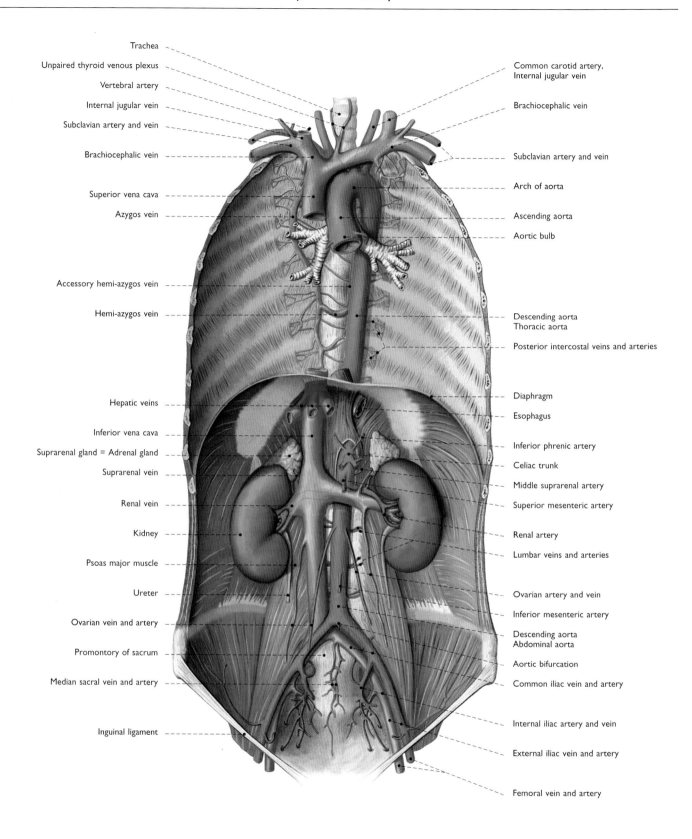

Trachea

Unpaired thyroid venous plexus

Vertebral artery

Internal jugular vein

Subclavian artery and vein

Brachiocephalic vein

Superior vena cava

Azygos vein

Accessory hemi-azygos vein

Hemi-azygos vein

Hepatic veins

Inferior vena cava

Suprarenal gland = Adrenal gland

Suprarenal vein

Renal vein

Kidney

Psoas major muscle

Ureter

Ovarian vein and artery

Promontory of sacrum

Median sacral vein and artery

Inguinal ligament

Common carotid artery,
Internal jugular vein

Brachiocephalic vein

Subclavian artery and vein

Arch of aorta

Ascending aorta

Aortic bulb

Descending aorta
Thoracic aorta

Posterior intercostal veins and arteries

Diaphragm

Esophagus

Inferior phrenic artery

Celiac trunk

Middle suprarenal artery

Superior mesenteric artery

Renal artery

Lumbar veins and arteries

Ovarian artery and vein

Inferior mesenteric artery

Descending aorta
Abdominal aorta

Aortic bifurcation

Common iliac vein and artery

Internal iliac artery and vein

External iliac vein and artery

Femoral vein and artery

14 Blood vessels of the trunk (30%)
Ventral aspect

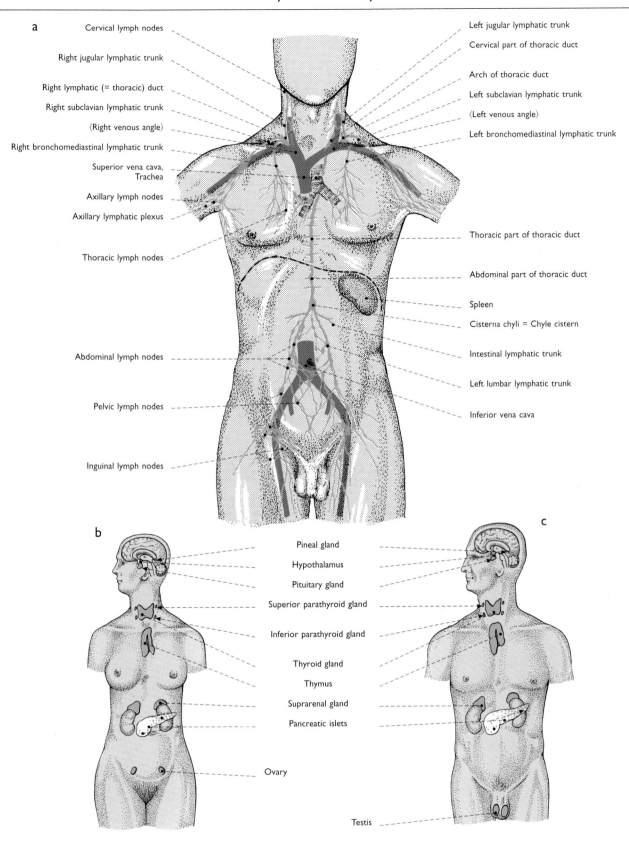

a

Cervical lymph nodes

Right jugular lymphatic trunk

Right lymphatic (= thoracic) duct

Right subclavian lymphatic trunk

⟨Right venous angle⟩

Right bronchomediastinal lymphatic trunk

Superior vena cava, Trachea

Axillary lymph nodes

Axillary lymphatic plexus

Thoracic lymph nodes

Abdominal lymph nodes

Pelvic lymph nodes

Inguinal lymph nodes

Left jugular lymphatic trunk

Cervical part of thoracic duct

Arch of thoracic duct

Left subclavian lymphatic trunk

⟨Left venous angle⟩

Left bronchomediastinal lymphatic trunk

Thoracic part of thoracic duct

Abdominal part of thoracic duct

Spleen

Cisterna chyli = Chyle cistern

Intestinal lymphatic trunk

Left lumbar lymphatic trunk

Inferior vena cava

b   c

Pineal gland

Hypothalamus

Pituitary gland

Superior parathyroid gland

Inferior parathyroid gland

Thyroid gland

Thymus

Suprarenal gland

Pancreatic islets

Ovary

Testis

15 Lymphoid system and endocrine glands

Ventral aspect
a Lymphatic trunks and ducts, lymphoid organs
b Female endocrine glands
c Male endocrine glands

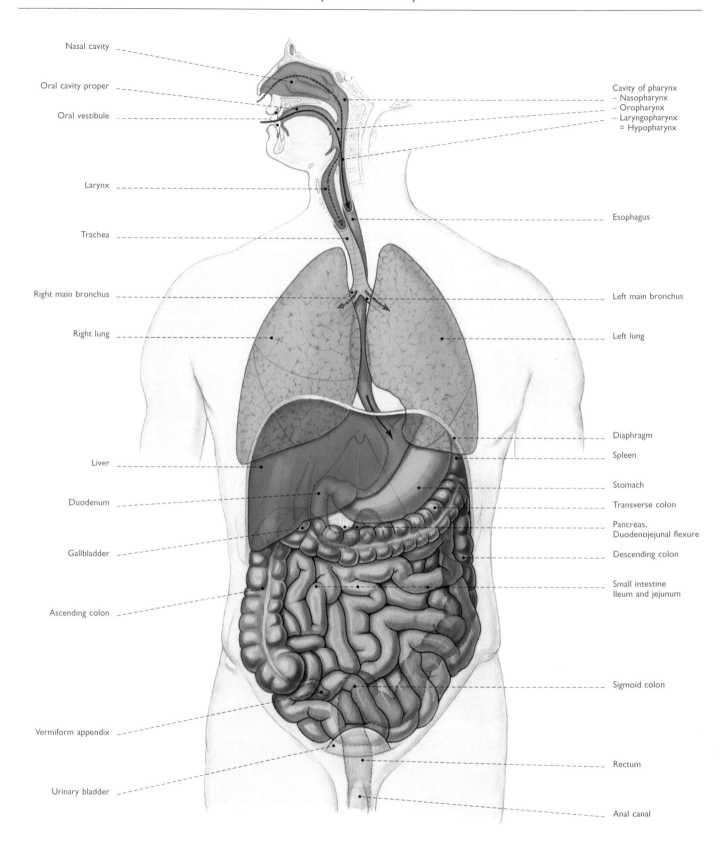

Nasal cavity

Oral cavity proper

Oral vestibule

Larynx

Trachea

Right main bronchus

Right lung

Liver

Duodenum

Gallbladder

Ascending colon

Vermiform appendix

Urinary bladder

Cavity of pharynx
– Nasopharynx
– Oropharynx
– Laryngopharynx
= Hypopharynx

Esophagus

Left main bronchus

Left lung

Diaphragm

Spleen

Stomach

Transverse colon

Pancreas,
Duodenojejunal flexure

Descending colon

Small intestine
Ileum and jejunum

Sigmoid colon

Rectum

Anal canal

16 Alimentary and respiratory systems (25%)
Ventral aspect

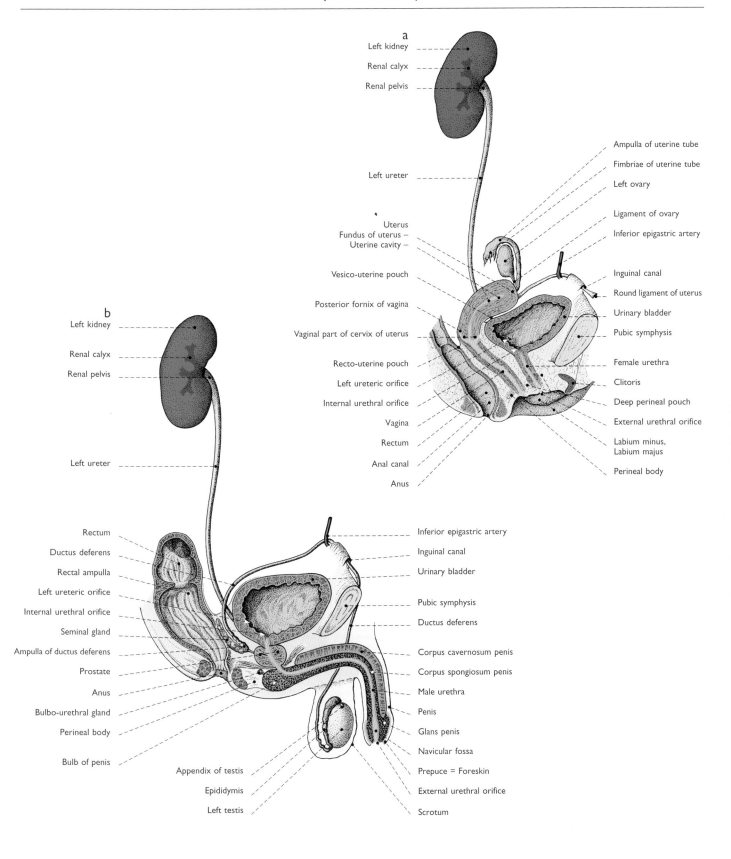

a

Left kidney

Renal calyx

Renal pelvis

Left ureter

Uterus
Fundus of uterus —
Uterine cavity —

Vesico-uterine pouch

Posterior fornix of vagina

Vaginal part of cervix of uterus

Recto-uterine pouch

Left ureteric orifice

Internal urethral orifice

Vagina

Rectum

Anal canal

Anus

Ampulla of uterine tube

Fimbriae of uterine tube

Left ovary

Ligament of ovary

Inferior epigastric artery

Inguinal canal

Round ligament of uterus

Urinary bladder

Pubic symphysis

Female urethra

Clitoris

Deep perineal pouch

External urethral orifice

Labium minus,
Labium majus

Perineal body

b

Left kidney

Renal calyx

Renal pelvis

Left ureter

Rectum

Ductus deferens

Rectal ampulla

Left ureteric orifice

Internal urethral orifice

Seminal gland

Ampulla of ductus deferens

Prostate

Anus

Bulbo-urethral gland

Perineal body

Bulb of penis

Appendix of testis

Epididymis

Left testis

Inferior epigastric artery

Inguinal canal

Urinary bladder

Pubic symphysis

Ductus deferens

Corpus cavernosum penis

Corpus spongiosum penis

Male urethra

Penis

Glans penis

Navicular fossa

Prepuce = Foreskin

External urethral orifice

Scrotum

17   Urinary and genital systems (40%)

Schematized median section, medial aspect of the left half
a   Female
b   Male

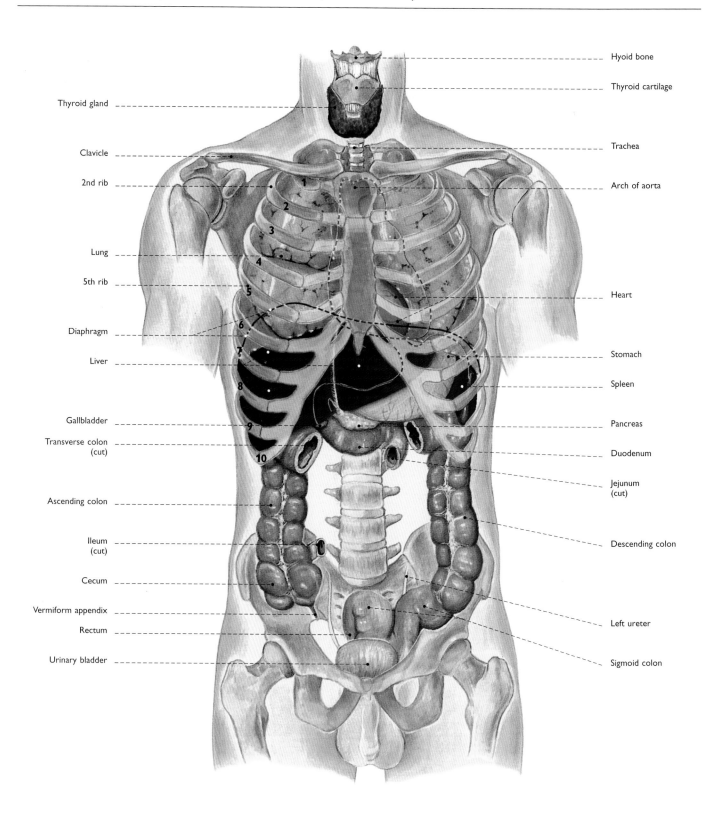

Hyoid bone

Thyroid cartilage

Thyroid gland

Clavicle

Trachea

2nd rib

Arch of aorta

Lung

5th rib

Heart

Diaphragm

Liver

Stomach

Spleen

Gallbladder

Pancreas

Transverse colon
(cut)

Duodenum

Jejunum
(cut)

Ascending colon

Descending colon

Ileum
(cut)

Cecum

Vermiform appendix

Rectum

Left ureter

Urinary bladder

Sigmoid colon

18 Surface projections of
thoracic and abdominal viscera (25%)
Jejunum, ileum, and transverse colon were removed. Ventral aspect

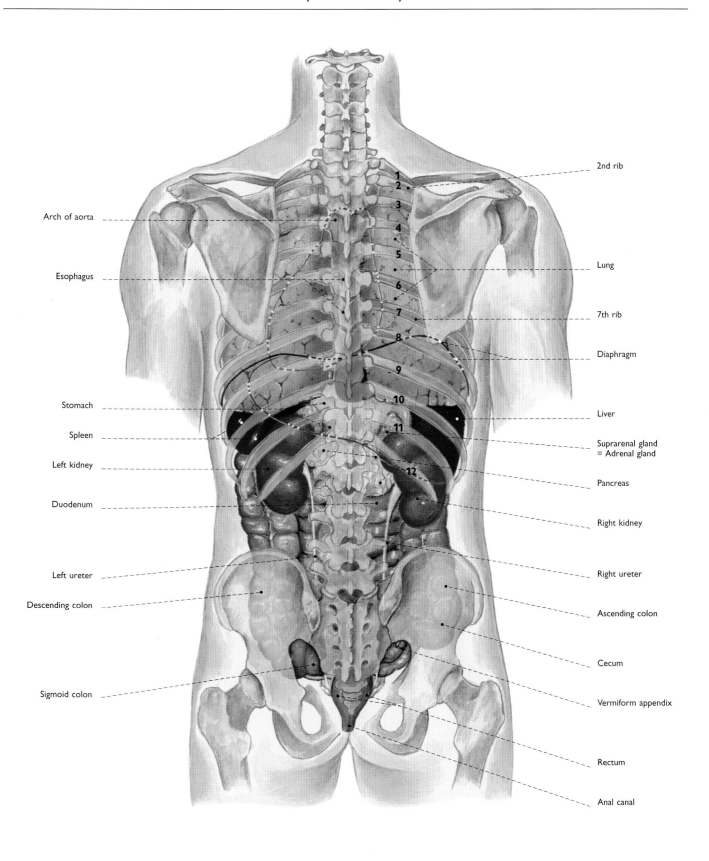

2nd rib

Arch of aorta

Esophagus

Lung

7th rib

Diaphragm

Stomach

Spleen

Liver

Left kidney

Suprarenal gland
= Adrenal gland

Duodenum

Pancreas

Right kidney

Left ureter

Right ureter

Descending colon

Ascending colon

Cecum

Sigmoid colon

Vermiform appendix

Rectum

Anal canal

**19   Surface projections of
thoracic and abdominal viscera** (25%)
Dorsal aspect

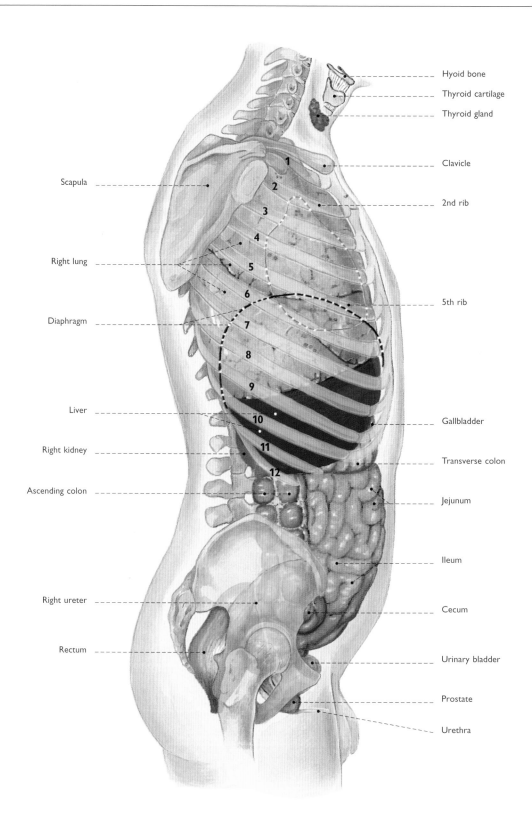

Hyoid bone

Thyroid cartilage

Thyroid gland

Clavicle

2nd rib

5th rib

Gallbladder

Transverse colon

Jejunum

Ileum

Cecum

Urinary bladder

Prostate

Urethra

Scapula

Right lung

Diaphragm

Liver

Right kidney

Ascending colon

Right ureter

Rectum

**20 Surface projections of
thoracic and abdominal viscera** (25%)
Right lateral aspect

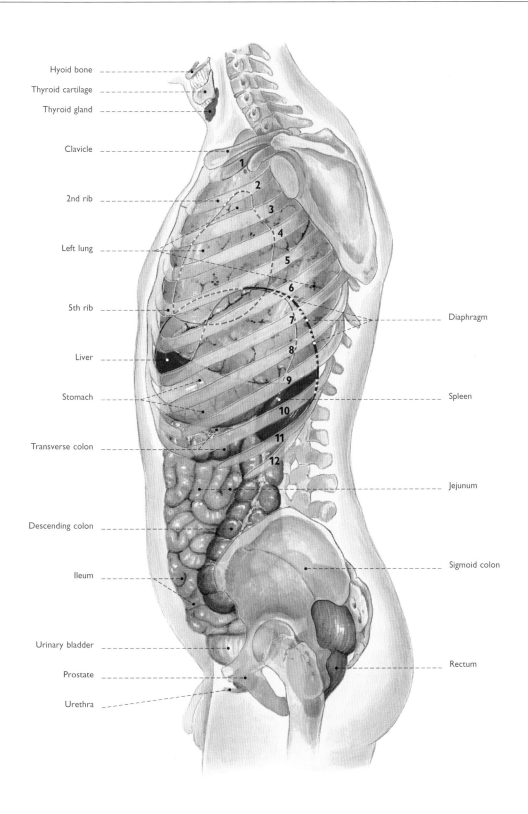

Hyoid bone

Thyroid cartilage

Thyroid gland

Clavicle

2nd rib

Left lung

5th rib

Liver

Stomach

Transverse colon

Descending colon

Ileum

Urinary bladder

Prostate

Urethra

1
2
3
4
5
6
7
8
9
10
11
12

Diaphragm

Spleen

Jejunum

Sigmoid colon

Rectum

21 Surface projections of
thoracic and abdominal viscera (25%)
Left lateral aspect

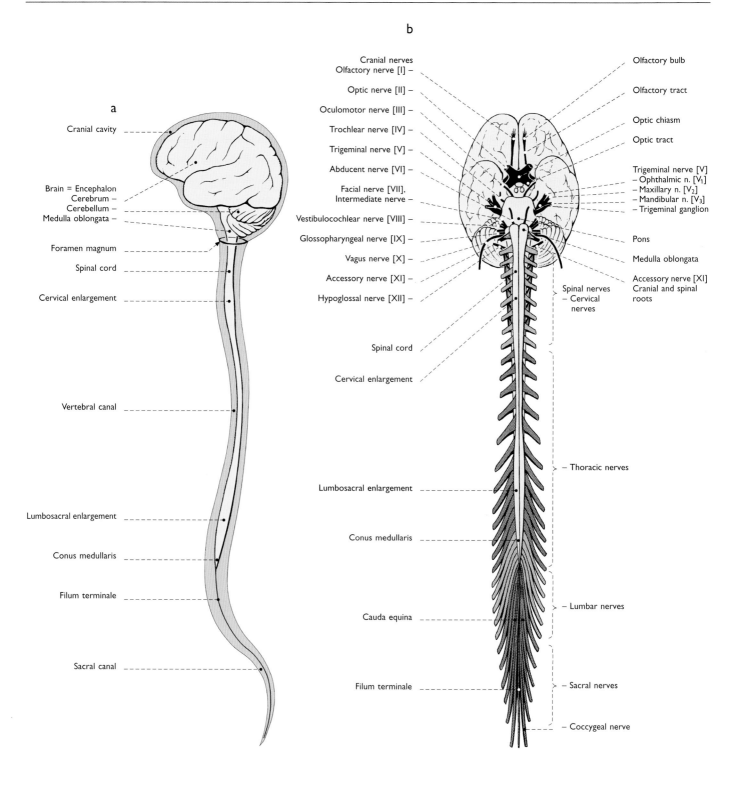

a

Cranial cavity

Brain = Encephalon
Cerebrum –
Cerebellum –
Medulla oblongata –

Foramen magnum

Spinal cord

Cervical enlargement

Vertebral canal

Lumbosacral enlargement

Conus medullaris

Filum terminale

Sacral canal

b

Cranial nerves
Olfactory nerve [I] –

Optic nerve [II] –

Oculomotor nerve [III] –

Trochlear nerve [IV] –

Trigeminal nerve [V] –

Abducent nerve [VI] –

Facial nerve [VII],
Intermediate nerve –

Vestibulocochlear nerve [VIII] –

Glossopharyngeal nerve [IX] –

Vagus nerve [X] –

Accessory nerve [XI] –

Hypoglossal nerve [XII] –

Spinal cord

Cervical enlargement

Lumbosacral enlargement

Conus medullaris

Cauda equina

Filum terminale

Olfactory bulb

Olfactory tract

Optic chiasm

Optic tract

Trigeminal nerve [V]
– Ophthalmic n. [V_1]
– Maxillary n. [V_2]
– Mandibular n. [V_3]
– Trigeminal ganglion

Pons

Medulla oblongata

Accessory nerve [XI]
Cranial and spinal
roots

Spinal nerves
– Cervical
nerves

– Thoracic nerves

– Lumbar nerves

– Sacral nerves

– Coccygeal nerve

22 Central and peripheral nervous systems
a Central nervous system, left lateral aspect
b Cranial and spinal nerves, ventral aspect

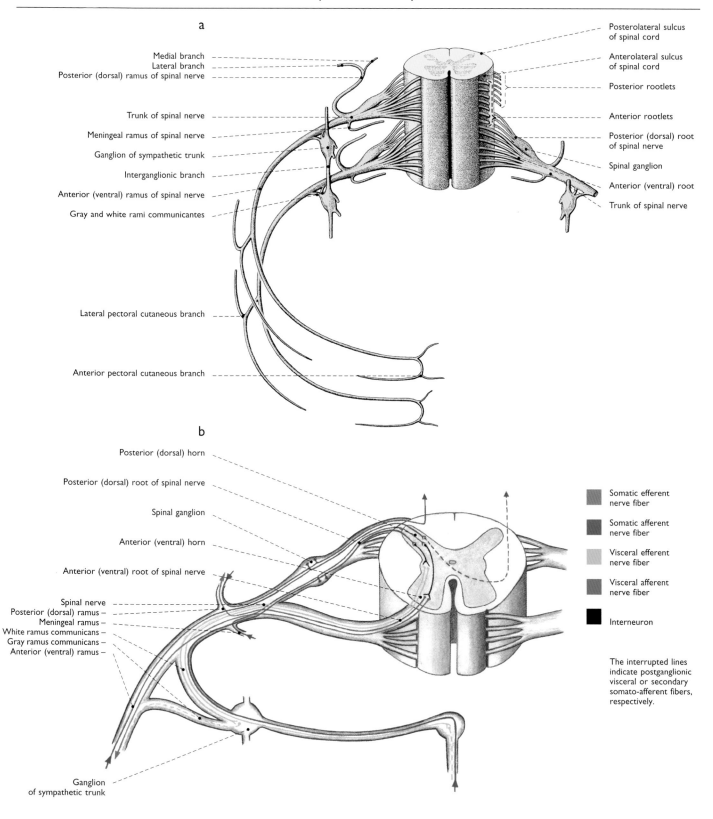

a

Medial branch
Lateral branch
Posterior (dorsal) ramus of spinal nerve

Trunk of spinal nerve

Meningeal ramus of spinal nerve

Ganglion of sympathetic trunk

Interganglionic branch

Anterior (ventral) ramus of spinal nerve

Gray and white rami communicantes

Lateral pectoral cutaneous branch

Anterior pectoral cutaneous branch

Posterolateral sulcus of spinal cord

Anterolateral sulcus of spinal cord

Posterior rootlets

Anterior rootlets

Posterior (dorsal) root of spinal nerve

Spinal ganglion

Anterior (ventral) root

Trunk of spinal nerve

b

Posterior (dorsal) horn

Posterior (dorsal) root of spinal nerve

Spinal ganglion

Anterior (ventral) horn

Anterior (ventral) root of spinal nerve

Spinal nerve
Posterior (dorsal) ramus –
Meningeal ramus –
White ramus communicans –
Gray ramus communicans –
Anterior (ventral) ramus –

Ganglion
of sympathetic trunk

Somatic efferent nerve fiber

Somatic afferent nerve fiber

Visceral efferent nerve fiber

Visceral afferent nerve fiber

Interneuron

The interrupted lines indicate postganglionic visceral or secondary somato-afferent fibers, respectively.

23 Spinal cord and spinal nerves
Ventral aspect
a Distribution and
b Construction
of typical spinal nerves (thoracic nerves)

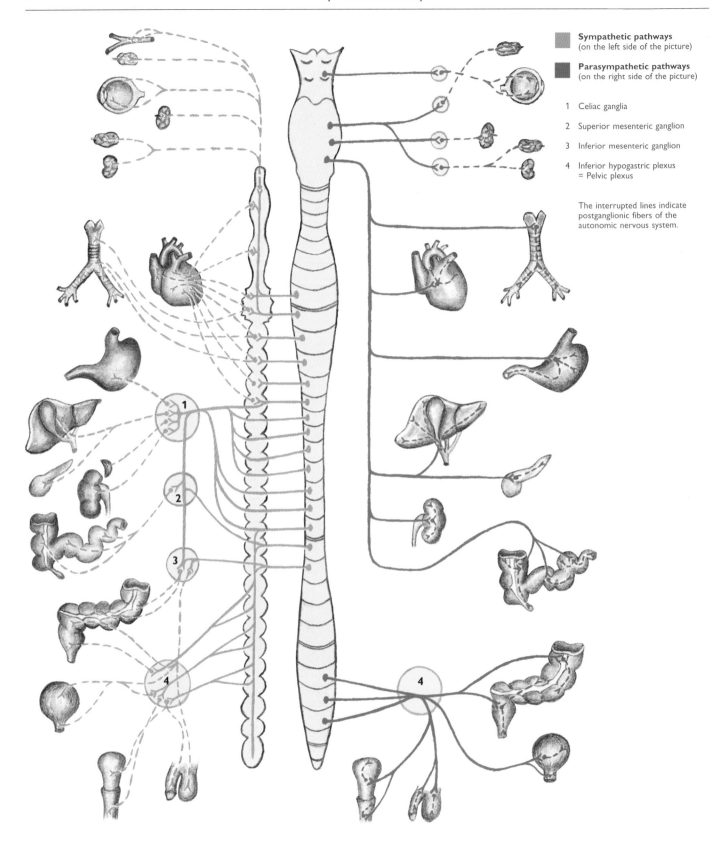

Sympathetic pathways
(on the left side of the picture)

Parasympathetic pathways
(on the right side of the picture)

1 Celiac ganglia

2 Superior mesenteric ganglion

3 Inferior mesenteric ganglion

4 Inferior hypogastric plexus
   = Pelvic plexus

The interrupted lines indicate
postganglionic fibers of the
autonomic nervous system.

24 Autonomic division
of the peripheral nervous system
Origins, essential circuitry, and peripheral innervation
of the sympathetic and parasympathetic nervous systems.
Schematic representation, ventral aspect

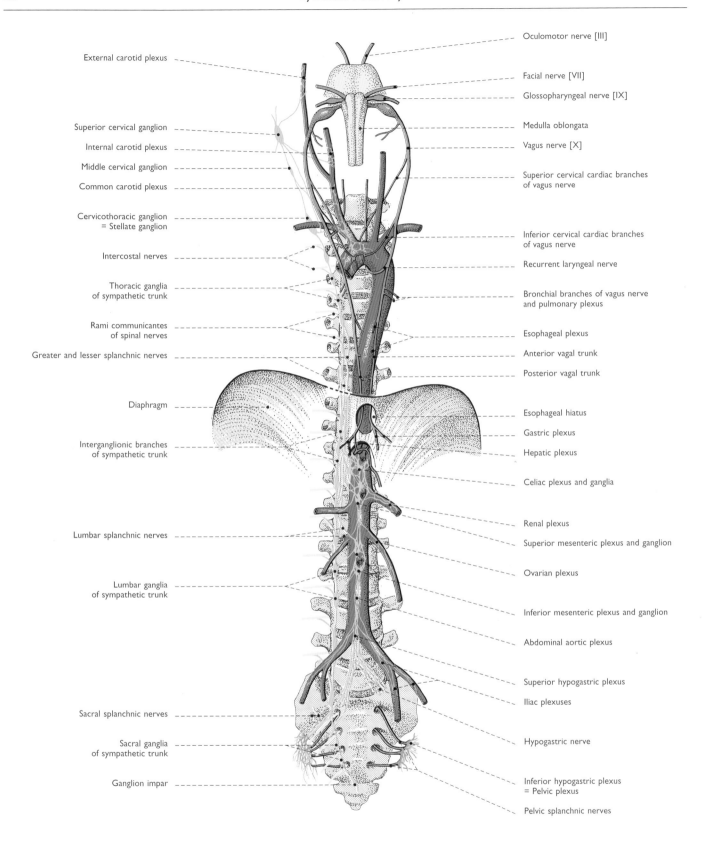

External carotid plexus

Superior cervical ganglion

Internal carotid plexus

Middle cervical ganglion

Common carotid plexus

Cervicothoracic ganglion
= Stellate ganglion

Intercostal nerves

Thoracic ganglia
of sympathetic trunk

Rami communicantes
of spinal nerves

Greater and lesser splanchnic nerves

Diaphragm

Interganglionic branches
of sympathetic trunk

Lumbar splanchnic nerves

Lumbar ganglia
of sympathetic trunk

Sacral splanchnic nerves

Sacral ganglia
of sympathetic trunk

Ganglion impar

Oculomotor nerve [III]

Facial nerve [VII]

Glossopharyngeal nerve [IX]

Medulla oblongata

Vagus nerve [X]

Superior cervical cardiac branches
of vagus nerve

Inferior cervical cardiac branches
of vagus nerve

Recurrent laryngeal nerve

Bronchial branches of vagus nerve
and pulmonary plexus

Esophageal plexus

Anterior vagal trunk

Posterior vagal trunk

Esophageal hiatus

Gastric plexus

Hepatic plexus

Celiac plexus and ganglia

Renal plexus

Superior mesenteric plexus and ganglion

Ovarian plexus

Inferior mesenteric plexus and ganglion

Abdominal aortic plexus

Superior hypogastric plexus

Iliac plexuses

Hypogastric nerve

Inferior hypogastric plexus
= Pelvic plexus

Pelvic splanchnic nerves

**25   Autonomic division
of the peripheral nervous system** (25%)
Peripheral sympathetic (**orange**) and parasympathetic (**brown**)
nerves and ganglia. The sympathetic components are shown
only on the left side of the picture. Ventral aspect

Body Wall

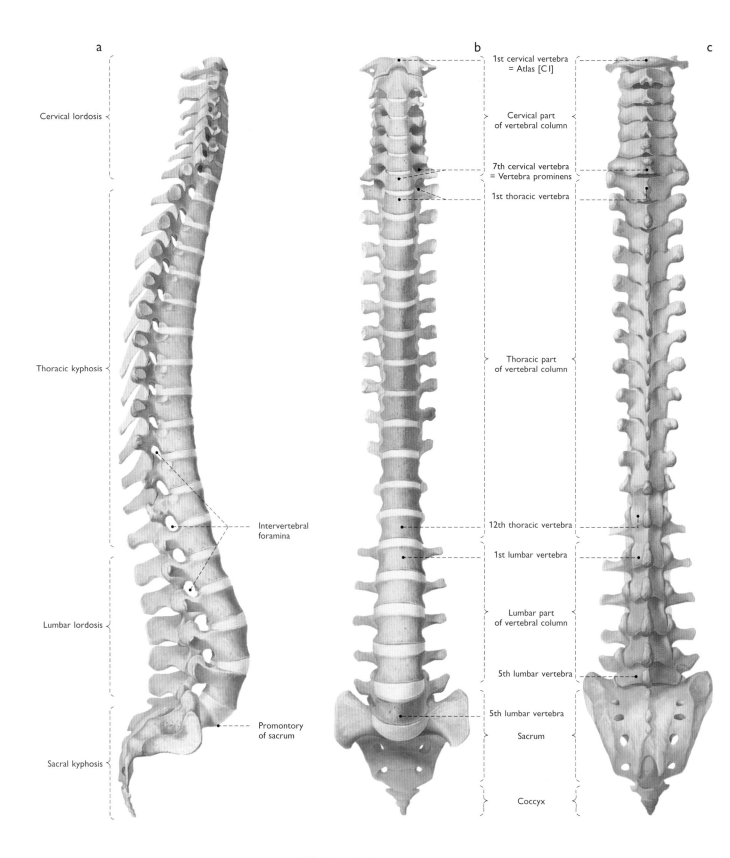

a

Cervical lordosis

Thoracic kyphosis

Intervertebral foramina

Lumbar lordosis

Promontory of sacrum

Sacral kyphosis

b

1st cervical vertebra = Atlas [C I]

Cervical part of vertebral column

7th cervical vertebra = Vertebra prominens

1st thoracic vertebra

Thoracic part of vertebral column

12th thoracic vertebra

1st lumbar vertebra

Lumbar part of vertebral column

5th lumbar vertebra

5th lumbar vertebra

Sacrum

Coccyx

c

28 Vertebral column (30%)

a Right lateral aspect
b Ventral aspect
c Dorsal aspect

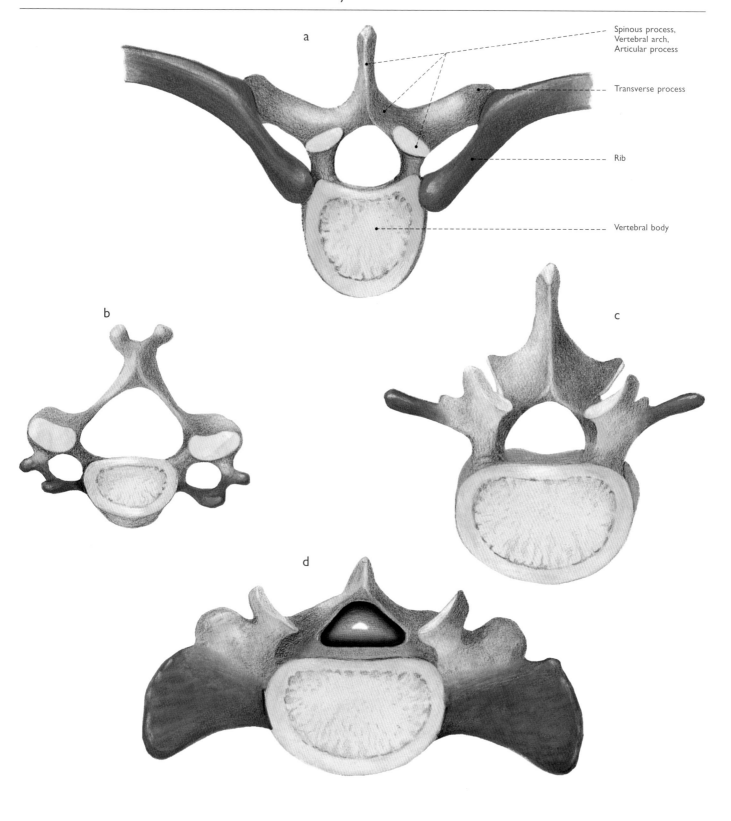

Spinous process,
Vertebral arch,
Articular process

Transverse process

Rib

Vertebral body

a

b

c

d

29 Homology of parts of vertebrae

Homologous parts of vertebrae are represented by the same color.
Cranial aspect
a Thoracic vertebra with ribs
b Cervical vertebra
c Lumbar vertebra
d Sacrum

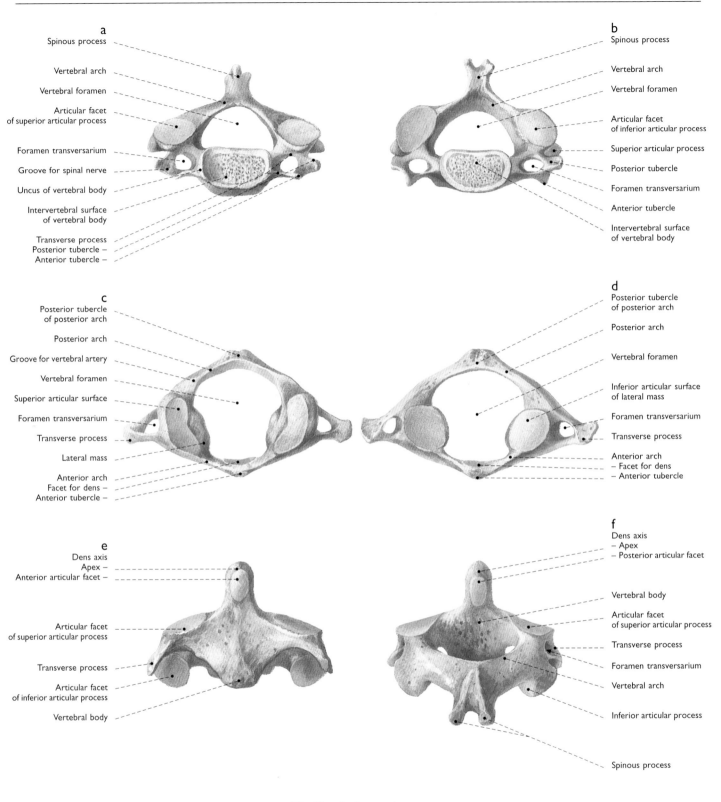

a
Spinous process
Vertebral arch
Vertebral foramen
Articular facet
of superior articular process
Foramen transversarium
Groove for spinal nerve
Uncus of vertebral body
Intervertebral surface
of vertebral body
Transverse process
Posterior tubercle –
Anterior tubercle –

b
Spinous process
Vertebral arch
Vertebral foramen
Articular facet
of inferior articular process
Superior articular process
Posterior tubercle
Foramen transversarium
Anterior tubercle
Intervertebral surface
of vertebral body

c
Posterior tubercle
of posterior arch
Posterior arch
Groove for vertebral artery
Vertebral foramen
Superior articular surface
Foramen transversarium
Transverse process
Lateral mass
Anterior arch
Facet for dens –
Anterior tubercle –

d
Posterior tubercle
of posterior arch
Posterior arch
Vertebral foramen
Inferior articular surface
of lateral mass
Foramen transversarium
Transverse process
Anterior arch
– Facet for dens
– Anterior tubercle

e
Dens axis
Apex –
Anterior articular facet –
Articular facet
of superior articular process
Transverse process
Articular facet
of inferior articular process
Vertebral body

f
Dens axis
– Apex
– Posterior articular facet
Vertebral body
Articular facet
of superior articular process
Transverse process
Foramen transversarium
Vertebral arch
Inferior articular process
Spinous process

30 Cervical vertebrae (90%)
a, b Middle cervical vertebra
   a Cranial aspect
   b Caudal aspect
c, d First cervical vertebra = atlas [C I]
   c Cranial aspect
   d Caudal aspect
e, f Second cervical vertebra = axis [C II]
   e Ventral aspect
   f Dorsal aspect

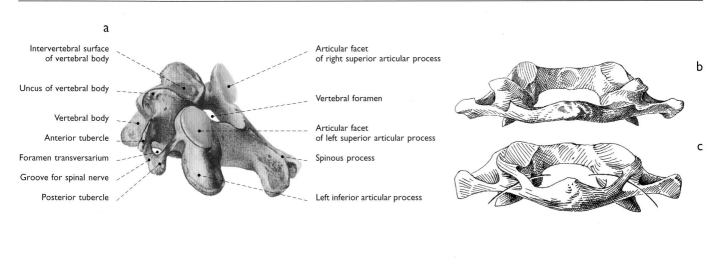

a

Intervertebral surface of vertebral body

Uncus of vertebral body

Vertebral body

Anterior tubercle

Foramen transversarium

Groove for spinal nerve

Posterior tubercle

Articular facet of right superior articular process

Vertebral foramen

Articular facet of left superior articular process

Spinous process

Left inferior articular process

b

c

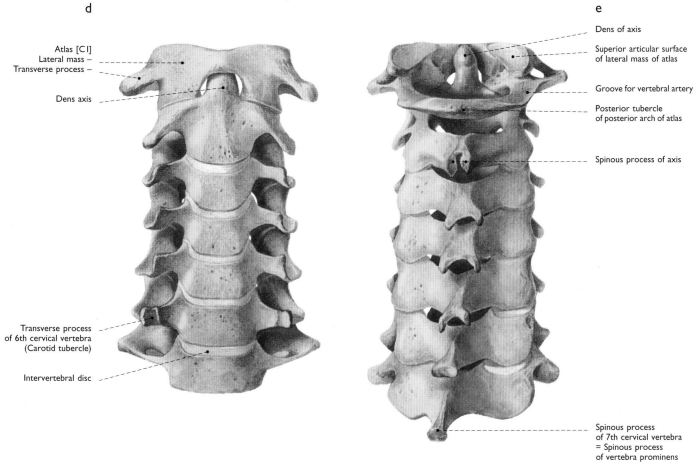

d

Atlas [C I]
Lateral mass –
Transverse process –

Dens axis

Transverse process of 6th cervical vertebra (Carotid tubercle)

Intervertebral disc

e

Dens of axis

Superior articular surface of lateral mass of atlas

Groove for vertebral artery

Posterior tubercle of posterior arch of atlas

Spinous process of axis

Spinous process of 7th cervical vertebra = Spinous process of vertebra prominens

31 Cervical vertebrae and cervical spine

a Middle cervical vertebra (90%), left lateral aspect
b, c First cervical vertebra = atlas [C I], dorsal aspect
b Deep groove for the vertebral artery on both sides
c Canal for the vertebral artery on both sides
d, e Cervical spine with intervertebral discs (100%)
d Ventral aspect
e Dorsal aspect

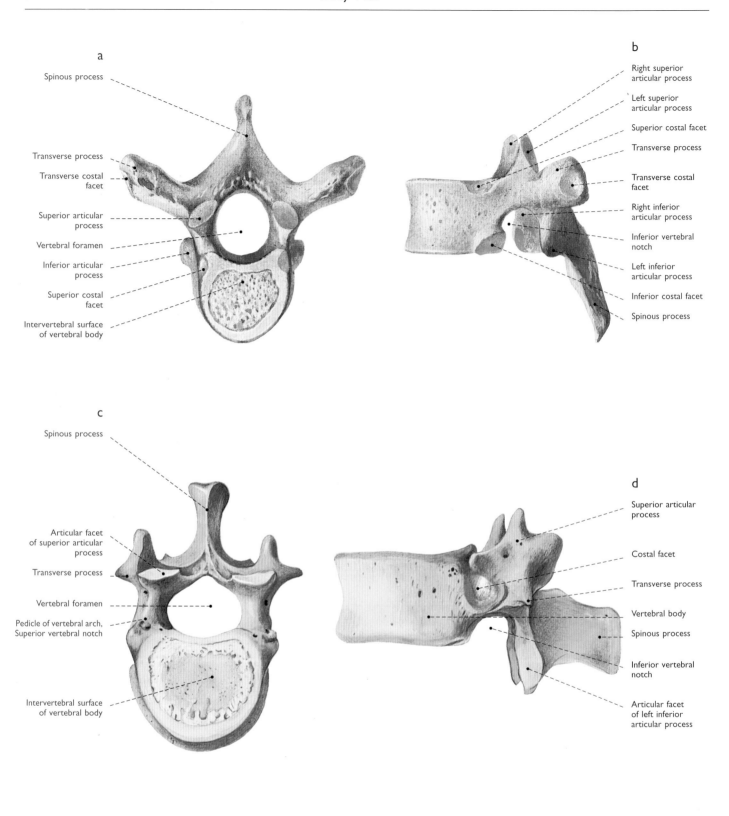

a

Spinous process

Transverse process

Transverse costal
facet

Superior articular
process

Vertebral foramen

Inferior articular
process

Superior costal
facet

Intervertebral surface
of vertebral body

b

Right superior
articular process

Left superior
articular process

Superior costal facet

Transverse process

Transverse costal
facet

Right inferior
articular process

Inferior vertebral
notch

Left inferior
articular process

Inferior costal facet

Spinous process

c

Spinous process

Articular facet
of superior articular
process

Transverse process

Vertebral foramen

Pedicle of vertebral arch,
Superior vertebral notch

Intervertebral surface
of vertebral body

d

Superior articular
process

Costal facet

Transverse process

Vertebral body

Spinous process

Inferior vertebral
notch

Articular facet
of left inferior
articular process

32   Thoracic vertebrae (100%)

a, b   Sixth thoracic vertebra
     a   Cranial aspect
     b   Left lateral aspect
c, d   Twelfth thoracic vertebra
     c   Cranial aspect
     d   Left lateral aspect

a

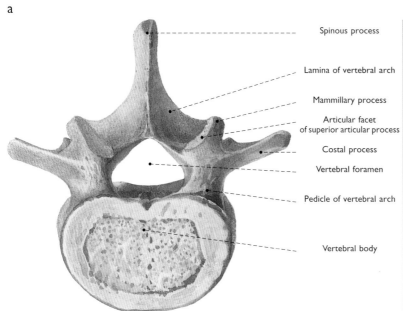

Spinous process

Lamina of vertebral arch

Mammillary process

Articular facet
of superior articular process

Costal process

Vertebral foramen

Pedicle of vertebral arch

Vertebral body

b

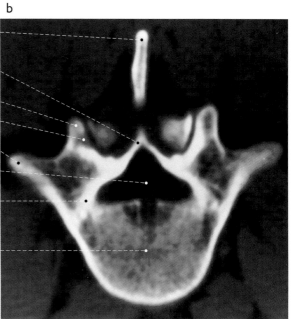

c

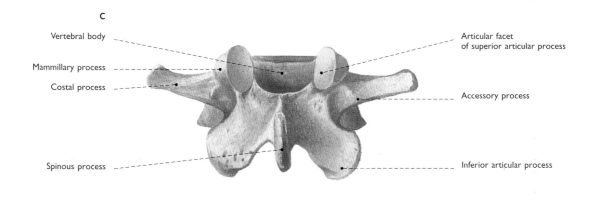

Vertebral body

Mammillary process

Costal process

Spinous process

Articular facet
of superior articular process

Accessory process

Inferior articular process

d

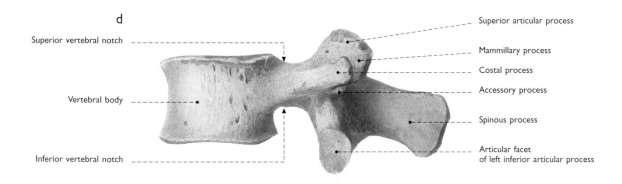

Superior vertebral notch

Vertebral body

Inferior vertebral notch

Superior articular process

Mammillary process

Costal process

Accessory process

Spinous process

Articular facet
of left inferior articular process

33 Middle lumbar vertebra (100%)

a Cranial aspect
b Transverse computed tomogram (CT)
c Dorsal aspect
d Left lateral aspect

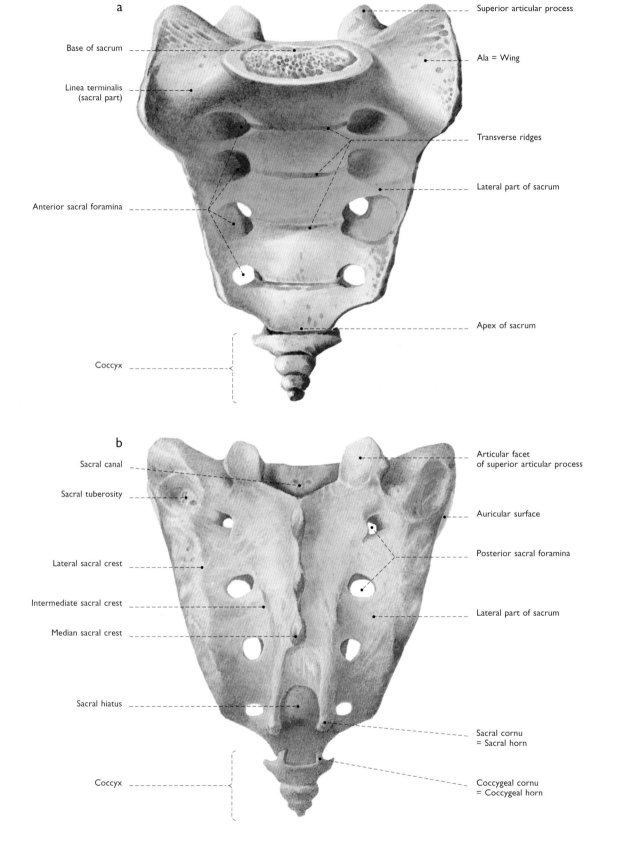

a

Base of sacrum

Linea terminalis
(sacral part)

Anterior sacral foramina

Coccyx

Superior articular process

Ala = Wing

Transverse ridges

Lateral part of sacrum

Apex of sacrum

b

Sacral canal

Sacral tuberosity

Lateral sacral crest

Intermediate sacral crest

Median sacral crest

Sacral hiatus

Coccyx

Articular facet
of superior articular process

Auricular surface

Posterior sacral foramina

Lateral part of sacrum

Sacral cornu
= Sacral horn

Coccygeal cornu
= Coccygeal horn

34 Sacrum and coccyx (80%)

    a   Ventral aspect
    b   Dorsal aspect

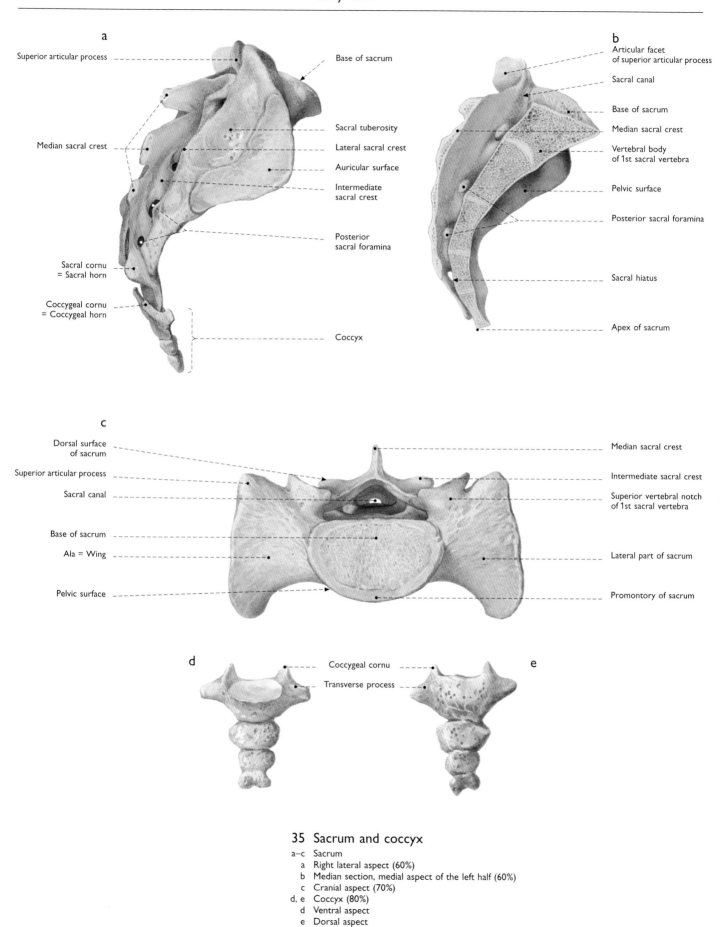

a

Superior articular process

Median sacral crest

Sacral cornu = Sacral horn

Coccygeal cornu = Coccygeal horn

Base of sacrum

Sacral tuberosity

Lateral sacral crest

Auricular surface

Intermediate sacral crest

Posterior sacral foramina

Coccyx

b

Articular facet of superior articular process

Sacral canal

Base of sacrum

Median sacral crest

Vertebral body of 1st sacral vertebra

Pelvic surface

Posterior sacral foramina

Sacral hiatus

Apex of sacrum

c

Dorsal surface of sacrum

Superior articular process

Sacral canal

Base of sacrum

Ala = Wing

Pelvic surface

Median sacral crest

Intermediate sacral crest

Superior vertebral notch of 1st sacral vertebra

Lateral part of sacrum

Promontory of sacrum

d

e

Coccygeal cornu

Transverse process

35 Sacrum and coccyx

a–c Sacrum
  a Right lateral aspect (60%)
  b Median section, medial aspect of the left half (60%)
  c Cranial aspect (70%)
d, e Coccyx (80%)
  d Ventral aspect
  e Dorsal aspect

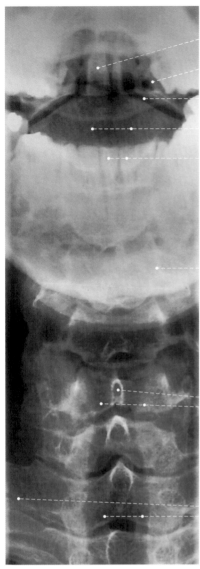

a

Dens axis

Lateral mass of atlas

Lateral atlanto-axial joint

Vertebral body of axis

Incisor teeth

Body of mandible

6th cervical vertebra
– Spinous process
– Vertebral body

1st thoracic vertebra
– Transverse process
– Vertebral body

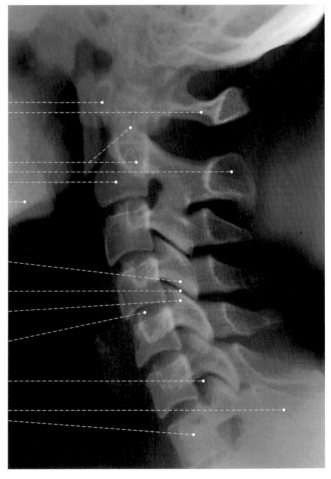

b

1st cervical vertebra
= Atlas [C I]
Anterior arch –
Posterior arch –

2nd cervical vertebra
= Axis [C II]
Dens –
Spinous process –
Vertebral body –

Mandible

Inferior articular process
of 4th cervical vertebra

Zygapophysial joint

Superior articular process
of 5th cervical vertebra

Intervertebral disc

Intervertebral foramen

7th cervical vertebra
Spinous process –
Vertebral body –

36 Cervical spine (100%)
a Anteroposterior radiograph
b Lateral radiograph

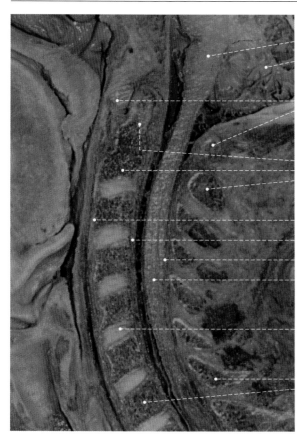

a

Medulla oblongata

Cerebellum

1st cervical vertebra = Atlas [C I]
– Anterior arch
– Posterior arch

2nd cervical vertebra = Axis [C II]
– Dens
– Vertebral body
– Spinous process

Anterior longitudinal ligament

Posterior longitudinal ligament

Ligamentum flavum

Spinal cord

Intervertebral disc

7th cervical vertebra
= Vertebra prominens
– Spinous process
– Vertebral body

Basilar part of occipital bone

Medulla oblongata

Squamous part of occipital bone

1st cervical vertebra = Atlas [C I]
Anterior arch –
Posterior arch –

2nd cervical vertebra = Axis [C II]
Dens –
Vertebral body –
Spinous process –

Anterior longitudinal ligament

Posterior longitudinal ligament

Intervertebral disc

Ligamentum flavum

Spinal cord

7th cervical vertebra
= Vertebra prominens
Spinous process –
Vertebral body –

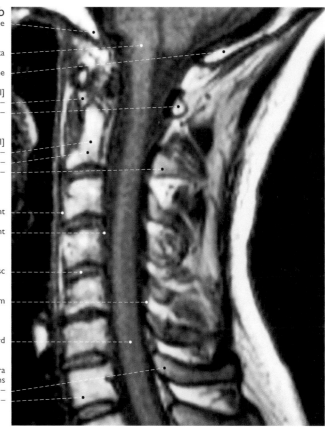

b

37 Cervical spine (90%)

Midsagittal section
a Anatomical section
b Magnetic resonance image (MRI, T$_1$-weighted)

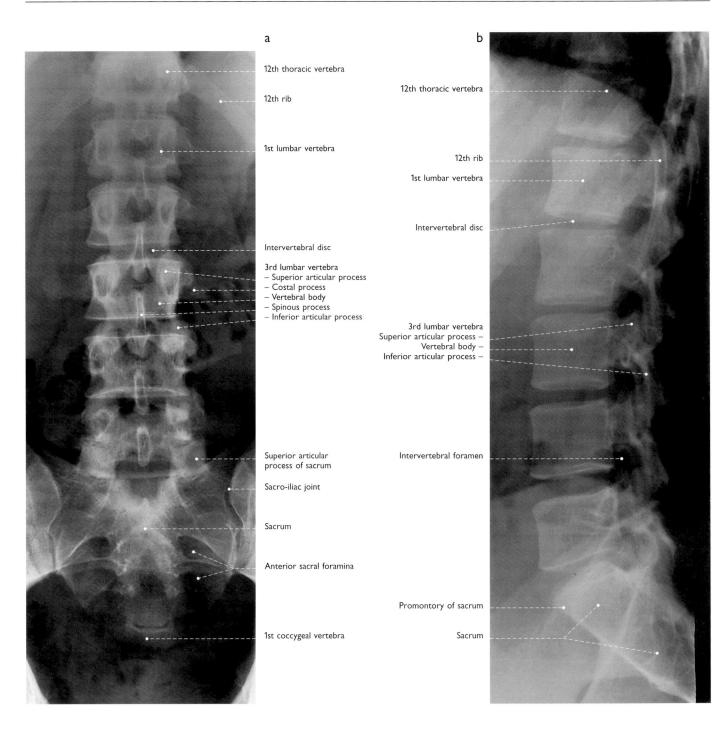

a

12th thoracic vertebra

12th rib

1st lumbar vertebra

Intervertebral disc

3rd lumbar vertebra
– Superior articular process
– Costal process
– Vertebral body
– Spinous process
– Inferior articular process

Superior articular
process of sacrum

Sacro-iliac joint

Sacrum

Anterior sacral foramina

1st coccygeal vertebra

b

12th thoracic vertebra

12th rib

1st lumbar vertebra

Intervertebral disc

3rd lumbar vertebra
Superior articular process –
Vertebral body –
Inferior articular process –

Intervertebral foramen

Promontory of sacrum

Sacrum

38 Lumbar spine, sacrum, and coccyx (50%)

a   Anteroposterior radiograph
b   Lateral radiograph

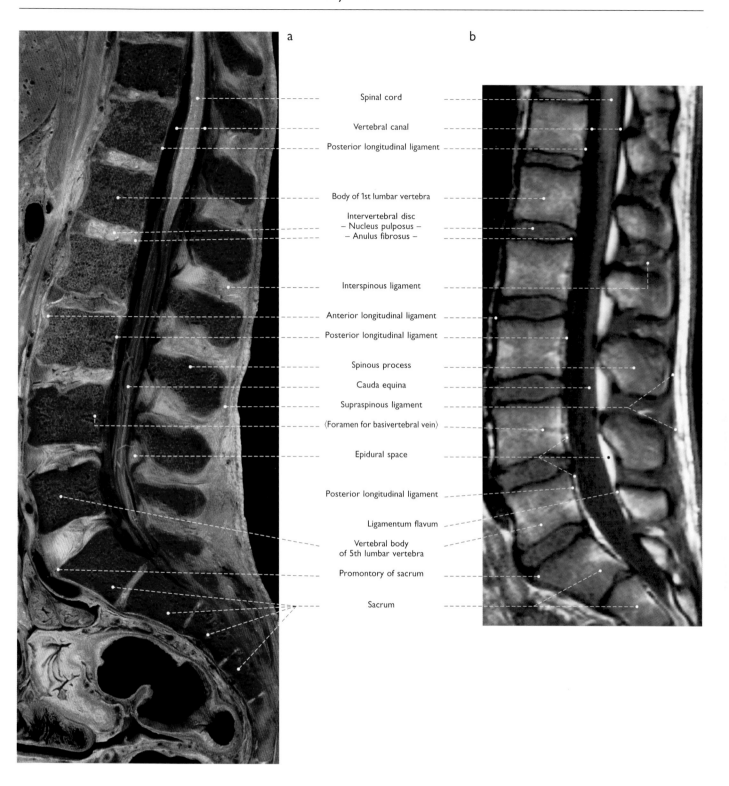

a

b

Spinal cord

Vertebral canal

Posterior longitudinal ligament

Body of 1st lumbar vertebra

Intervertebral disc
– Nucleus pulposus –
– Anulus fibrosus –

Interspinous ligament

Anterior longitudinal ligament

Posterior longitudinal ligament

Spinous process

Cauda equina

Supraspinous ligament

⟨Foramen for basivertebral vein⟩

Epidural space

Posterior longitudinal ligament

Ligamentum flavum

Vertebral body
of 5th lumbar vertebra

Promontory of sacrum

Sacrum

39 Lumbar spine, sacrum, and coccyx (50%)

Midsagittal section
a Anatomical section
b Magnetic resonance image (MRI, T$_1$-weighted)

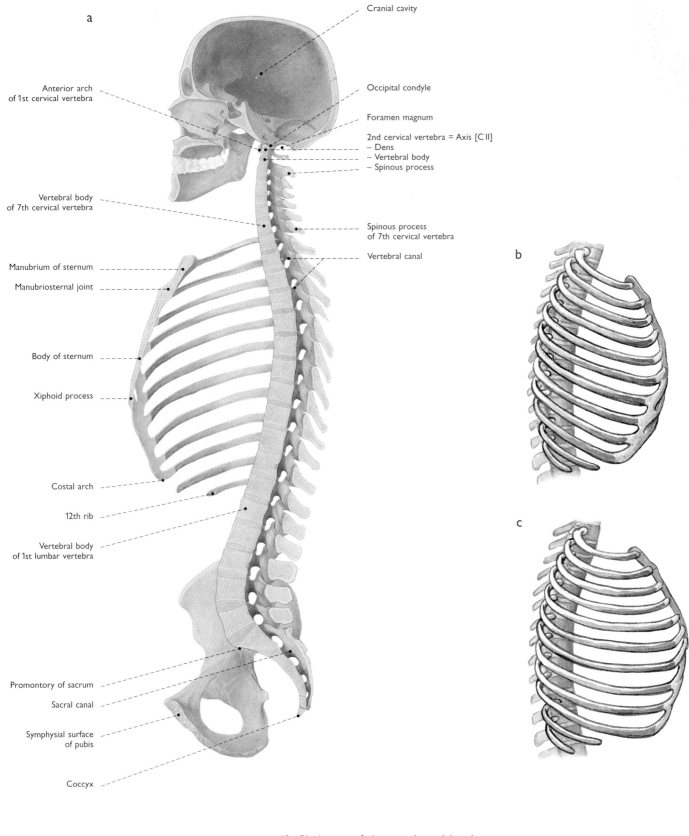

a

Cranial cavity

Anterior arch
of 1st cervical vertebra

Occipital condyle

Foramen magnum

2nd cervical vertebra = Axis [C II]
– Dens
– Vertebral body
– Spinous process

Vertebral body
of 7th cervical vertebra

Spinous process
of 7th cervical vertebra

Vertebral canal

b

Manubrium of sternum

Manubriosternal joint

Body of sternum

Xiphoid process

Costal arch

12th rib

Vertebral body
of 1st lumbar vertebra

c

Promontory of sacrum

Sacral canal

Symphysial surface
of pubis

Coccyx

40 Skeleton of the trunk and hip bone

a Median section (25%), medial aspect
b, c Alterations of the shape of thorax during respiration,
right lateral aspect
b Phase of expiration
c Phase of inspiration

a

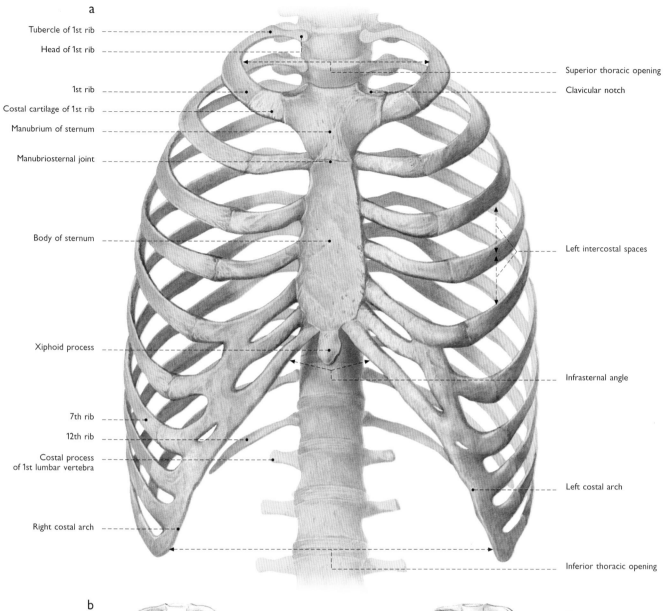

Tubercle of 1st rib

Head of 1st rib

1st rib

Costal cartilage of 1st rib

Manubrium of sternum

Manubriosternal joint

Body of sternum

Xiphoid process

7th rib

12th rib

Costal process
of 1st lumbar vertebra

Right costal arch

Superior thoracic opening

Clavicular notch

Left intercostal spaces

Infrasternal angle

Left costal arch

Inferior thoracic opening

b

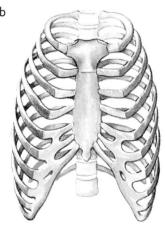

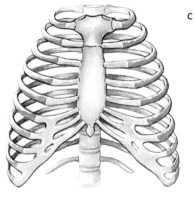

c

41   Thorax

a   Ventral aspect (45%)
b, c   Alterations of the shape of thorax during respiration,
        ventral aspect
b   Phase of expiration
c   Phase of inspiration

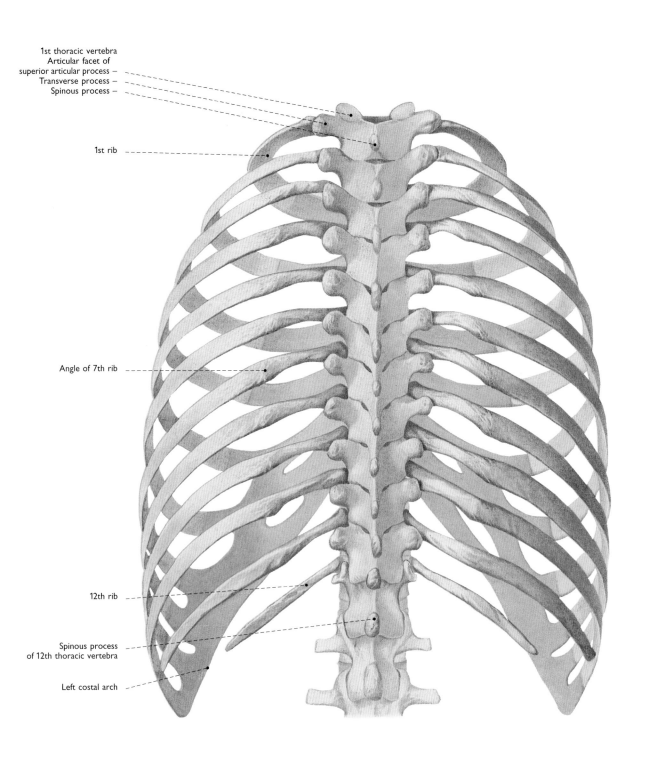

1st thoracic vertebra
Articular facet of
superior articular process —
Transverse process —
Spinous process —

1st rib

Angle of 7th rib

12th rib

Spinous process
of 12th thoracic vertebra

Left costal arch

42 Thorax (50%)
Dorsal aspect

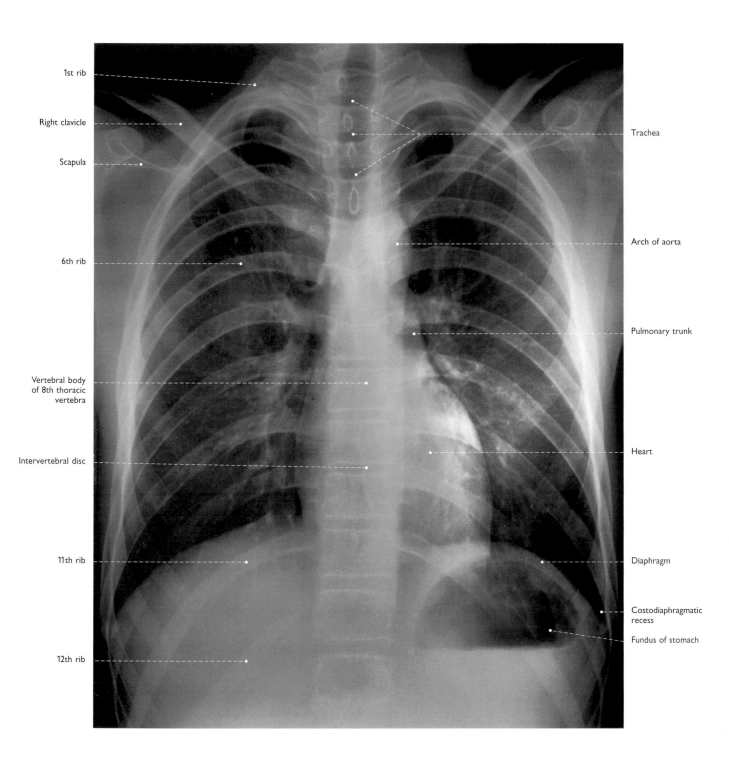

1st rib

Right clavicle

Scapula

6th rib

Vertebral body
of 8th thoracic
vertebra

Intervertebral disc

11th rib

12th rib

Trachea

Arch of aorta

Pulmonary trunk

Heart

Diaphragm

Costodiaphragmatic
recess

Fundus of stomach

43 Thorax (50%)

Postero-anterior radiograph of the thorax and
the pectoral girdle. The arms are elevated.

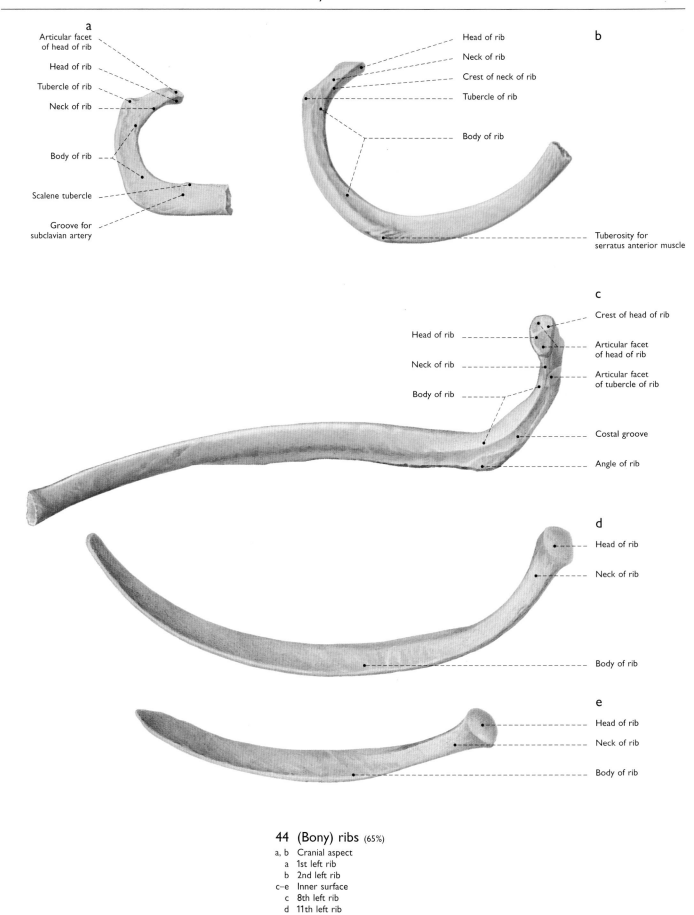

a
Articular facet of head of rib
Head of rib
Tubercle of rib
Neck of rib
Body of rib
Scalene tubercle
Groove for subclavian artery

b
Head of rib
Neck of rib
Crest of neck of rib
Tubercle of rib
Body of rib
Tuberosity for serratus anterior muscle

c
Crest of head of rib
Head of rib
Articular facet of head of rib
Neck of rib
Articular facet of tubercle of rib
Body of rib
Costal groove
Angle of rib

d
Head of rib
Neck of rib
Body of rib

e
Head of rib
Neck of rib
Body of rib

44 (Bony) ribs (65%)

a, b Cranial aspect
a 1st left rib
b 2nd left rib
c–e Inner surface
c 8th left rib
d 11th left rib
e 12th left rib

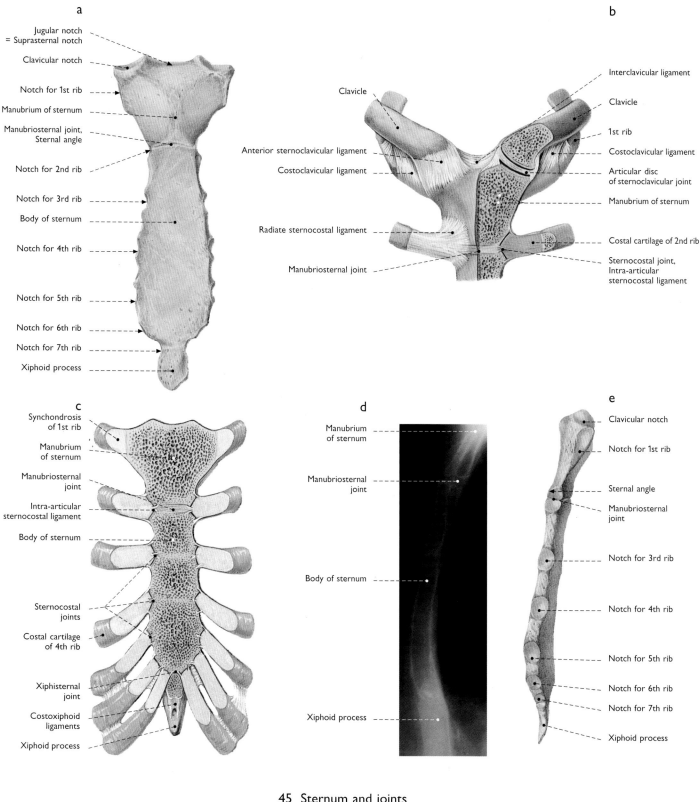

a

Jugular notch
= Suprasternal notch

Clavicular notch

Notch for 1st rib

Manubrium of sternum

Manubriosternal joint,
Sternal angle

Notch for 2nd rib

Notch for 3rd rib

Body of sternum

Notch for 4th rib

Notch for 5th rib

Notch for 6th rib

Notch for 7th rib

Xiphoid process

b

Clavicle

Anterior sternoclavicular ligament

Costoclavicular ligament

Radiate sternocostal ligament

Manubriosternal joint

Interclavicular ligament

Clavicle

1st rib

Costoclavicular ligament

Articular disc
of sternoclavicular joint

Manubrium of sternum

Costal cartilage of 2nd rib

Sternocostal joint,
Intra-articular
sternocostal ligament

c

Synchondrosis
of 1st rib

Manubrium
of sternum

Manubriosternal
joint

Intra-articular
sternocostal ligament

Body of sternum

Sternocostal
joints

Costal cartilage
of 4th rib

Xiphisternal
joint

Costoxiphoid
ligaments

Xiphoid process

d

Manubrium
of sternum

Manubriosternal
joint

Body of sternum

Xiphoid process

e

Clavicular notch

Notch for 1st rib

Sternal angle

Manubriosternal
joint

Notch for 3rd rib

Notch for 4th rib

Notch for 5th rib

Notch for 6th rib

Notch for 7th rib

Xiphoid process

45 Sternum and joints

a Sternum (45%), ventral aspect
b Sternoclavicular joint (70%), ventral aspect.
   The sternoclavicular and sternocostal joints were
   exposed on the left side of the body by a frontal section.
c Sternocostal joints (45%), exposed by a frontal section,
   ventral aspect
d, e Sternum (50%)
   d Lateral radiograph
   e Left lateral aspect

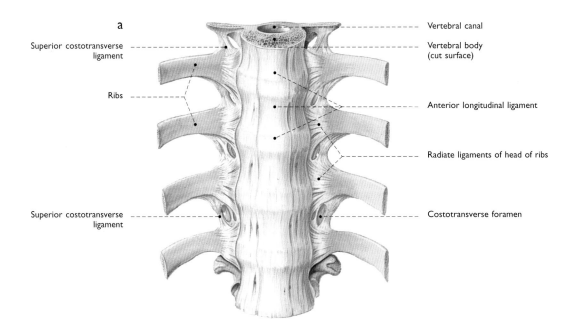

a

Superior costotransverse ligament

Ribs

Superior costotransverse ligament

Vertebral canal

Vertebral body (cut surface)

Anterior longitudinal ligament

Radiate ligaments of head of ribs

Costotransverse foramen

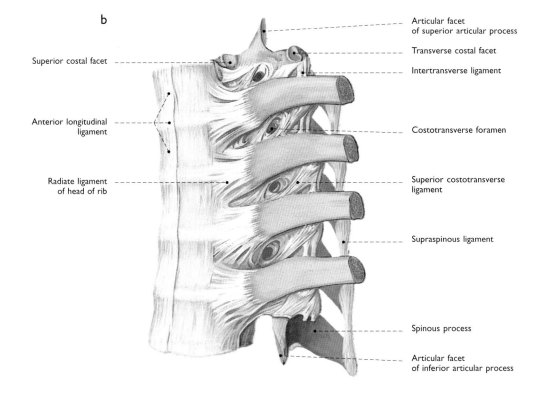

b

Superior costal facet

Anterior longitudinal ligament

Radiate ligament of head of rib

Articular facet of superior articular process

Transverse costal facet

Intertransverse ligament

Costotransverse foramen

Superior costotransverse ligament

Supraspinous ligament

Spinous process

Articular facet of inferior articular process

46 Costovertebral joints
a Ventral aspect (60%)
b Left lateral aspect (70%)

a

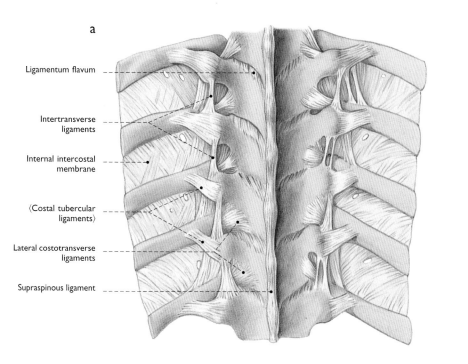

Ligamentum flavum

Intertransverse
ligaments

Internal intercostal
membrane

⟨Costal tubercular
ligaments⟩

Lateral costotransverse
ligaments

Supraspinous ligament

b

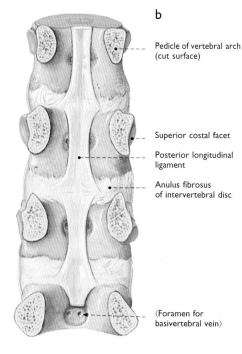

Pedicle of vertebral arch
(cut surface)

Superior costal facet

Posterior longitudinal
ligament

Anulus fibrosus
of intervertebral disc

⟨Foramen for
basivertebral vein⟩

c

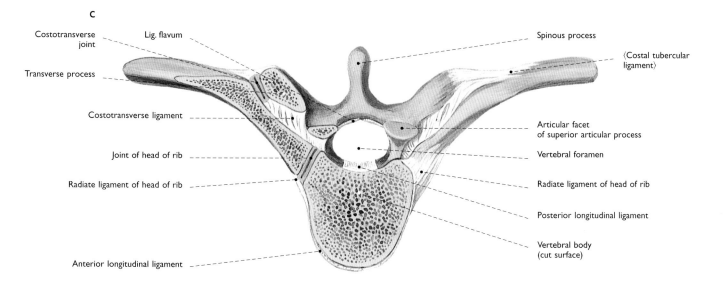

Costotransverse
joint

Transverse process

Costotransverse ligament

Joint of head of rib

Radiate ligament of head of rib

Anterior longitudinal ligament

Lig. flavum

Spinous process

⟨Costal tubercular
ligament⟩

Articular facet
of superior articular process

Vertebral foramen

Radiate ligament of head of rib

Posterior longitudinal ligament

Vertebral body
(cut surface)

47 Thoracic spine and costovertebral joints

a   Costovertebral joints (60%), dorsal aspect
b   Thoracic spine (70%), dorsal aspect of the ventral wall of
    the vertebral canal after removal of the vertebral arches
c   Middle thoracic vertebra and its ribs (100%), oblique section,
    cranial aspect

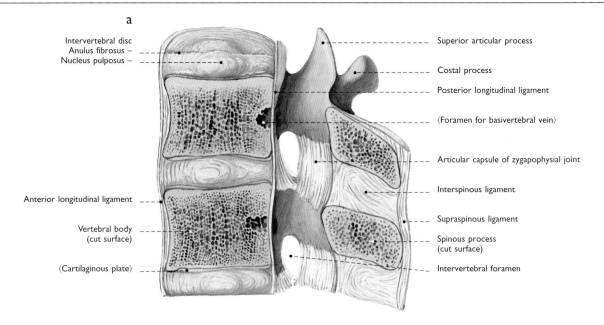

Intervertebral disc
Anulus fibrosus –
Nucleus pulposus –

Anterior longitudinal ligament

Vertebral body
(cut surface)

〈Cartilaginous plate〉

Superior articular process

Costal process

Posterior longitudinal ligament

〈Foramen for basivertebral vein〉

Articular capsule of zygapophysial joint

Interspinous ligament

Supraspinous ligament

Spinous process
(cut surface)

Intervertebral foramen

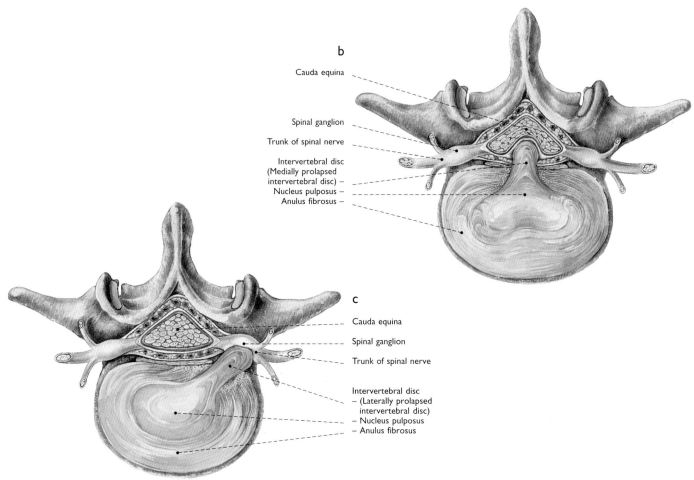

Cauda equina

Spinal ganglion

Trunk of spinal nerve

Intervertebral disc
(Medially prolapsed
intervertebral disc) –
Nucleus pulposus –
Anulus fibrosus –

Cauda equina

Spinal ganglion

Trunk of spinal nerve

Intervertebral disc
– (Laterally prolapsed
intervertebral disc)
– Nucleus pulposus
– Anulus fibrosus

48 Intervertebral disc

  a   Middle lumbar vertebrae with intervertebral discs (80%),
       median section, medial aspect
b, c   Lower lumbar vertebra with intervertebral disc,
       cauda equina and spinal nerves (100%), cranial aspect
  b   Medial prolapse of the disc
  c   Lateral prolapse of the disc

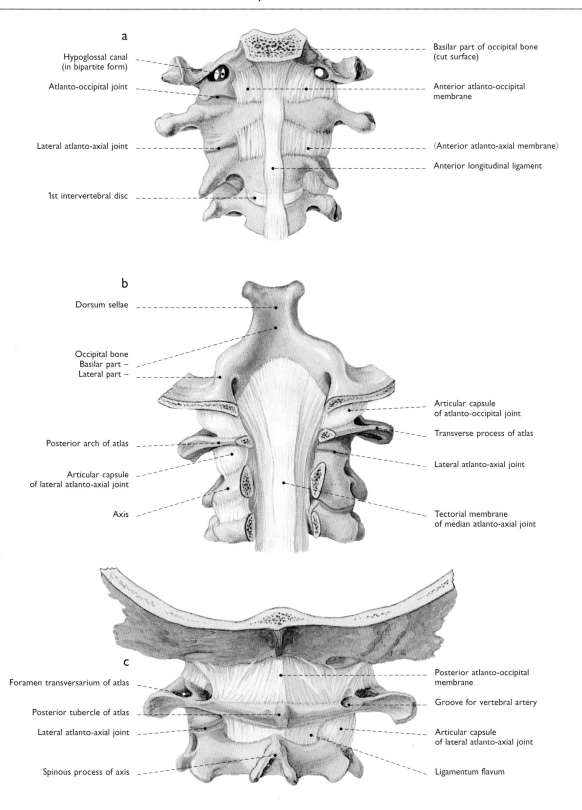

a

Hypoglossal canal
(in bipartite form)

Atlanto-occipital joint

Lateral atlanto-axial joint

1st intervertebral disc

Basilar part of occipital bone
(cut surface)

Anterior atlanto-occipital
membrane

⟨Anterior atlanto-axial membrane⟩

Anterior longitudinal ligament

b

Dorsum sellae

Occipital bone
Basilar part –
Lateral part –

Posterior arch of atlas

Articular capsule
of lateral atlanto-axial joint

Axis

Articular capsule
of atlanto-occipital joint

Transverse process of atlas

Lateral atlanto-axial joint

Tectorial membrane
of median atlanto-axial joint

c

Foramen transversarium of atlas

Posterior tubercle of atlas

Lateral atlanto-axial joint

Spinous process of axis

Posterior atlanto-occipital
membrane

Groove for vertebral artery

Articular capsule
of lateral atlanto-axial joint

Ligamentum flavum

49 Atlanto-occipital and atlanto-axial joints

  a   Ventral aspect (90%)
  b   Dorsal aspect (90%) after removal of the posterior part of
      the occipital bone and the arches of the upper cervical vertebrae.
      The vertebral canal was opened.
  c   Dorsal aspect with remaining vertebral arches (110%)

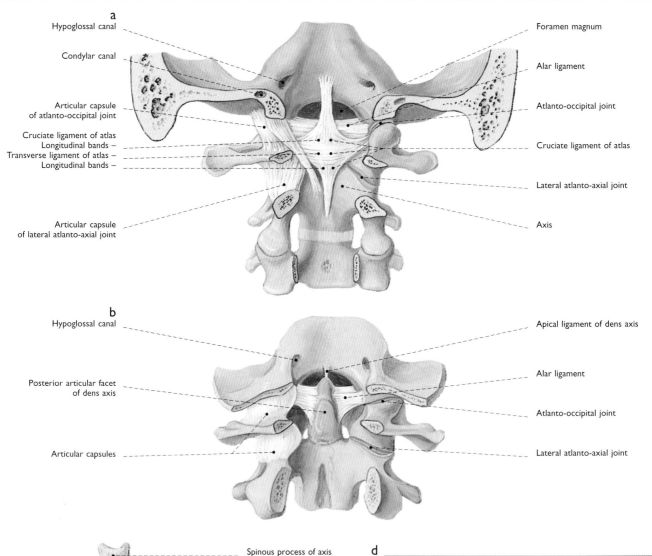

a

Hypoglossal canal

Condylar canal

Articular capsule
of atlanto-occipital joint

Cruciate ligament of atlas
Longitudinal bands –
Transverse ligament of atlas –
Longitudinal bands –

Articular capsule
of lateral atlanto-axial joint

Foramen magnum

Alar ligament

Atlanto-occipital joint

Cruciate ligament of atlas

Lateral atlanto-axial joint

Axis

b

Hypoglossal canal

Posterior articular facet
of dens axis

Articular capsules

Apical ligament of dens axis

Alar ligament

Atlanto-occipital joint

Lateral atlanto-axial joint

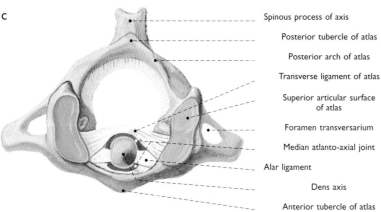

c

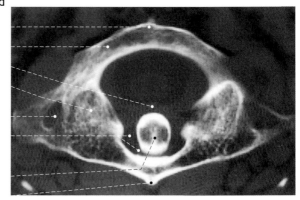

d

Spinous process of axis

Posterior tubercle of atlas

Posterior arch of atlas

Transverse ligament of atlas

Superior articular surface
of atlas

Foramen transversarium

Median atlanto-axial joint

Alar ligament

Dens axis

Anterior tubercle of atlas

50 Atlanto-occipital and atlanto-axial joints (100%)

a Dorsal aspect after removal of the posterior part
of the occipital bone and the arches of the upper cervical
vertebrae. The vertebral canal was opened.
b Dorsal aspect after additional removal
of the cruciate ligament of atlas
c Cranial aspect of the median atlanto-axial joint
d Transverse computed tomogram (CT) of the atlas and
the median atlanto-axial joint

a

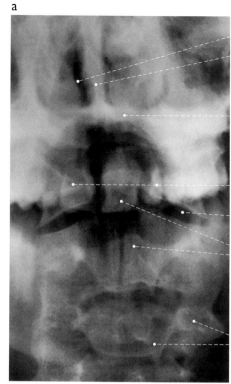

Nasal cavity

Nasal septum

Hard palate

Lateral masses of atlas

Lateral atlanto-axial joint

Axis
– Dens
– Vertebral body

3rd cervical vertebra
– Transverse process
– Vertebral body

b

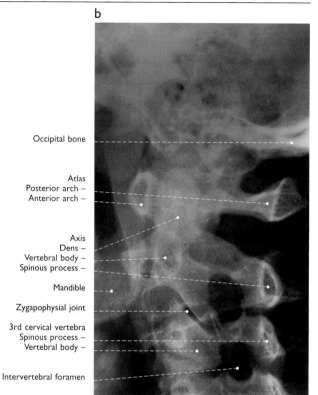

Occipital bone

Atlas
Posterior arch –
Anterior arch –

Axis
Dens –
Vertebral body –
Spinous process –

Mandible

Zygapophysial joint

3rd cervical vertebra
Spinous process –
Vertebral body –

Intervertebral foramen

c

Sphenoidal bone

Cranial dura mater

〈Anterior atlanto-occipital
membrane〉

Apical ligament of dens axis

Apical bursa of dens axis

Tectorial membrane

Median atlanto-axial joint

Transverse ligament of atlas

〈Anterior atlanto-axial membrane〉

Vertebral body of axis

Anterior longitudinal ligament

1st intervertebral disc

Basilar (venous) plexus

Vestibulocochlear nerve [VIII],
Facial nerve [VII]

Glossopharyngeal nerve [IX],
Vagus nerve [X],
Accessory nerve [XI]

Hypoglossal nerve [XII]

Squamous part of occipital bone

Vertebral artery,
Roots of 1st cervical nerve

Synovial bursa

51 Median atlanto-axial joint

a   Anteroposterior radiograph of the upper cervical spine
    (mouth opened) (70%)
b   Lateral radiograph of the upper cervical spine (70%)
c   Medial aspect of a median section through the occipital bone
    and the first cervical vertebrae (90%)

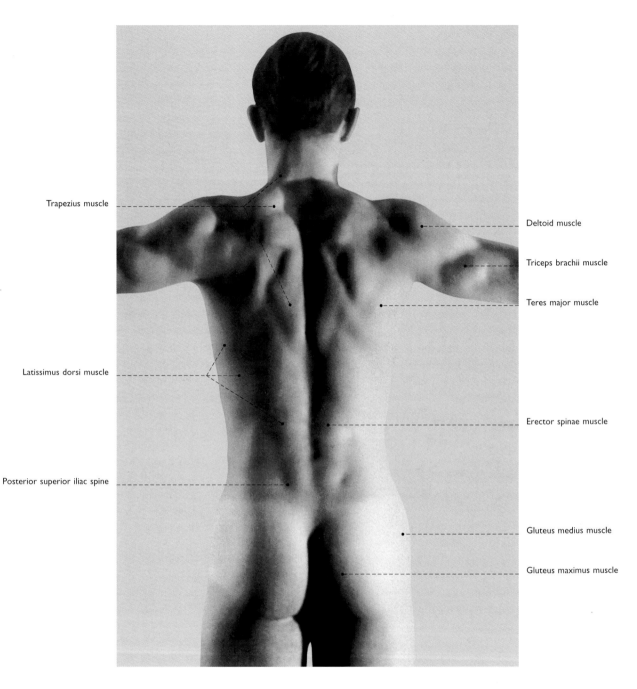

Trapezius muscle

Deltoid muscle

Triceps brachii muscle

Teres major muscle

Latissimus dorsi muscle

Erector spinae muscle

Posterior superior iliac spine

Gluteus medius muscle

Gluteus maximus muscle

52 Surface anatomy of the back of a male (20%)
Dorsal aspect

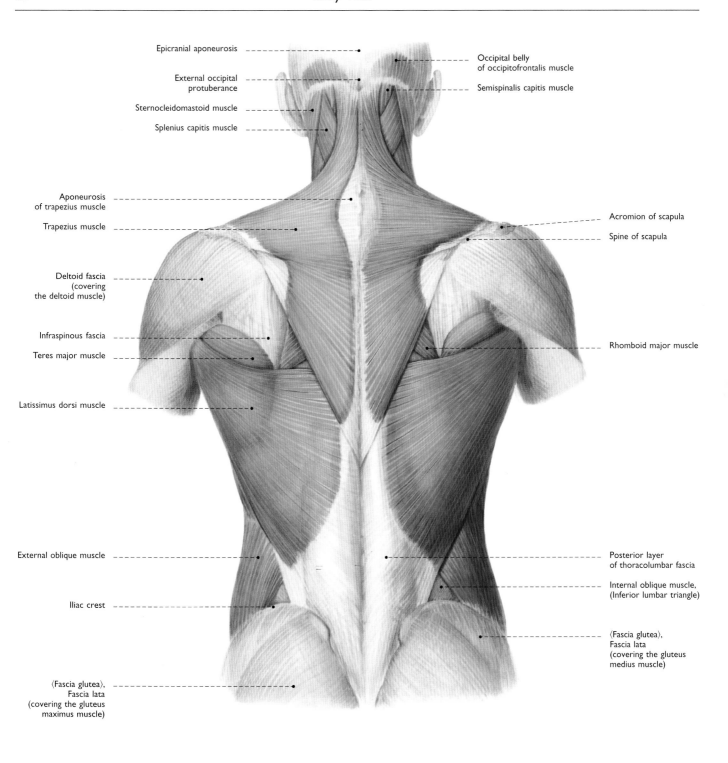

Epicranial aponeurosis

External occipital protuberance

Sternocleidomastoid muscle

Splenius capitis muscle

Occipital belly of occipitofrontalis muscle

Semispinalis capitis muscle

Aponeurosis of trapezius muscle

Trapezius muscle

Deltoid fascia (covering the deltoid muscle)

Infraspinous fascia

Teres major muscle

Latissimus dorsi muscle

Acromion of scapula

Spine of scapula

Rhomboid major muscle

External oblique muscle

Iliac crest

⟨Fascia glutea⟩, Fascia lata (covering the gluteus maximus muscle)

Posterior layer of thoracolumbar fascia

Internal oblique muscle, (Inferior lumbar triangle)

⟨Fascia glutea⟩, Fascia lata (covering the gluteus medius muscle)

53 Muscles of the back (25%)
Superficial layer

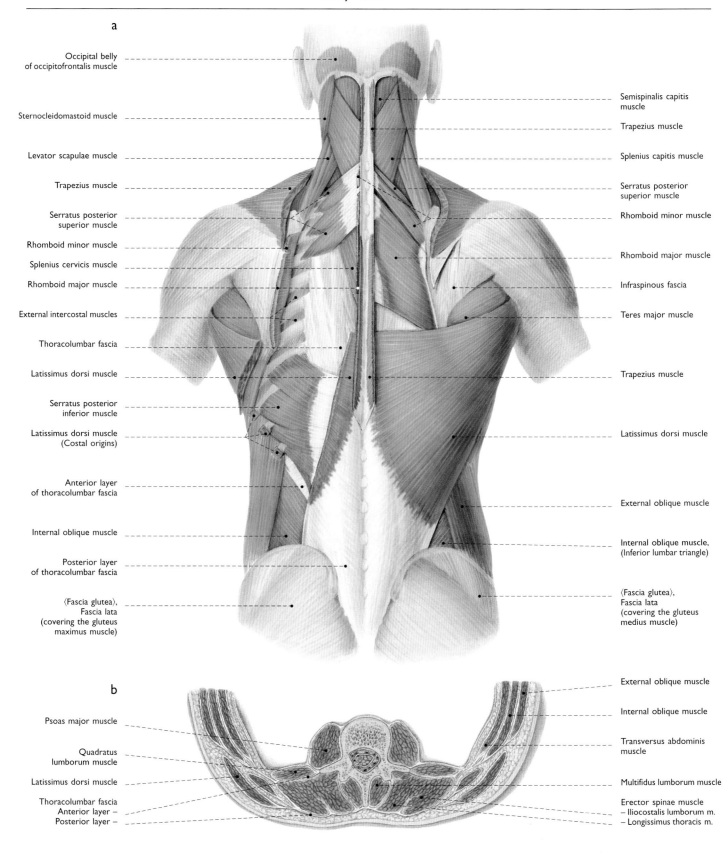

a

Occipital belly
of occipitofrontalis muscle

Sternocleidomastoid muscle

Levator scapulae muscle

Trapezius muscle

Serratus posterior
superior muscle

Rhomboid minor muscle

Splenius cervicis muscle

Rhomboid major muscle

External intercostal muscles

Thoracolumbar fascia

Latissimus dorsi muscle

Serratus posterior
inferior muscle

Latissimus dorsi muscle
(Costal origins)

Anterior layer
of thoracolumbar fascia

Internal oblique muscle

Posterior layer
of thoracolumbar fascia

⟨Fascia glutea⟩,
Fascia lata
(covering the gluteus
maximus muscle)

Semispinalis capitis
muscle

Trapezius muscle

Splenius capitis muscle

Serratus posterior
superior muscle

Rhomboid minor muscle

Rhomboid major muscle

Infraspinous fascia

Teres major muscle

Trapezius muscle

Latissimus dorsi muscle

External oblique muscle

Internal oblique muscle,
(Inferior lumbar triangle)

⟨Fascia glutea⟩,
Fascia lata
(covering the gluteus
medius muscle)

b

Psoas major muscle

Quadratus
lumborum muscle

Latissimus dorsi muscle

Thoracolumbar fascia
Anterior layer –
Posterior layer –

External oblique muscle

Internal oblique muscle

Transversus abdominis
muscle

Multifidus lumborum muscle

Erector spinae muscle
– Iliocostalis lumborum m.
– Longissimus thoracis m.

54 Muscles of the back

a Deeper layer (25%)
b Schematized transverse section through the posterior and
lateral abdominal wall in the lumbar region (35%)

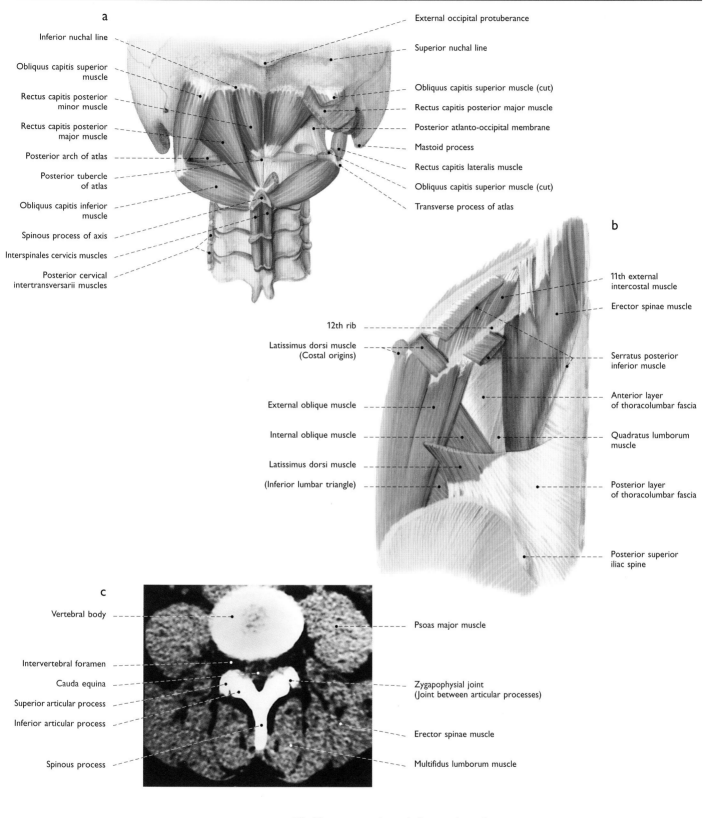

a

External occipital protuberance

Inferior nuchal line

Superior nuchal line

Obliquus capitis superior muscle

Obliquus capitis superior muscle (cut)

Rectus capitis posterior minor muscle

Rectus capitis posterior major muscle

Rectus capitis posterior major muscle

Posterior atlanto-occipital membrane

Posterior arch of atlas

Mastoid process

Posterior tubercle of atlas

Rectus capitis lateralis muscle

Obliquus capitis inferior muscle

Obliquus capitis superior muscle (cut)

Spinous process of axis

Transverse process of atlas

Interspinales cervicis muscles

Posterior cervical intertransversarii muscles

b

11th external intercostal muscle

Erector spinae muscle

12th rib

Latissimus dorsi muscle (Costal origins)

Serratus posterior inferior muscle

External oblique muscle

Anterior layer of thoracolumbar fascia

Internal oblique muscle

Quadratus lumborum muscle

Latissimus dorsi muscle

Posterior layer of thoracolumbar fascia

(Inferior lumbar triangle)

Posterior superior iliac spine

c

Vertebral body

Psoas major muscle

Intervertebral foramen

Cauda equina

Zygapophysial joint (Joint between articular processes)

Superior articular process

Inferior articular process

Erector spinae muscle

Spinous process

Multifidus lumborum muscle

55 Deep muscles of the neck and muscles of the lumbar region

a Deep muscles of the neck (50%), dorsal aspect
b Muscles of the lumbar region (40%), left dorsolateral aspect.
  The latissimus dorsi and serratus posterior inferior muscles
  were partially removed.
c Transverse computed tomogram (CT) of the fifth lumbar vertebra
  with adjacent muscles (40%)

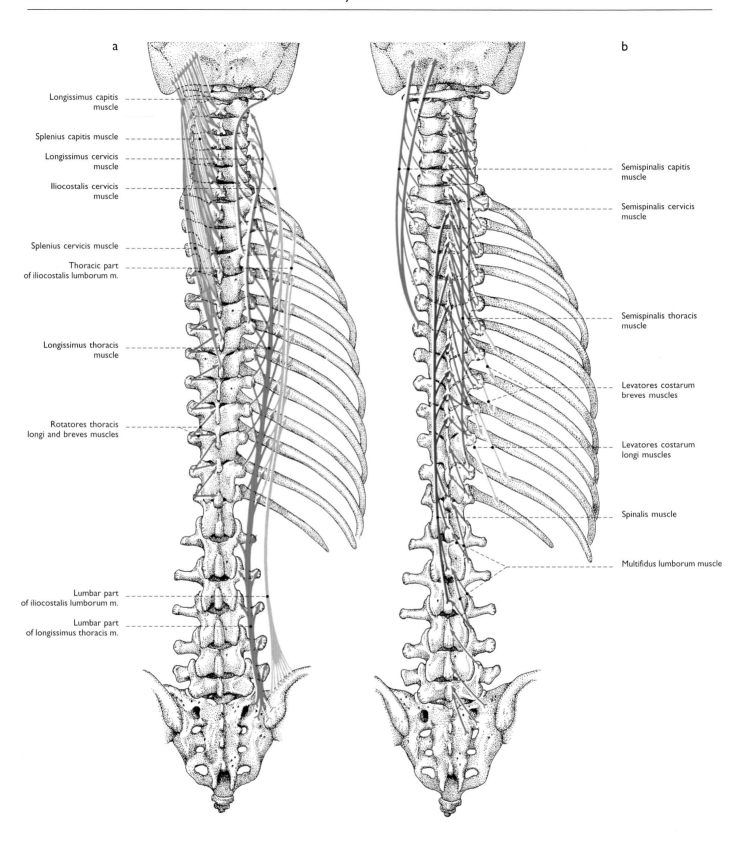

a

Longissimus capitis muscle

Splenius capitis muscle

Longissimus cervicis muscle

Iliocostalis cervicis muscle

Splenius cervicis muscle

Thoracic part of iliocostalis lumborum m.

Longissimus thoracis muscle

Rotatores thoracis longi and breves muscles

Lumbar part of iliocostalis lumborum m.

Lumbar part of longissimus thoracis m.

b

Semispinalis capitis muscle

Semispinalis cervicis muscle

Semispinalis thoracis muscle

Levatores costarum breves muscles

Levatores costarum longi muscles

Spinalis muscle

Multifidus lumborum muscle

56 Muscles of the back proper (30%)

Schematic course
The muscles of the medial tract of the erector spinae are colored
in red to brown, the muscles of the lateral tract in blue,
the splenii and levatores costarum muscles are given in green.

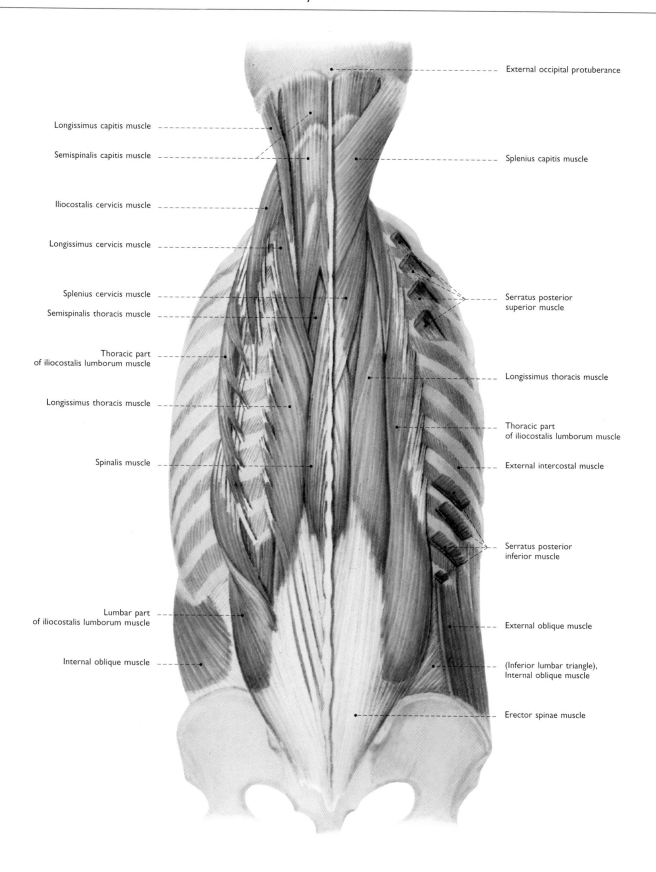

Longissimus capitis muscle

Semispinalis capitis muscle

Iliocostalis cervicis muscle

Longissimus cervicis muscle

Splenius cervicis muscle

Semispinalis thoracis muscle

Thoracic part
of iliocostalis lumborum muscle

Longissimus thoracis muscle

Spinalis muscle

Lumbar part
of iliocostalis lumborum muscle

Internal oblique muscle

External occipital protuberance

Splenius capitis muscle

Serratus posterior
superior muscle

Longissimus thoracis muscle

Thoracic part
of iliocostalis lumborum muscle

External intercostal muscle

Serratus posterior
inferior muscle

External oblique muscle

(Inferior lumbar triangle),
Internal oblique muscle

Erector spinae muscle

57 Muscles of the back proper (30%)
Superficial layer

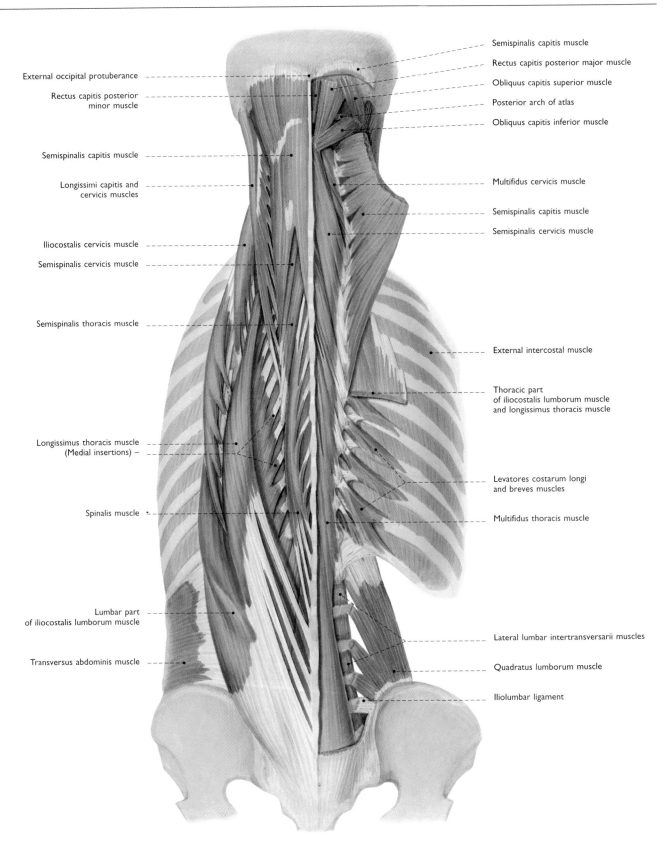

Semispinalis capitis muscle

Rectus capitis posterior major muscle

Obliquus capitis superior muscle

Posterior arch of atlas

Obliquus capitis inferior muscle

Multifidus cervicis muscle

Semispinalis capitis muscle

Semispinalis cervicis muscle

External intercostal muscle

Thoracic part
of iliocostalis lumborum muscle
and longissimus thoracis muscle

Levatores costarum longi
and breves muscles

Multifidus thoracis muscle

Lateral lumbar intertransversarii muscles

Quadratus lumborum muscle

Iliolumbar ligament

External occipital protuberance

Rectus capitis posterior
minor muscle

Semispinalis capitis muscle

Longissimi capitis and
cervicis muscles

Iliocostalis cervicis muscle

Semispinalis cervicis muscle

Semispinalis thoracis muscle

Longissimus thoracis muscle
(Medial insertions)

Spinalis muscle

Lumbar part
of iliocostalis lumborum muscle

Transversus abdominis muscle

58 Muscles of the back proper (30%)
Deeper layer

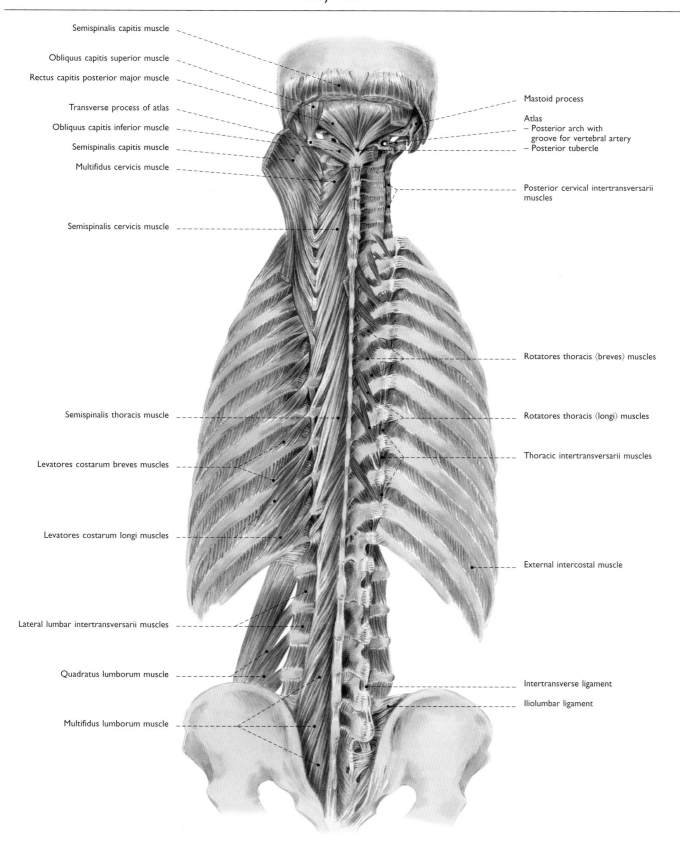

Semispinalis capitis muscle

Obliquus capitis superior muscle

Rectus capitis posterior major muscle

Transverse process of atlas

Obliquus capitis inferior muscle

Semispinalis capitis muscle

Multifidus cervicis muscle

Semispinalis cervicis muscle

Semispinalis thoracis muscle

Levatores costarum breves muscles

Levatores costarum longi muscles

Lateral lumbar intertransversarii muscles

Quadratus lumborum muscle

Multifidus lumborum muscle

Mastoid process

Atlas
– Posterior arch with
  groove for vertebral artery
– Posterior tubercle

Posterior cervical intertransversarii
muscles

Rotatores thoracis ⟨breves⟩ muscles

Rotatores thoracis ⟨longi⟩ muscles

Thoracic intertransversarii muscles

External intercostal muscle

Intertransverse ligament

Iliolumbar ligament

59 Muscles of the back proper (30%)
Deep layer

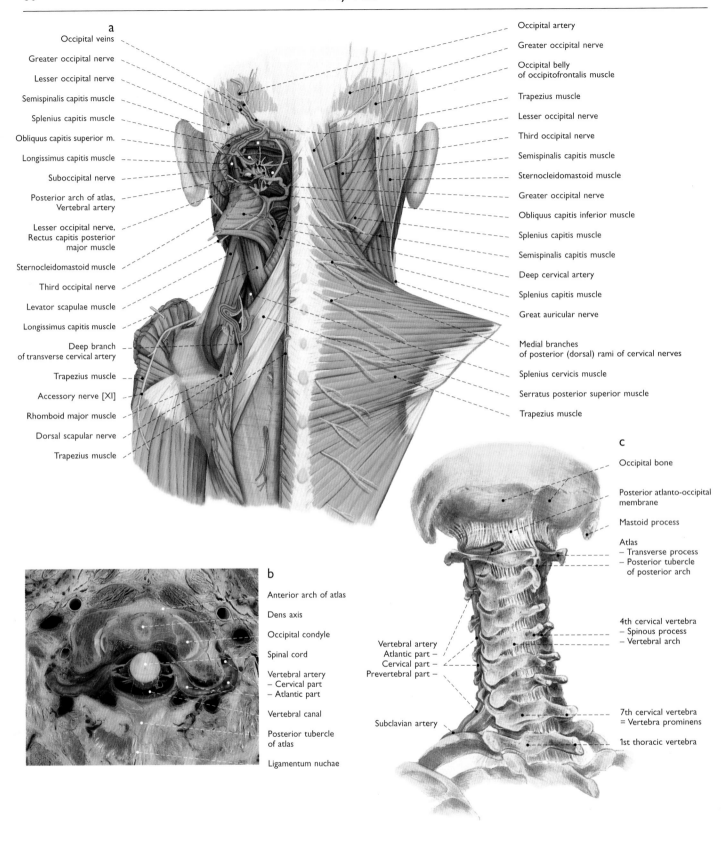

a

Occipital veins

Greater occipital nerve

Lesser occipital nerve

Semispinalis capitis muscle

Splenius capitis muscle

Obliquus capitis superior m.

Longissimus capitis muscle

Suboccipital nerve

Posterior arch of atlas,
Vertebral artery

Lesser occipital nerve,
Rectus capitis posterior
major muscle

Sternocleidomastoid muscle

Third occipital nerve

Levator scapulae muscle

Longissimus capitis muscle

Deep branch
of transverse cervical artery

Trapezius muscle

Accessory nerve [XI]

Rhomboid major muscle

Dorsal scapular nerve

Trapezius muscle

Occipital artery

Greater occipital nerve

Occipital belly
of occipitofrontalis muscle

Trapezius muscle

Lesser occipital nerve

Third occipital nerve

Semispinalis capitis muscle

Sternocleidomastoid muscle

Greater occipital nerve

Obliquus capitis inferior muscle

Splenius capitis muscle

Semispinalis capitis muscle

Deep cervical artery

Splenius capitis muscle

Great auricular nerve

Medial branches
of posterior (dorsal) rami of cervical nerves

Splenius cervicis muscle

Serratus posterior superior muscle

Trapezius muscle

b

Anterior arch of atlas

Dens axis

Occipital condyle

Spinal cord

Vertebral artery
− Cervical part
− Atlantic part

Vertebral canal

Posterior tubercle
of atlas

Ligamentum nuchae

c

Occipital bone

Posterior atlanto-occipital
membrane

Mastoid process

Atlas
− Transverse process
− Posterior tubercle
  of posterior arch

4th cervical vertebra
− Spinous process
− Vertebral arch

7th cervical vertebra
= Vertebra prominens

1st thoracic vertebra

Vertebral artery
Atlantic part −
Cervical part −
Prevertebral part −

Subclavian artery

60 Neck and shoulder regions

a Right, superficial layer; left, deeper layer (40%). Dorsal aspect
b Horizontal section at the level of the first cervical vertebra (= atlas)
(60%). Cranial aspect
c Course of the vertebral artery (60%). Left dorsolateral aspect

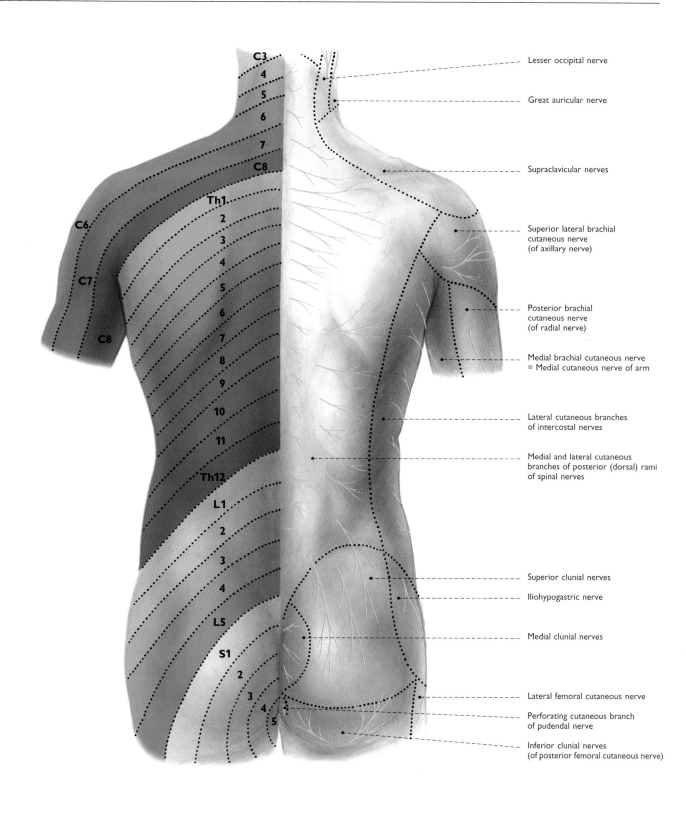

**61 Cutaneous and segmental innervation
of the dorsal body wall** (25%)
Schematic representation

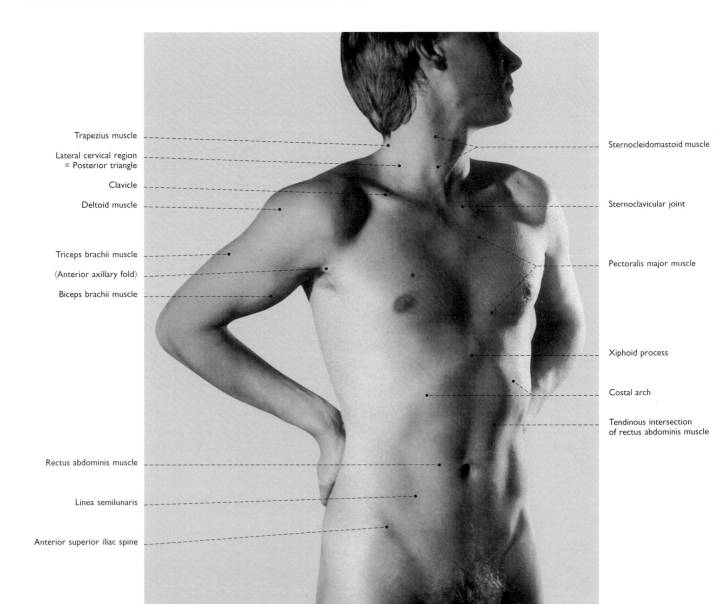

Trapezius muscle

Lateral cervical region = Posterior triangle

Clavicle

Deltoid muscle

Triceps brachii muscle

⟨Anterior axillary fold⟩

Biceps brachii muscle

Rectus abdominis muscle

Linea semilunaris

Anterior superior iliac spine

Sternocleidomastoid muscle

Sternoclavicular joint

Pectoralis major muscle

Xiphoid process

Costal arch

Tendinous intersection of rectus abdominis muscle

62 **Surface anatomy of the thorax and abdomen of a male** (20%)
Ventral aspect

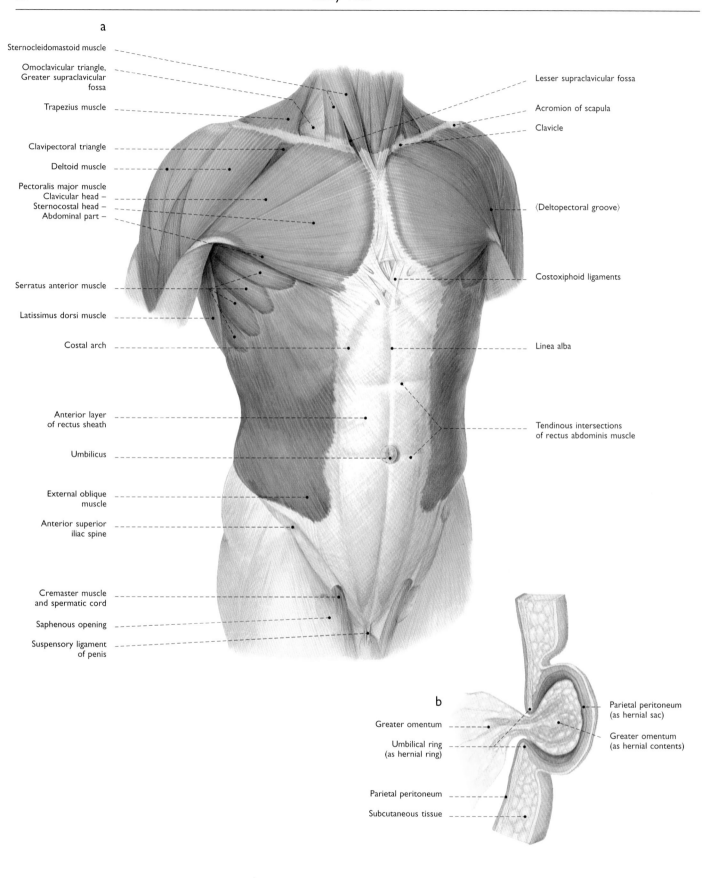

a

Sternocleidomastoid muscle

Omoclavicular triangle, Greater supraclavicular fossa

Trapezius muscle

Clavipectoral triangle

Deltoid muscle

Pectoralis major muscle
Clavicular head –
Sternocostal head –
Abdominal part –

Serratus anterior muscle

Latissimus dorsi muscle

Costal arch

Anterior layer of rectus sheath

Umbilicus

External oblique muscle

Anterior superior iliac spine

Cremaster muscle and spermatic cord

Saphenous opening

Suspensory ligament of penis

Lesser supraclavicular fossa

Acromion of scapula

Clavicle

⟨Deltopectoral groove⟩

Costoxiphoid ligaments

Linea alba

Tendinous intersections of rectus abdominis muscle

b

Greater omentum

Umbilical ring (as hernial ring)

Parietal peritoneum

Subcutaneous tissue

Parietal peritoneum (as hernial sac)

Greater omentum (as hernial contents)

63 Ventral muscles of the trunk
a Superficial layer (25%)
b Schematic representation of an umbilical hernia

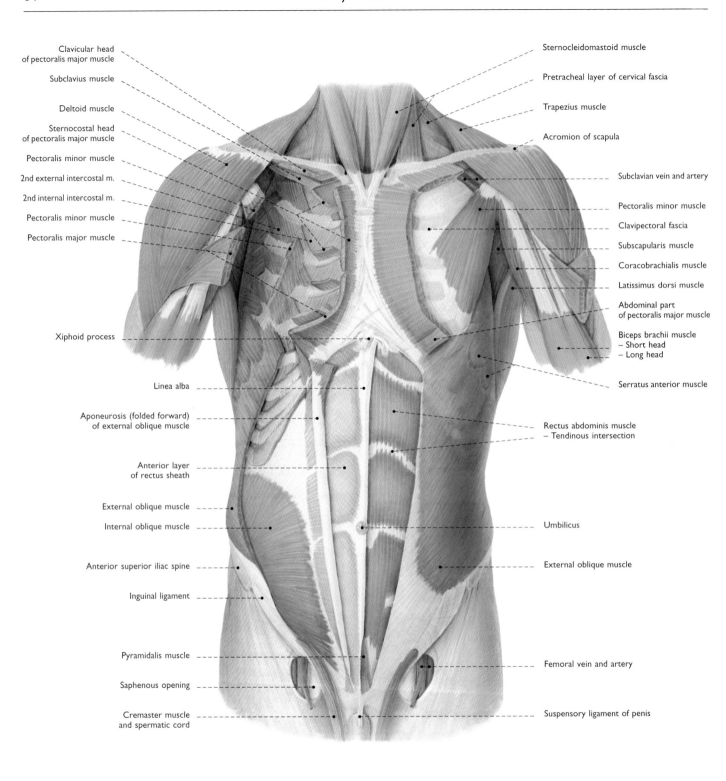

Clavicular head
of pectoralis major muscle

Subclavius muscle

Deltoid muscle

Sternocostal head
of pectoralis major muscle

Pectoralis minor muscle

2nd external intercostal m.

2nd internal intercostal m.

Pectoralis minor muscle

Pectoralis major muscle

Xiphoid process

Linea alba

Aponeurosis (folded forward)
of external oblique muscle

Anterior layer
of rectus sheath

External oblique muscle

Internal oblique muscle

Anterior superior iliac spine

Inguinal ligament

Pyramidalis muscle

Saphenous opening

Cremaster muscle
and spermatic cord

Sternocleidomastoid muscle

Pretracheal layer of cervical fascia

Trapezius muscle

Acromion of scapula

Subclavian vein and artery

Pectoralis minor muscle

Clavipectoral fascia

Subscapularis muscle

Coracobrachialis muscle

Latissimus dorsi muscle

Abdominal part
of pectoralis major muscle

Biceps brachii muscle
– Short head
– Long head

Serratus anterior muscle

Rectus abdominis muscle
– Tendinous intersection

Umbilicus

External oblique muscle

Femoral vein and artery

Suspensory ligament of penis

64 Ventral muscles of the trunk (25%)
Deeper layer

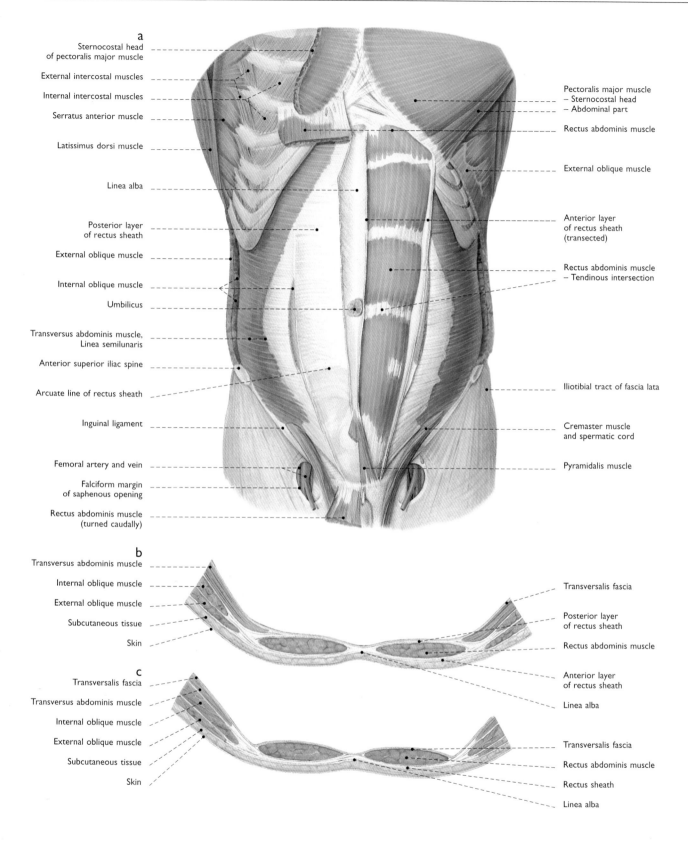

a
Sternocostal head of pectoralis major muscle
External intercostal muscles
Internal intercostal muscles
Serratus anterior muscle
Latissimus dorsi muscle
Linea alba
Posterior layer of rectus sheath
External oblique muscle
Internal oblique muscle
Umbilicus
Transversus abdominis muscle, Linea semilunaris
Anterior superior iliac spine
Arcuate line of rectus sheath
Inguinal ligament
Femoral artery and vein
Falciform margin of saphenous opening
Rectus abdominis muscle (turned caudally)

Pectoralis major muscle
– Sternocostal head
– Abdominal part
Rectus abdominis muscle
External oblique muscle
Anterior layer of rectus sheath (transected)
Rectus abdominis muscle – Tendinous intersection
Iliotibial tract of fascia lata
Cremaster muscle and spermatic cord
Pyramidalis muscle

b
Transversus abdominis muscle
Internal oblique muscle
External oblique muscle
Subcutaneous tissue
Skin

Transversalis fascia
Posterior layer of rectus sheath
Rectus abdominis muscle
Anterior layer of rectus sheath
Linea alba

c
Transversalis fascia
Transversus abdominis muscle
Internal oblique muscle
External oblique muscle
Subcutaneous tissue
Skin

Transversalis fascia
Rectus abdominis muscle
Rectus sheath
Linea alba

65 Muscles of the abdomen
a   Deepest layer (30%)
b, c Schematized transverse sections through
     the anterior abdominal wall (50%)
b   above the umbilical region
c   below the arcuate line of rectus sheath

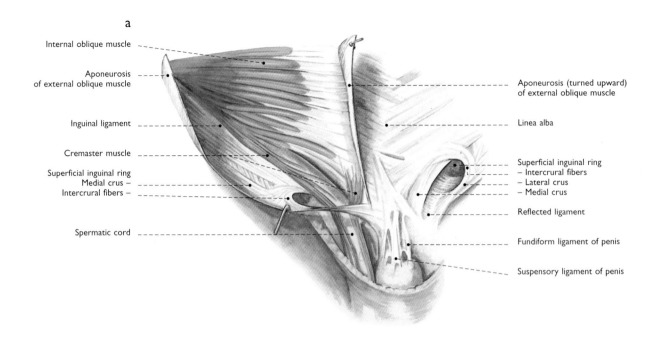

a

Internal oblique muscle

Aponeurosis
of external oblique muscle

Inguinal ligament

Cremaster muscle

Superficial inguinal ring
Medial crus –
Intercrural fibers –

Spermatic cord

Aponeurosis (turned upward)
of external oblique muscle

Linea alba

Superficial inguinal ring
– Intercrural fibers
– Lateral crus
– Medial crus

Reflected ligament

Fundiform ligament of penis

Suspensory ligament of penis

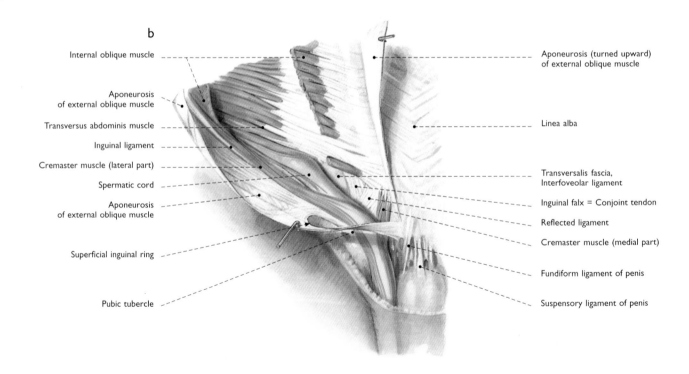

b

Internal oblique muscle

Aponeurosis
of external oblique muscle

Transversus abdominis muscle

Inguinal ligament

Cremaster muscle (lateral part)

Spermatic cord

Aponeurosis
of external oblique muscle

Superficial inguinal ring

Pubic tubercle

Aponeurosis (turned upward)
of external oblique muscle

Linea alba

Transversalis fascia,
Interfoveolar ligament

Inguinal falx = Conjoint tendon

Reflected ligament

Cremaster muscle (medial part)

Fundiform ligament of penis

Suspensory ligament of penis

66 Inguinal region of a male (60%)

a   Superficial layer
b   Deep layer
a, b   The two portions of the dissected aponeurosis of the external
oblique muscle were retracted on the right side of the body.
In fig. b, the internal oblique muscle was additionally removed partially.
On the left side of the body in fig. a, the spermatic cord was taken away
to demonstrate the inguinal canal.

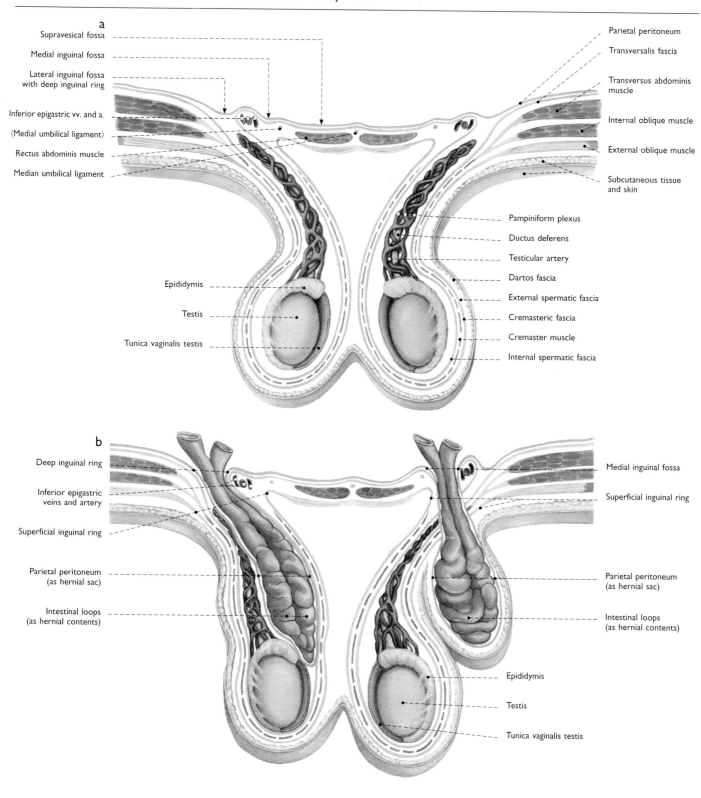

a

Supravesical fossa

Medial inguinal fossa

Lateral inguinal fossa
with deep inguinal ring

Inferior epigastric vv. and a.
⟨Medial umbilical ligament⟩

Rectus abdominis muscle

Median umbilical ligament

Parietal peritoneum

Transversalis fascia

Transversus abdominis
muscle

Internal oblique muscle

External oblique muscle

Subcutaneous tissue
and skin

Pampiniform plexus

Ductus deferens

Testicular artery

Dartos fascia

External spermatic fascia

Cremasteric fascia

Cremaster muscle

Internal spermatic fascia

Epididymis

Testis

Tunica vaginalis testis

b

Deep inguinal ring

Inferior epigastric
veins and artery

Superficial inguinal ring

Parietal peritoneum
(as hernial sac)

Intestinal loops
(as hernial contents)

Medial inguinal fossa

Superficial inguinal ring

Parietal peritoneum
(as hernial sac)

Intestinal loops
(as hernial contents)

Epididymis

Testis

Tunica vaginalis testis

67 Inguinal region of a male

a, b Schematized sections through the anterior abdominal wall
on the level of the inguinal canal and through the scrotum
(according to Benninghoff, 1985).
a Normal situation
b Inguinal herniae. On the right side of the body, a lateral indirect
hernia through the inguinal canal; the inner hernial ring is the
deep inguinal ring lateral to the inferior epigastric vessels.
On the left side of the body, a medial direct hernia; the inner hernial ring
is the medial inguinal fossa medial to the inferior epigastric vessels.

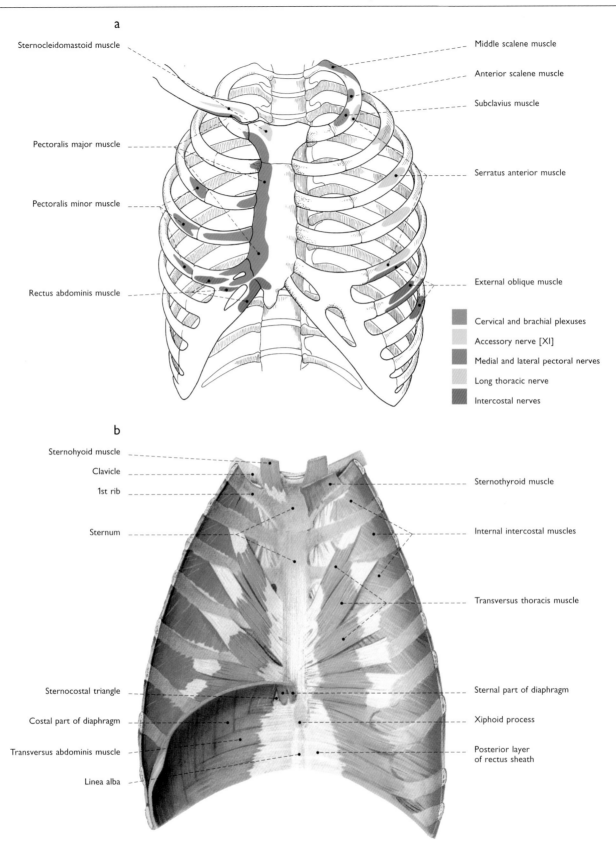

a

Sternocleidomastoid muscle

Middle scalene muscle

Anterior scalene muscle

Subclavius muscle

Pectoralis major muscle

Pectoralis minor muscle

Serratus anterior muscle

External oblique muscle

Rectus abdominis muscle

Cervical and brachial plexuses

Accessory nerve [XI]

Medial and lateral pectoral nerves

Long thoracic nerve

Intercostal nerves

b

Sternohyoid muscle

Clavicle

1st rib

Sternum

Sternothyroid muscle

Internal intercostal muscles

Transversus thoracis muscle

Sternocostal triangle

Costal part of diaphragm

Transversus abdominis muscle

Linea alba

Sternal part of diaphragm

Xiphoid process

Posterior layer
of rectus sheath

68 Ventral muscles of the trunk

a Muscle attachments on the ventrolateral thorax.
  The colors indicate the innervation.
b Internal aspect of the anterior chest wall and
  the genuine muscles of the thorax (35%)

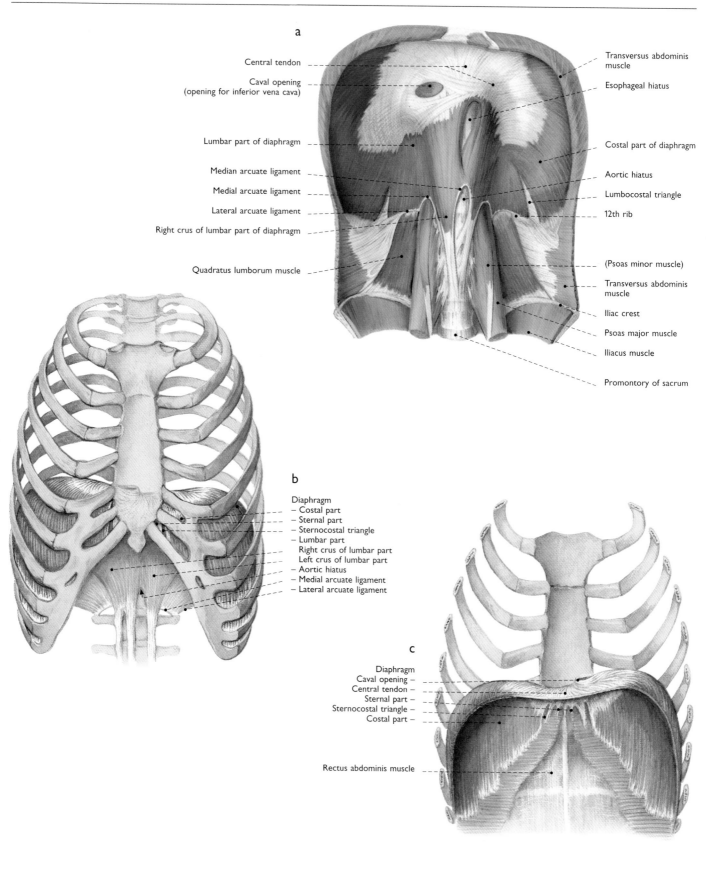

a

Central tendon

Caval opening
(opening for inferior vena cava)

Lumbar part of diaphragm

Median arcuate ligament

Medial arcuate ligament

Lateral arcuate ligament

Right crus of lumbar part of diaphragm

Quadratus lumborum muscle

Transversus abdominis
muscle

Esophageal hiatus

Costal part of diaphragm

Aortic hiatus

Lumbocostal triangle

12th rib

(Psoas minor muscle)

Transversus abdominis
muscle

Iliac crest

Psoas major muscle

Iliacus muscle

Promontory of sacrum

b

Diaphragm
– Costal part
– Sternal part
– Sternocostal triangle
– Lumbar part
  Right crus of lumbar part
  Left crus of lumbar part
– Aortic hiatus
– Medial arcuate ligament
– Lateral arcuate ligament

c

Diaphragm
Caval opening –
Central tendon –
Sternal part –
Sternocostal triangle –
Costal part –

Rectus abdominis muscle

69 Diaphragm (30%)
a Caudal aspect
b Ventral aspect
c Dorsal aspect

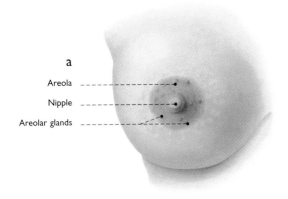

a

Areola

Nipple

Areolar glands

b

Lobes of mammary gland

Lactiferous ducts

Nipple

Skin
(cut edges)

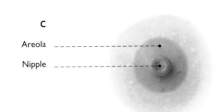

c

Areola

Nipple

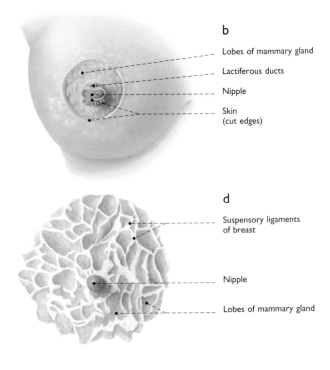

d

Suspensory ligaments
of breast

Nipple

Lobes of mammary gland

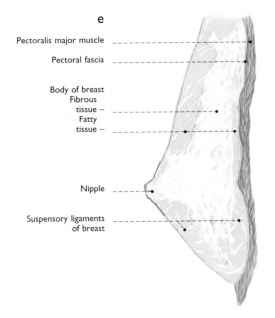

e

Pectoralis major muscle

Pectoral fascia

Body of breast
Fibrous
tissue –
Fatty
tissue –

Nipple

Suspensory ligaments
of breast

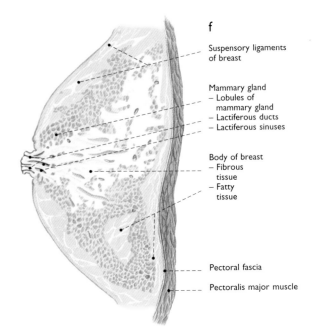

f

Suspensory ligaments
of breast

Mammary gland
– Lobules of
mammary gland
– Lactiferous ducts
– Lactiferous sinuses

Body of breast
– Fibrous
tissue
– Fatty
tissue

Pectoral fascia

Pectoralis major muscle

70 Breast

a Ventral aspect (40%)
b Ventral aspect (40%). The skin around the nipple was removed.
c Depressed nipple (70%)
d Parenchyma of the mammary gland after removal of
   the skin and the subcutaneous tissue (40%)
e Sagittal section through the breast of a 16-year-old
   non-pregnant nullipara (60%)
f Sagittal section through the breast of a 28-year-old
   woman immediately before lactation (60%)

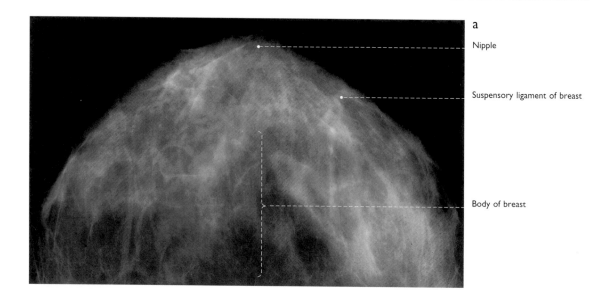

a

Nipple

Suspensory ligament of breast

Body of breast

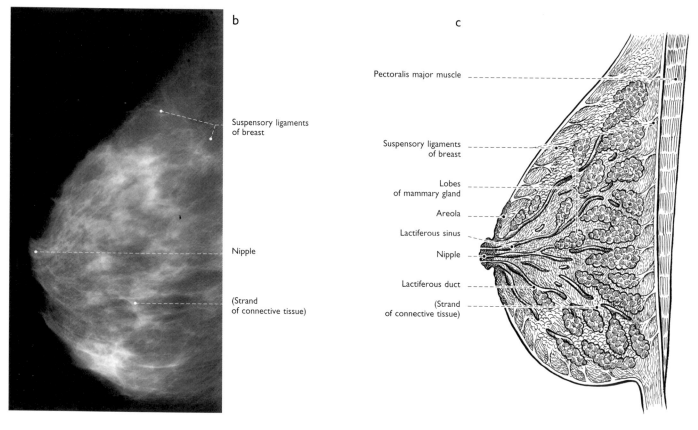

b

Suspensory ligaments
of breast

Nipple

(Strand
of connective tissue)

c

Pectoralis major muscle

Suspensory ligaments
of breast

Lobes
of mammary gland

Areola

Lactiferous sinus

Nipple

Lactiferous duct

(Strand
of connective tissue)

71 Breast

a, b Mammograms
  a Craniocaudal radiogram
  b Lateral radiogram
  c Construction of the breast,
    schematized representation of a sagittal section

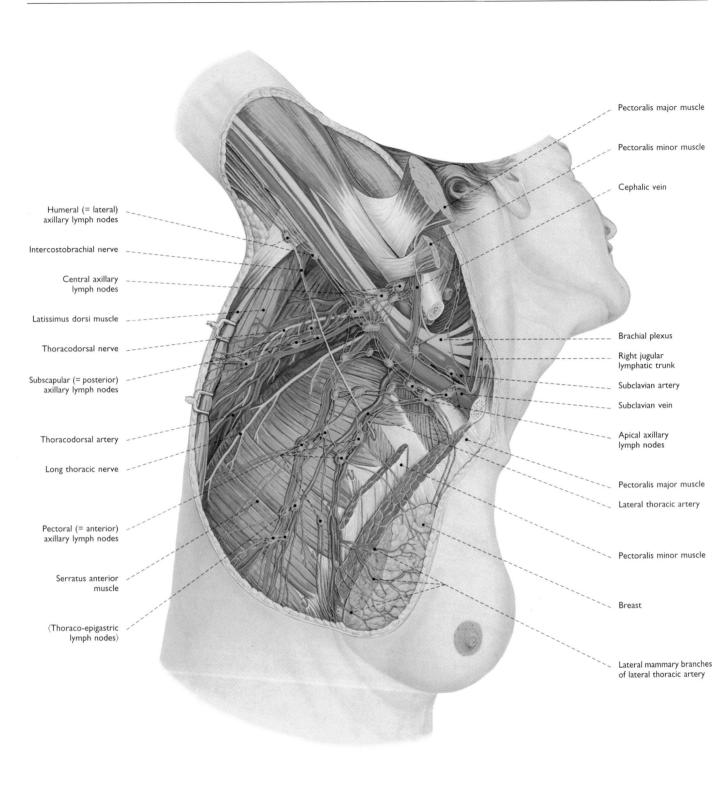

Pectoralis major muscle

Pectoralis minor muscle

Cephalic vein

Humeral (= lateral)
axillary lymph nodes

Intercostobrachial nerve

Central axillary
lymph nodes

Latissimus dorsi muscle

Thoracodorsal nerve

Subscapular (= posterior)
axillary lymph nodes

Thoracodorsal artery

Long thoracic nerve

Pectoral (= anterior)
axillary lymph nodes

Serratus anterior
muscle

(Thoraco-epigastric
lymph nodes)

Brachial plexus

Right jugular
lymphatic trunk

Subclavian artery

Subclavian vein

Apical axillary
lymph nodes

Pectoralis major muscle

Lateral thoracic artery

Pectoralis minor muscle

Breast

Lateral mammary branches
of lateral thoracic artery

**72 Lymphatic vessels and lymph nodes
of the axilla and the anterior chest wall** (50%)
Lateral aspect

a

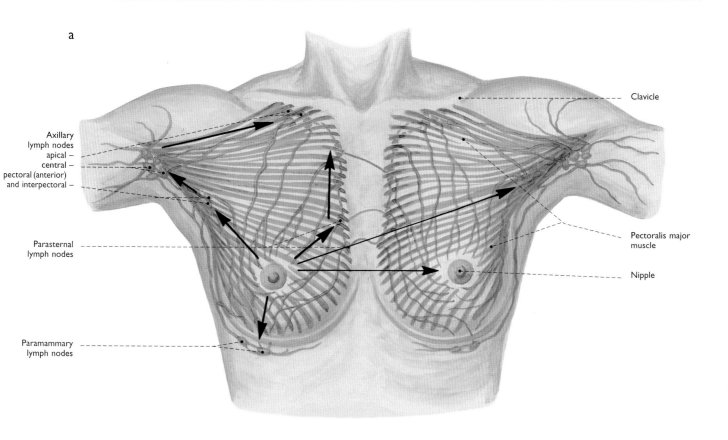

Clavicle

Axillary
lymph nodes
apical –
central –
pectoral (anterior) –
and interpectoral –

Parasternal
lymph nodes

Paramammary
lymph nodes

Pectoralis major
muscle

Nipple

b

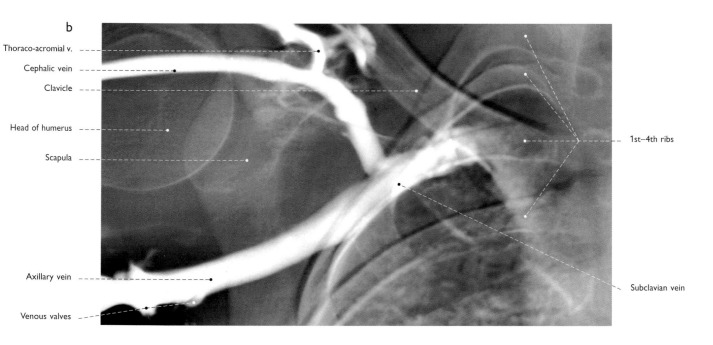

Thoraco-acromial v.

Cephalic vein

Clavicle

Head of humerus

Scapula

1st–4th ribs

Axillary vein

Subclavian vein

Venous valves

**73 Lymphatic vessels, lymph nodes, and veins
of the axilla and anterior chest wall**

a Schematic representation of the lymphatic drainage from the right breast (30%).
The arrows illustrate the main ways of drainage.
b Venogram of the veins of the axilla after injection of contrast medium,
postero-anterior radiogram (80%)

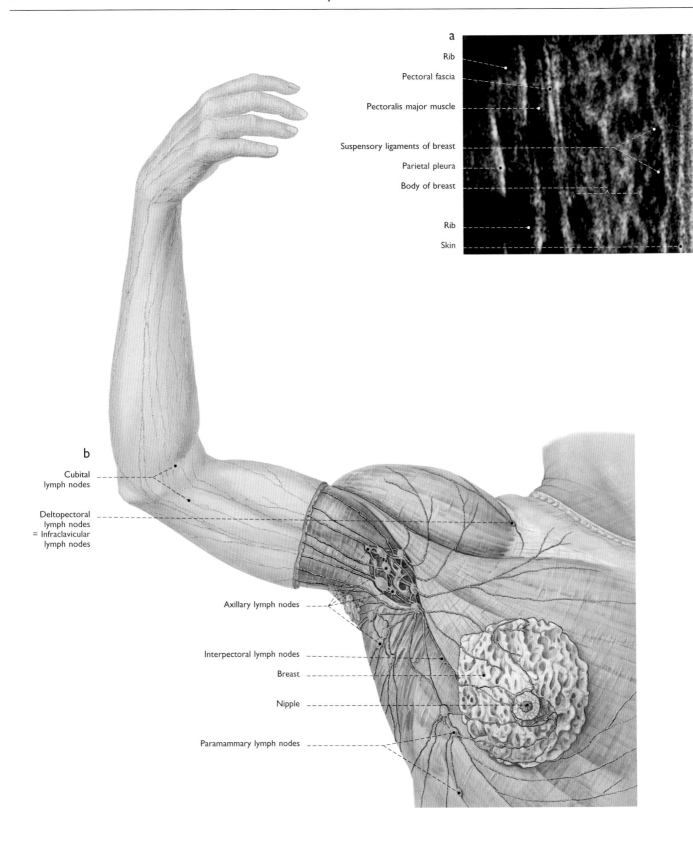

a
Rib
Pectoral fascia
Pectoralis major muscle

Suspensory ligaments of breast
Parietal pleura
Body of breast

Rib
Skin

b
Cubital
lymph nodes

Deltopectoral
lymph nodes
= Infraclavicular
lymph nodes

Axillary lymph nodes

Interpectoral lymph nodes

Breast

Nipple

Paramammary lymph nodes

**74 Breast, lymphatic vessels and lymph nodes
of the upper limb and the breast**

a Sonogram (ultrasonic image) of the breast, sagittal section
b Lymphatic drainage from the upper limb and the breast (35%),
ventral aspect

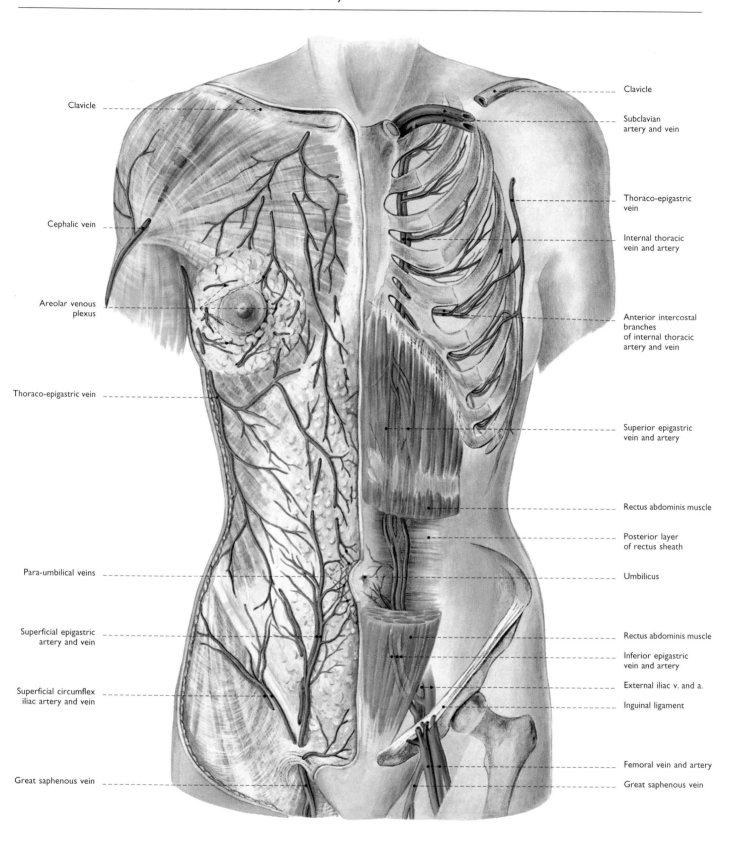

Clavicle

Clavicle

Cephalic vein

Subclavian
artery and vein

Areolar venous
plexus

Thoraco-epigastric
vein

Thoraco-epigastric vein

Internal thoracic
vein and artery

Para-umbilical veins

Anterior intercostal
branches
of internal thoracic
artery and vein

Superficial epigastric
artery and vein

Superior epigastric
vein and artery

Superficial circumflex
iliac artery and vein

Rectus abdominis muscle

Great saphenous vein

Posterior layer
of rectus sheath

Umbilicus

Rectus abdominis muscle

Inferior epigastric
vein and artery

External iliac v. and a.

Inguinal ligament

Femoral vein and artery

Great saphenous vein

75 Blood vessels of the ventral body wall (35%)
On the right side of the body, superficial vessels in the subcutaneous fatty tissue;
on the left side of the body, deep vessels shining through the covering layers
(the rectus abdominis muscle is cut above and below the umbilical region)

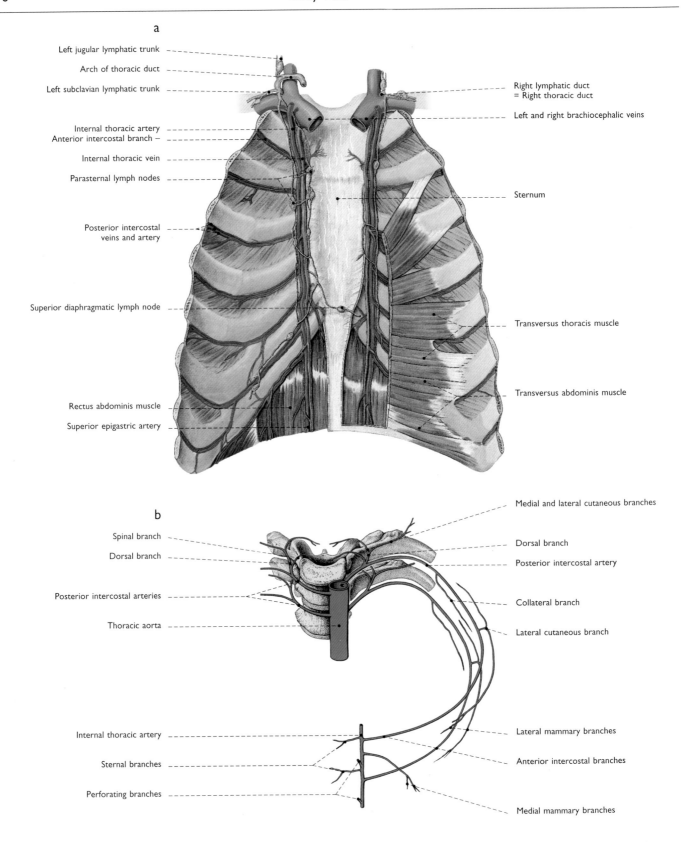

a

Left jugular lymphatic trunk

Arch of thoracic duct

Left subclavian lymphatic trunk

Internal thoracic artery
Anterior intercostal branch

Internal thoracic vein

Parasternal lymph nodes

Posterior intercostal
veins and artery

Superior diaphragmatic lymph node

Rectus abdominis muscle

Superior epigastric artery

Right lymphatic duct
= Right thoracic duct

Left and right brachiocephalic veins

Sternum

Transversus thoracis muscle

Transversus abdominis muscle

b

Spinal branch

Dorsal branch

Posterior intercostal arteries

Thoracic aorta

Internal thoracic artery

Sternal branches

Perforating branches

Medial and lateral cutaneous branches

Dorsal branch

Posterior intercostal artery

Collateral branch

Lateral cutaneous branch

Lateral mammary branches

Anterior intercostal branches

Medial mammary branches

76 Blood and lymphatic vessels of the thorax

a Internal aspect of the anterior chest wall (35%)
b Segmental arteries of the body wall,
   cranioventral aspect of the left half (30%)

a

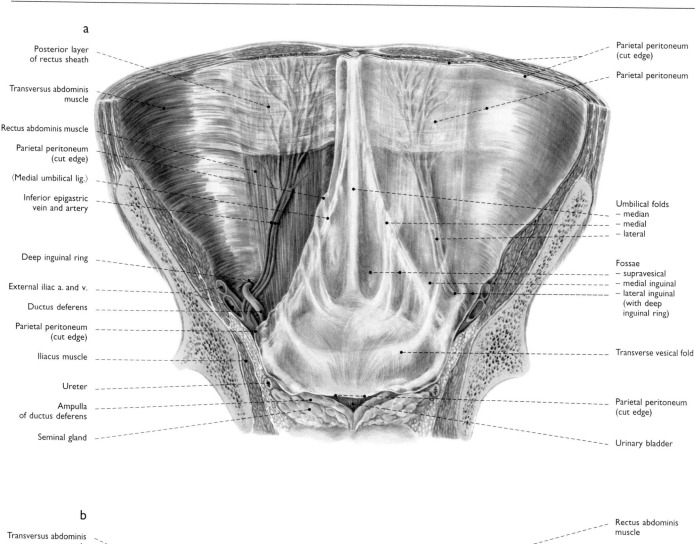

Posterior layer
of rectus sheath

Transversus abdominis
muscle

Rectus abdominis muscle

Parietal peritoneum
(cut edge)

⟨Medial umbilical lig.⟩

Inferior epigastric
vein and artery

Deep inguinal ring

External iliac a. and v.

Ductus deferens

Parietal peritoneum
(cut edge)

Iliacus muscle

Ureter

Ampulla
of ductus deferens

Seminal gland

Parietal peritoneum
(cut edge)

Parietal peritoneum

Umbilical folds
– median
– medial
– lateral

Fossae
– supravesical
– medial inguinal
– lateral inguinal
 (with deep
 inguinal ring)

Transverse vesical fold

Parietal peritoneum
(cut edge)

Urinary bladder

b

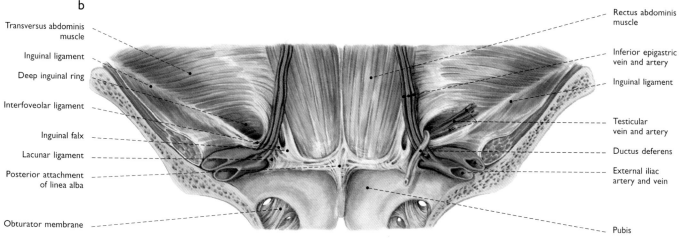

Transversus abdominis
muscle

Inguinal ligament

Deep inguinal ring

Interfoveolar ligament

Inguinal falx

Lacunar ligament

Posterior attachment
of linea alba

Obturator membrane

Rectus abdominis
muscle

Inferior epigastric
vein and artery

Inguinal ligament

Testicular
vein and artery

Ductus deferens

External iliac
artery and vein

Pubis

77 Inner surface of the anterior abdominal wall (50%)
Dorsal aspect
a Area between the umbilical region and the lesser pelvis,
   covered completely by peritoneum on the right side,
   but only partially on the left side
b Inguinal and pubic regions without peritoneal covering;
   on the right, the ductus deferens is additionally shown.

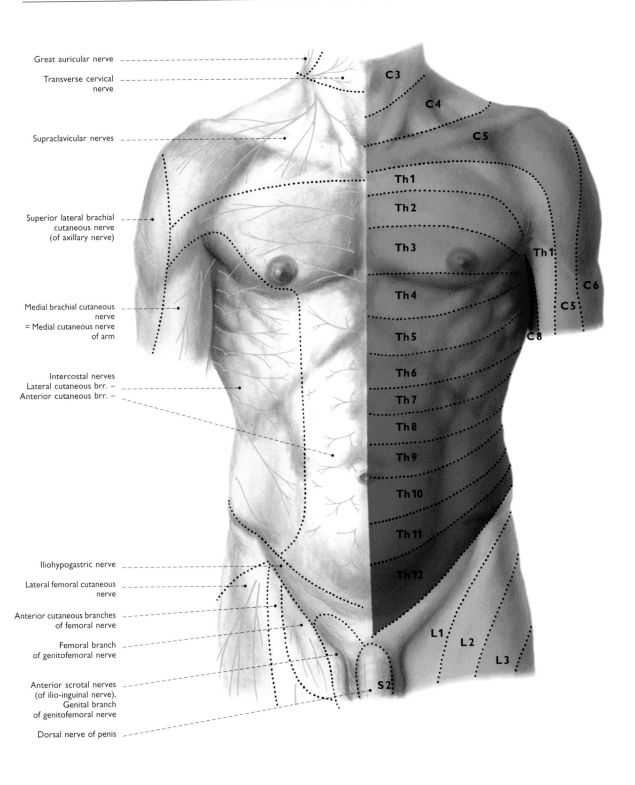

Great auricular nerve

Transverse cervical nerve

Supraclavicular nerves

Superior lateral brachial cutaneous nerve (of axillary nerve)

Medial brachial cutaneous nerve = Medial cutaneous nerve of arm

Intercostal nerves
Lateral cutaneous brr. –
Anterior cutaneous brr. –

Iliohypogastric nerve

Lateral femoral cutaneous nerve

Anterior cutaneous branches of femoral nerve

Femoral branch of genitofemoral nerve

Anterior scrotal nerves (of ilio-inguinal nerve), Genital branch of genitofemoral nerve

Dorsal nerve of penis

C3
C4
C5
Th1
Th2
Th3
Th4
Th5
Th6
Th7
Th8
Th9
Th10
Th11
Th12
Th1
C6
C5
C8
L1
L2
L3
S2

78 Cutaneous and segmental innervation of the ventral body wall (25%)
Schematic representation

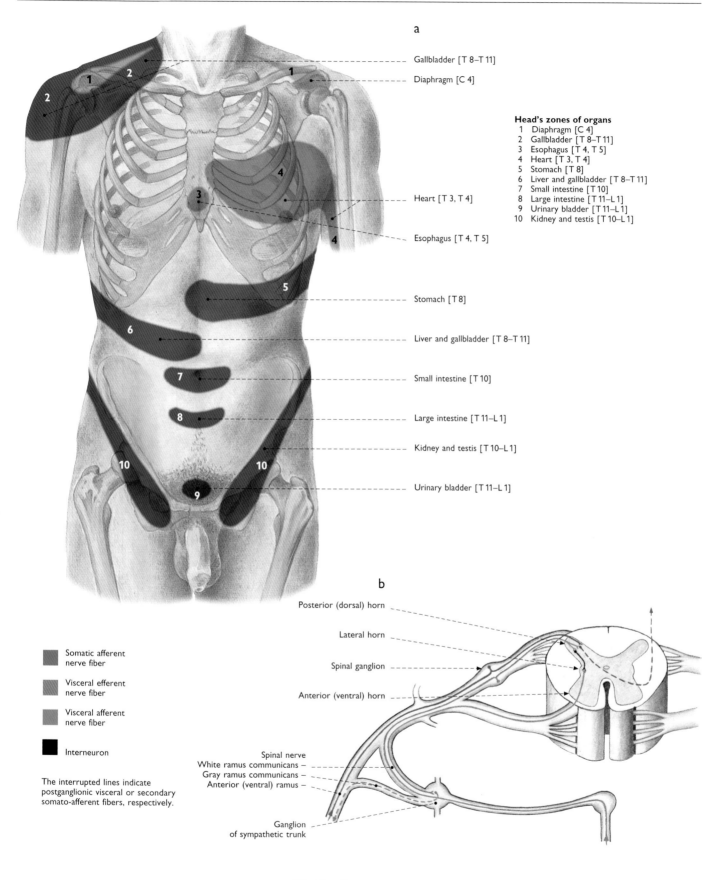

a

Gallbladder [T 8–T 11]

Diaphragm [C 4]

Head's zones of organs
1   Diaphragm [C 4]
2   Gallbladder [T 8–T 11]
3   Esophagus [T 4, T 5]
4   Heart [T 3, T 4]
5   Stomach [T 8]
6   Liver and gallbladder [T 8–T 11]
7   Small intestine [T 10]
8   Large intestine [T 11–L 1]
9   Urinary bladder [T 11–L 1]
10 Kidney and testis [T 10–L 1]

Heart [T 3, T 4]

Esophagus [T 4, T 5]

Stomach [T 8]

Liver and gallbladder [T 8–T 11]

Small intestine [T 10]

Large intestine [T 11–L 1]

Kidney and testis [T 10–L 1]

Urinary bladder [T 11–L 1]

b

Posterior (dorsal) horn

Lateral horn

Spinal ganglion

Anterior (ventral) horn

Spinal nerve
White ramus communicans
Gray ramus communicans
Anterior (ventral) ramus

Ganglion
of sympathetic trunk

Somatic afferent
nerve fiber

Visceral efferent
nerve fiber

Visceral afferent
nerve fiber

Interneuron

The interrupted lines indicate
postganglionic visceral or secondary
somato-afferent fibers, respectively.

79 Head's zones

a   Zones of hyperalgesia of diverse inner organs at the body surface (20%)
b   Scheme of circuitry of the radiated pain (Head's zones)

Upper Limb

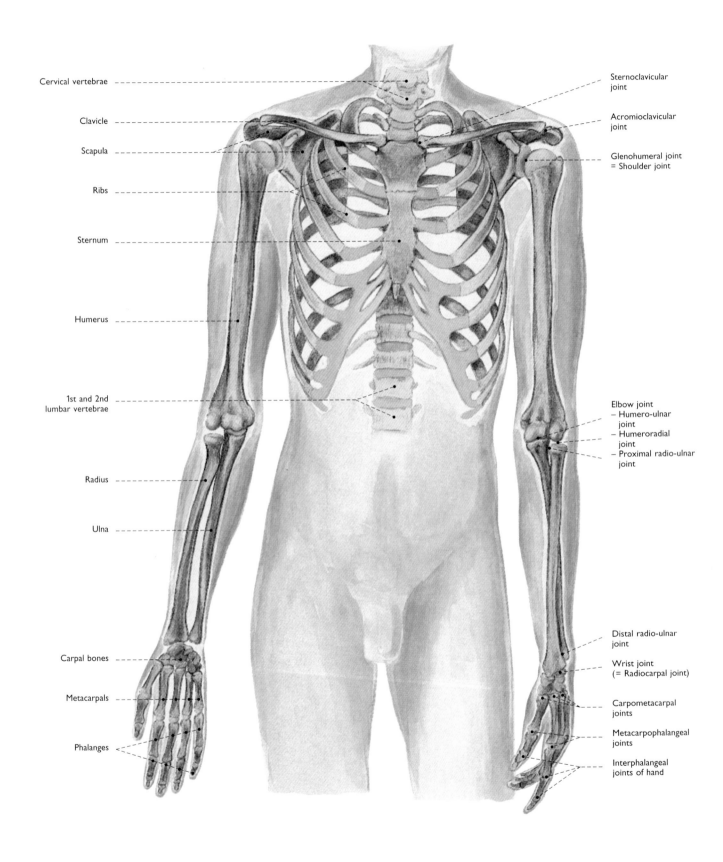

Cervical vertebrae

Clavicle

Scapula

Ribs

Sternum

Humerus

1st and 2nd
lumbar vertebrae

Radius

Ulna

Carpal bones

Metacarpals

Phalanges

Sternoclavicular
joint

Acromioclavicular
joint

Glenohumeral joint
= Shoulder joint

Elbow joint
– Humero-ulnar
  joint
– Humeroradial
  joint
– Proximal radio-ulnar
  joint

Distal radio-ulnar
joint

Wrist joint
(= Radiocarpal joint)

Carpometacarpal
joints

Metacarpophalangeal
joints

Interphalangeal
joints of hand

82 Upper limbs and thorax (25%)
Ventral aspect

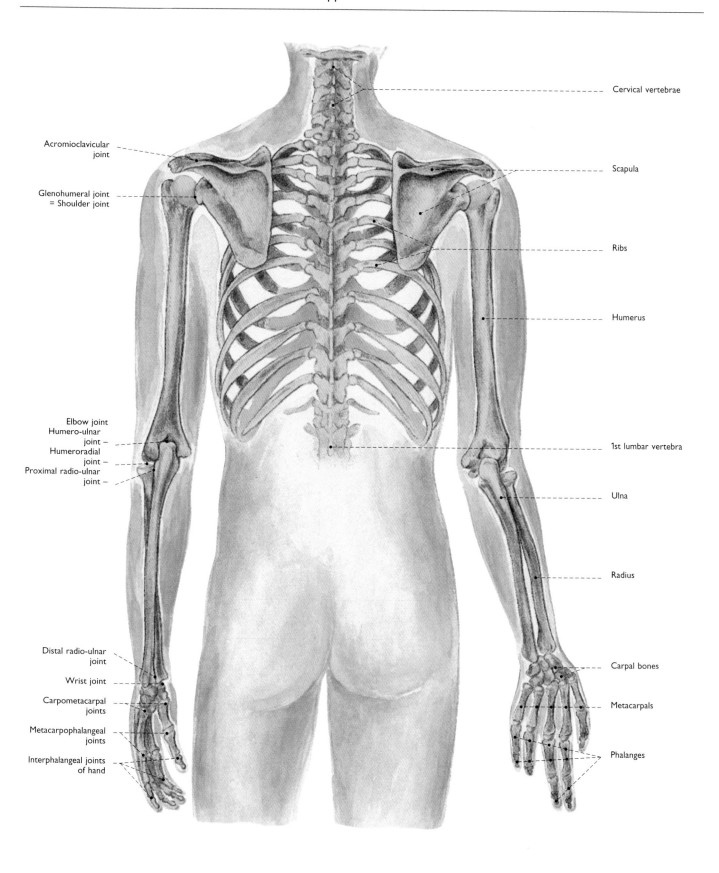

Cervical vertebrae

Acromioclavicular joint

Scapula

Glenohumeral joint = Shoulder joint

Ribs

Humerus

Elbow joint
Humero-ulnar joint
Humeroradial joint
Proximal radio-ulnar joint

1st lumbar vertebra

Ulna

Radius

Distal radio-ulnar joint

Wrist joint

Carpometacarpal joints

Metacarpophalangeal joints

Interphalangeal joints of hand

Carpal bones

Metacarpals

Phalanges

83 Upper limbs and thorax (25%)
Dorsal aspect

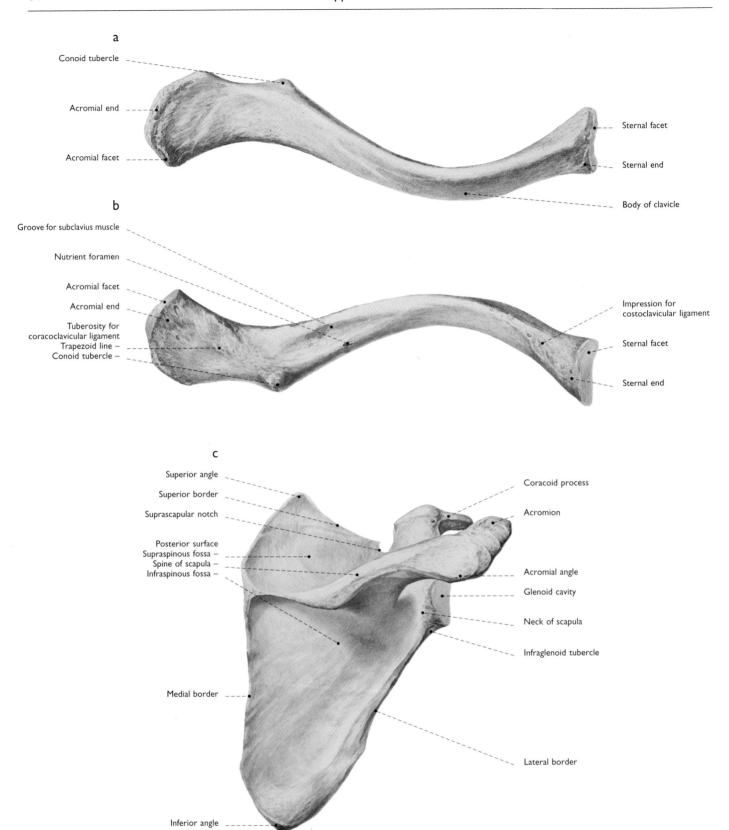

a

Conoid tubercle

Acromial end

Acromial facet

Sternal facet

Sternal end

Body of clavicle

b

Groove for subclavius muscle

Nutrient foramen

Acromial facet

Acromial end

Tuberosity for coracoclavicular ligament
Trapezoid line –
Conoid tubercle –

Impression for costoclavicular ligament

Sternal facet

Sternal end

c

Superior angle

Superior border

Suprascapular notch

Posterior surface
Supraspinous fossa –
Spine of scapula –
Infraspinous fossa –

Coracoid process

Acromion

Acromial angle

Glenoid cavity

Neck of scapula

Infraglenoid tubercle

Medial border

Lateral border

Inferior angle

84 Pectoral (= shoulder) girdle

a, b Right clavicle (90%)
a Superior aspect
b Inferior aspect
c Right scapula (50%), dorsal aspect

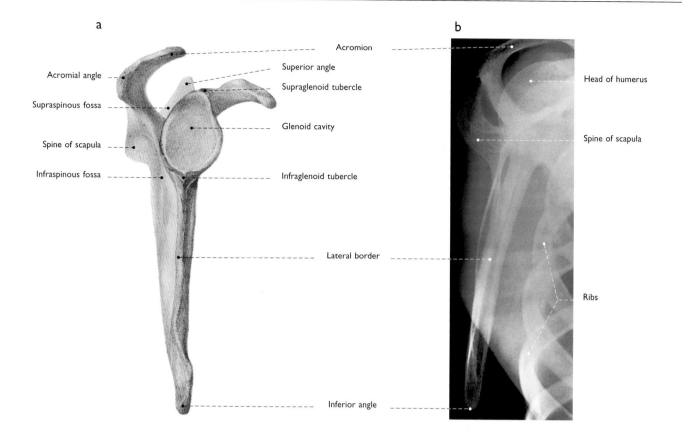

a

Acromial angle

Acromion

Superior angle

Supraglenoid tubercle

Supraspinous fossa

Spine of scapula

Glenoid cavity

Infraspinous fossa

Infraglenoid tubercle

Lateral border

Inferior angle

b

Head of humerus

Spine of scapula

Ribs

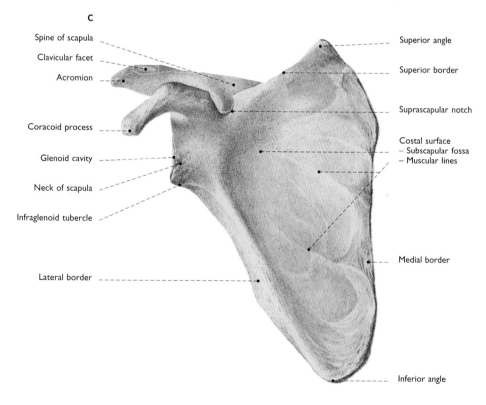

c

Spine of scapula

Clavicular facet

Acromion

Coracoid process

Glenoid cavity

Neck of scapula

Infraglenoid tubercle

Lateral border

Superior angle

Superior border

Suprascapular notch

Costal surface
− Subscapular fossa
− Muscular lines

Medial border

Inferior angle

85 Right scapula (50%)

  a   Lateral aspect
  b   Lateral radiograph
  c   Ventral aspect

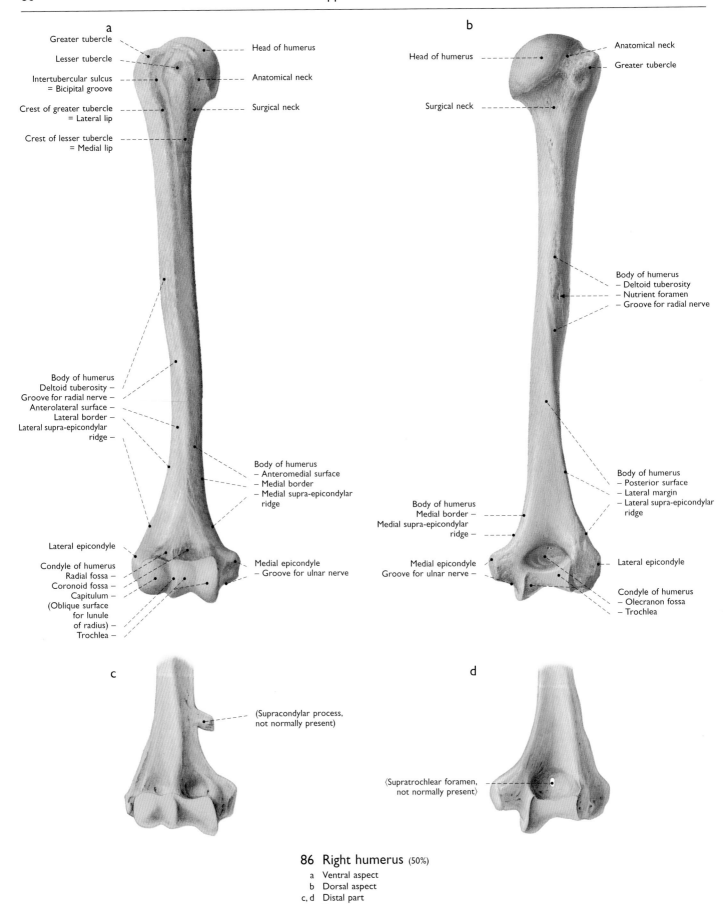

a

Greater tubercle
Lesser tubercle
Intertubercular sulcus
= Bicipital groove
Crest of greater tubercle
= Lateral lip
Crest of lesser tubercle
= Medial lip

Head of humerus
Anatomical neck
Surgical neck

Body of humerus
Deltoid tuberosity –
Groove for radial nerve –
Anterolateral surface –
Lateral border –
Lateral supra-epicondylar
ridge –

Body of humerus
– Anteromedial surface
– Medial border
– Medial supra-epicondylar
ridge

Lateral epicondyle
Condyle of humerus
Radial fossa –
Coronoid fossa –
Capitulum –
(Oblique surface
for lunule
of radius) –
Trochlea –

Medial epicondyle
– Groove for ulnar nerve

b

Head of humerus
Surgical neck

Anatomical neck
Greater tubercle

Body of humerus
– Deltoid tuberosity
– Nutrient foramen
– Groove for radial nerve

Body of humerus
Medial border –
Medial supra-epicondylar
ridge –

Body of humerus
– Posterior surface
– Lateral margin
– Lateral supra-epicondylar
ridge

Medial epicondyle
Groove for ulnar nerve –

Lateral epicondyle

Condyle of humerus
– Olecranon fossa
– Trochlea

c

(Supracondylar process,
not normally present)

d

⟨Supratrochlear foramen,
not normally present⟩

86   Right humerus (50%)

a   Ventral aspect
b   Dorsal aspect
c, d   Distal part
c   Ventral aspect
d   Dorsal aspect

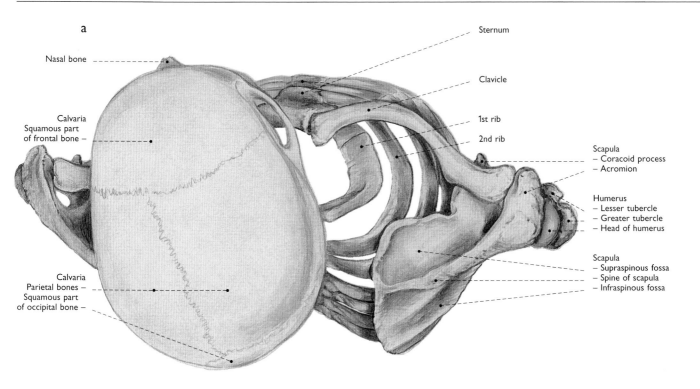

a

Nasal bone

Calvaria
Squamous part
of frontal bone –

Calvaria
Parietal bones –
Squamous part
of occipital bone –

Sternum

Clavicle

1st rib

2nd rib

Scapula
– Coracoid process
– Acromion

Humerus
– Lesser tubercle
– Greater tubercle
– Head of humerus

Scapula
– Supraspinous fossa
– Spine of scapula
– Infraspinous fossa

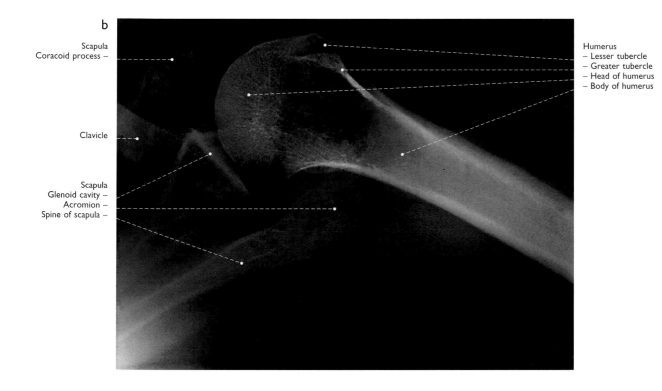

b

Scapula
Coracoid process –

Clavicle

Scapula
Glenoid cavity –
Acromion –
Spine of scapula –

Humerus
– Lesser tubercle
– Greater tubercle
– Head of humerus
– Body of humerus

87 Right pectoral girdle and humerus
a   Superior aspect (45%)
b   Supero-inferior radiograph

a

Head of radius
Articular facet –
Articular circumference –

Neck of radius – – – –

Body of radius
Tuberosity of radius –
Nutrient foramen –
Lateral surface –
Anterior border –
Anterior surface –
Interosseous border –

Radial styloid process – – –

Carpal articular surface –

b

Head of radius
– Articular facet
– ⟨Lunule⟩
– Articular circumference

Neck of radius

Body of radius
– Tuberosity of radius
– Posterior border
– Posterior surface
– Interosseous border
– Anterior surface
– Anterior border

Ulnar notch

Carpal articular surface

Radial styloid process

c

Head of radius
– Articular facet
– Articular circumference

Neck of radius

Body of radius
– Tuberosity of radius
– Lateral surface
– Posterior border
– Posterior surface
– Interosseous border

⟨Tendinous fossae⟩

Dorsal tubercle

Radial styloid process

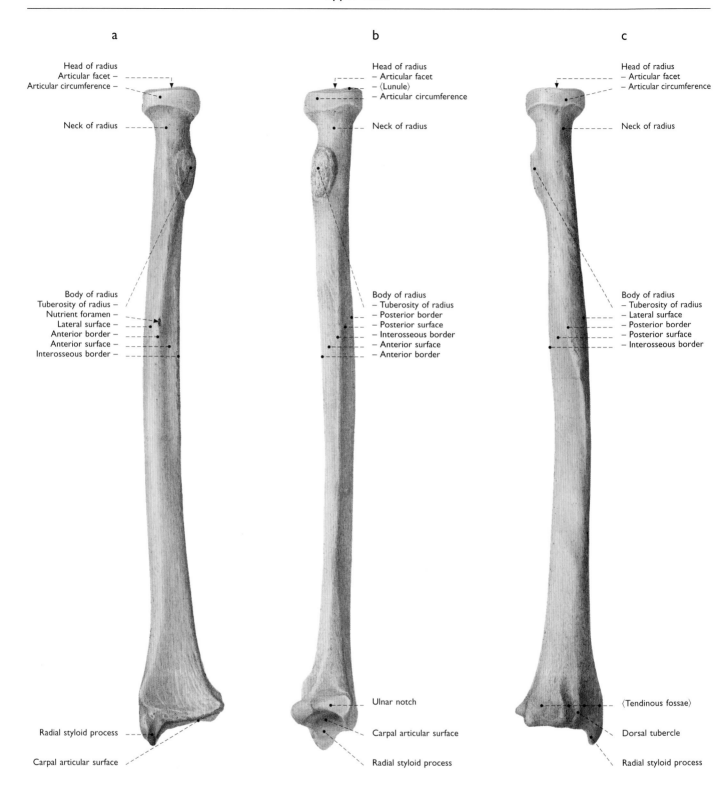

88　Right radius (70%)
a　Ventral aspect
b　Medial aspect
c　Dorsal aspect

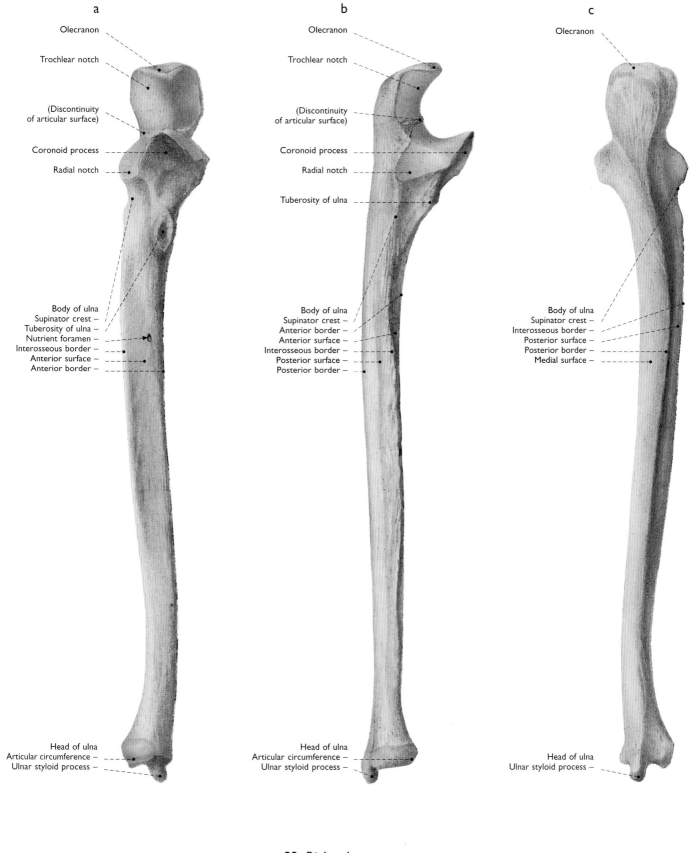

a

Olecranon

Trochlear notch

(Discontinuity
of articular surface)

Coronoid process

Radial notch

Body of ulna
Supinator crest —
Tuberosity of ulna —
Nutrient foramen —
Interosseous border —
Anterior surface —
Anterior border —

Head of ulna
Articular circumference —
Ulnar styloid process —

b

Olecranon

Trochlear notch

(Discontinuity
of articular surface)

Coronoid process

Radial notch

Tuberosity of ulna

Body of ulna
Supinator crest —
Anterior border —
Anterior surface —
Interosseous border —
Posterior surface —
Posterior border —

Head of ulna
Articular circumference —
Ulnar styloid process —

c

Olecranon

Body of ulna
Supinator crest —
Interosseous border —
Posterior surface —
Posterior border —
Medial surface —

Head of ulna
Ulnar styloid process —

89 Right ulna (70%)
a   Ventral aspect
b   Lateral aspect
c   Dorsal aspect

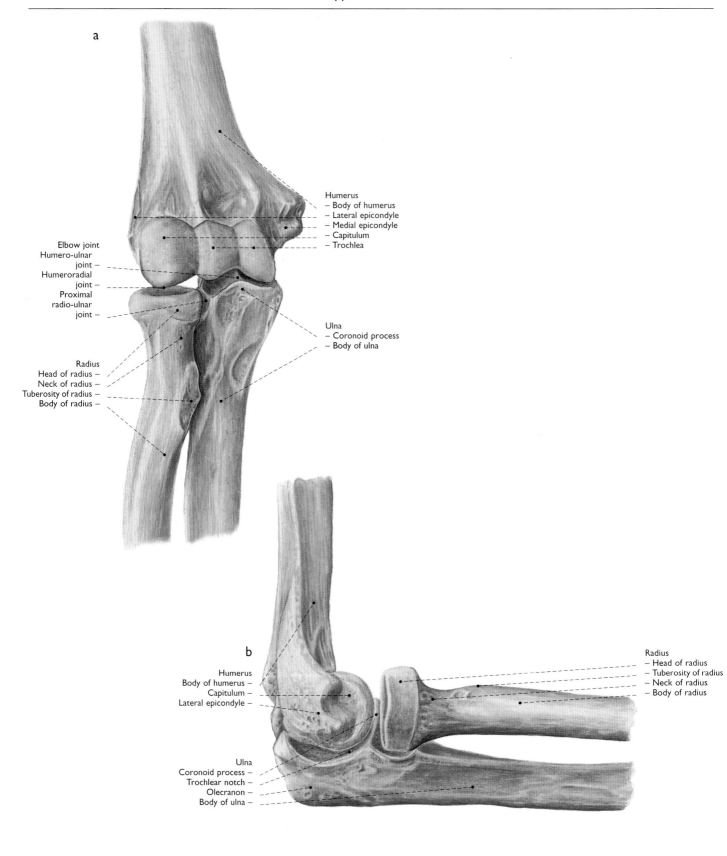

a

Humerus
– Body of humerus
– Lateral epicondyle
– Medial epicondyle
– Capitulum
– Trochlea

Elbow joint
Humero-ulnar
joint –
Humeroradial
joint –
Proximal
radio-ulnar
joint –

Ulna
– Coronoid process
– Body of ulna

Radius
Head of radius –
Neck of radius –
Tuberosity of radius –
Body of radius –

b

Radius
– Head of radius
– Tuberosity of radius
– Neck of radius
– Body of radius

Humerus
Body of humerus –
Capitulum –
Lateral epicondyle –

Ulna
Coronoid process –
Trochlear notch –
Olecranon –
Body of ulna –

90 Bones of the right elbow joint (90%)

a   Ventral aspect
b   Lateral (radial) aspect

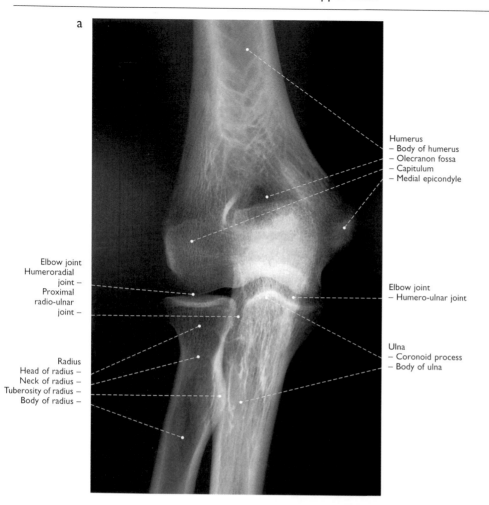

a

Humerus
– Body of humerus
– Olecranon fossa
– Capitulum
– Medial epicondyle

Elbow joint
Humeroradial
joint –
Proximal
radio-ulnar
joint –

Elbow joint
– Humero-ulnar joint

Radius
Head of radius –
Neck of radius –
Tuberosity of radius –
Body of radius –

Ulna
– Coronoid process
– Body of ulna

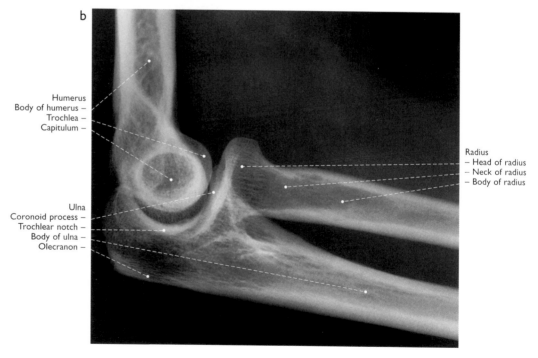

b

Humerus
Body of humerus –
Trochlea –
Capitulum –

Radius
– Head of radius
– Neck of radius
– Body of radius

Ulna
Coronoid process –
Trochlear notch –
Body of ulna –
Olecranon –

91 Right elbow joint (90%)

a Anteroposterior radiograph
b Radio-ulnar radiograph

a

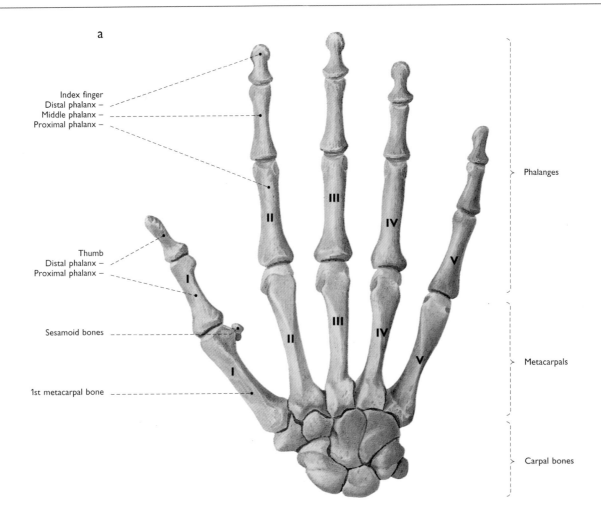

Index finger
Distal phalanx –
Middle phalanx –
Proximal phalanx –

II

III

IV

V

Thumb
Distal phalanx –
Proximal phalanx –

I

Sesamoid bones

I

II

III

IV

V

1st metacarpal bone

Phalanges

Metacarpals

Carpal bones

b

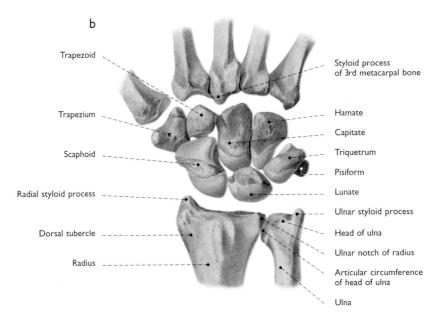

Trapezoid

Trapezium

Scaphoid

Radial styloid process

Dorsal tubercle

Radius

Styloid process
of 3rd metacarpal bone

Hamate

Capitate

Triquetrum

Pisiform

Lunate

Ulnar styloid process

Head of ulna

Ulnar notch of radius

Articular circumference
of head of ulna

Ulna

92 Bones of the right hand
  a   Dorsal aspect (60%)
  b   Carpal bones (70%), dorsal aspect

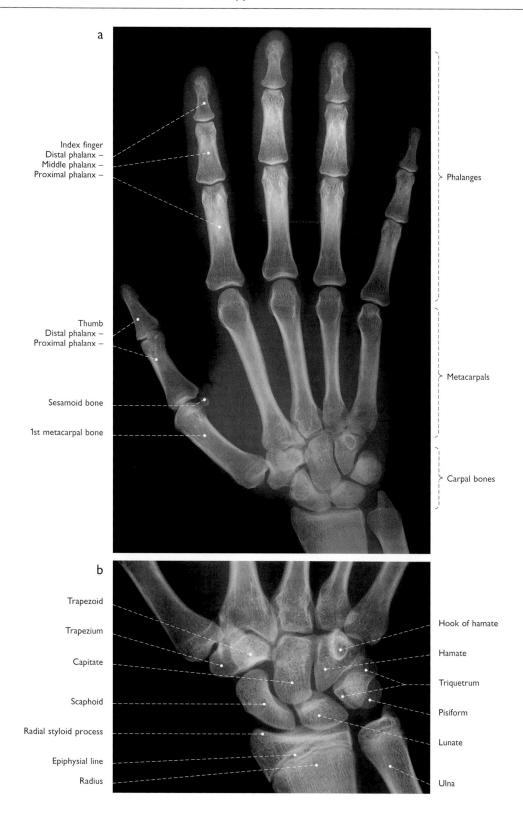

a

Index finger
Distal phalanx –
Middle phalanx –
Proximal phalanx –

Thumb
Distal phalanx –
Proximal phalanx –

Sesamoid bone

1st metacarpal bone

Phalanges

Metacarpals

Carpal bones

b

Trapezoid

Trapezium

Capitate

Scaphoid

Radial styloid process

Epiphysial line

Radius

Hook of hamate

Hamate

Triquetrum

Pisiform

Lunate

Ulna

93 Bones of the right hand
  a Dorsopalmar radiograph (60%)
  b Carpal bones (80%), dorsopalmar radiograph

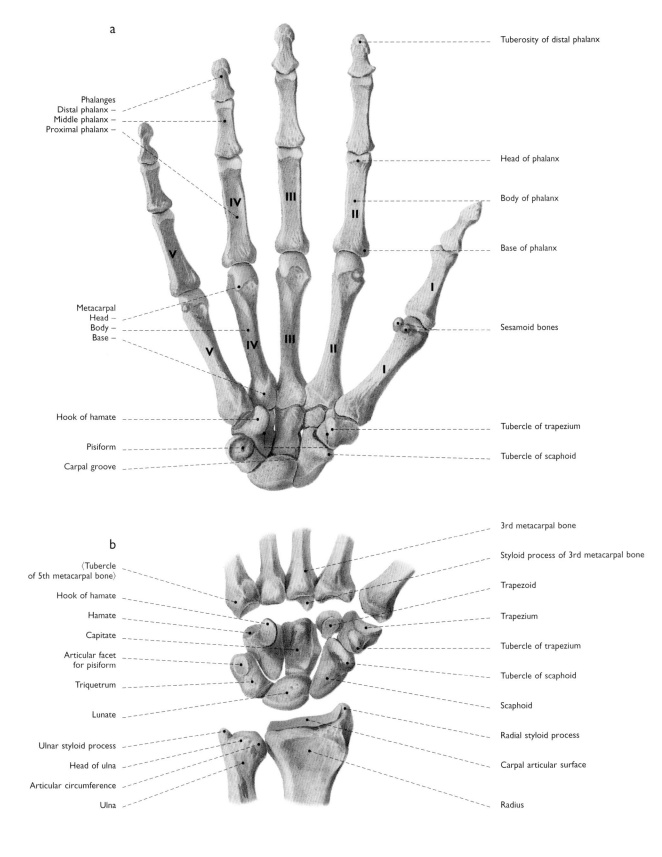

a

Tuberosity of distal phalanx

Phalanges
Distal phalanx —
Middle phalanx —
Proximal phalanx —

IV

III

II

Head of phalanx

Body of phalanx

Base of phalanx

V

I

Metacarpal
Head —
Body —
Base —

Sesamoid bones

V IV III II I

Hook of hamate

Tubercle of trapezium

Pisiform

Carpal groove

Tubercle of scaphoid

b

3rd metacarpal bone

Styloid process of 3rd metacarpal bone

⟨Tubercle
of 5th metacarpal bone⟩

Hook of hamate

Trapezoid

Hamate

Trapezium

Capitate

Articular facet
for pisiform

Tubercle of trapezium

Tubercle of scaphoid

Triquetrum

Lunate

Scaphoid

Ulnar styloid process

Head of ulna

Radial styloid process

Articular circumference

Carpal articular surface

Ulna

Radius

94 Bones of the right hand
a Palmar aspect (60%)
b Carpal bones (70%). The pisiform was removed.
    Palmar aspect

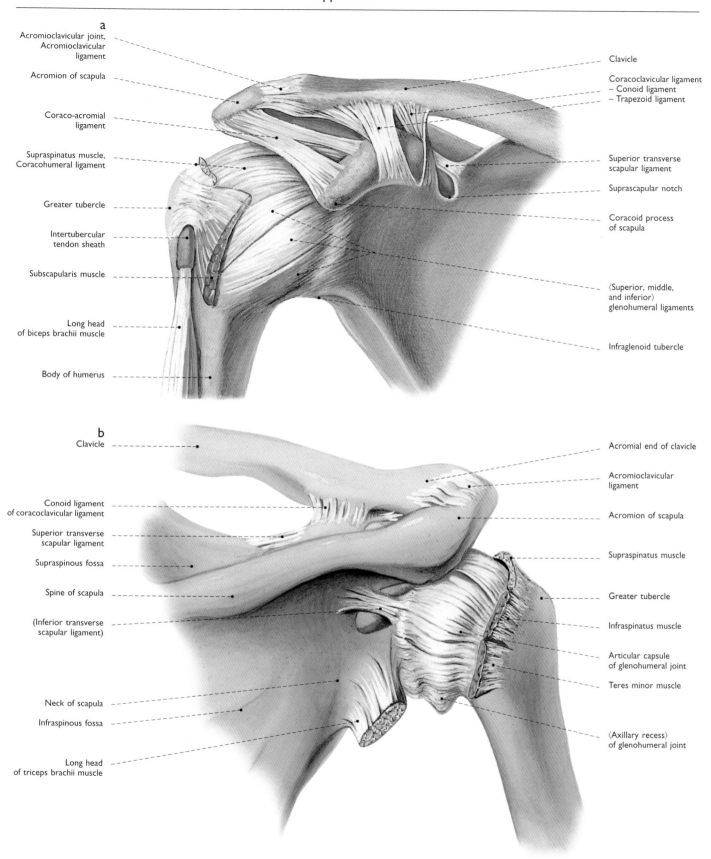

a
Acromioclavicular joint,
Acromioclavicular
ligament

Acromion of scapula

Coraco-acromial
ligament

Supraspinatus muscle,
Coracohumeral ligament

Greater tubercle

Intertubercular
tendon sheath

Subscapularis muscle

Long head
of biceps brachii muscle

Body of humerus

Clavicle

Coracoclavicular ligament
– Conoid ligament
– Trapezoid ligament

Superior transverse
scapular ligament

Suprascapular notch

Coracoid process
of scapula

⟨Superior, middle,
and inferior⟩
glenohumeral ligaments

Infraglenoid tubercle

b
Clavicle

Conoid ligament
of coracoclavicular ligament

Superior transverse
scapular ligament

Supraspinous fossa

Spine of scapula

(Inferior transverse
scapular ligament)

Neck of scapula

Infraspinous fossa

Long head
of triceps brachii muscle

Acromial end of clavicle

Acromioclavicular
ligament

Acromion of scapula

Supraspinatus muscle

Greater tubercle

Infraspinatus muscle

Articular capsule
of glenohumeral joint

Teres minor muscle

⟨Axillary recess⟩
of glenohumeral joint

95 Right glenohumeral (= shoulder) joint (80%)
a Ventral aspect
b Dorsal aspect

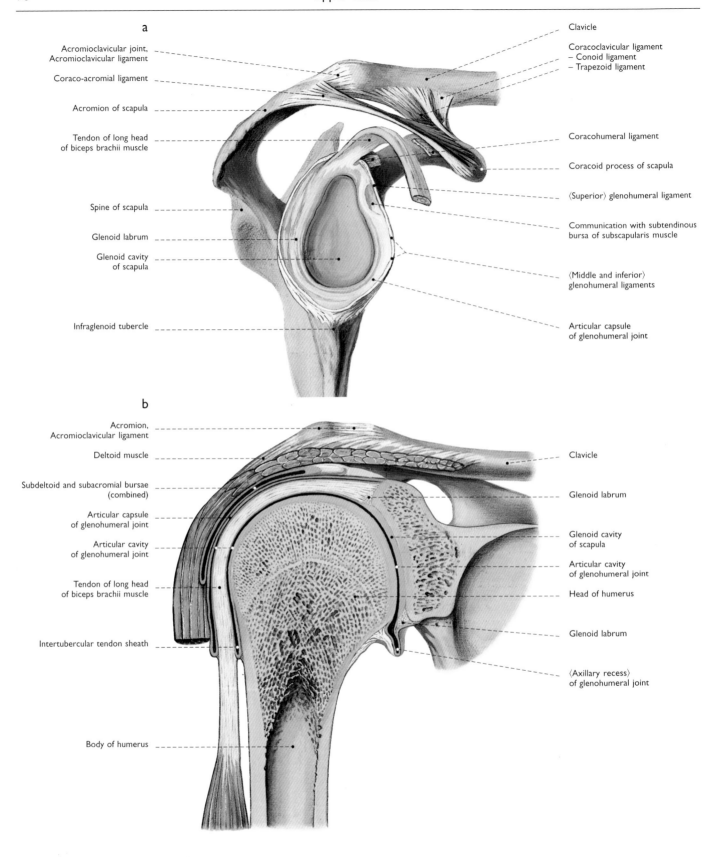

a

Acromioclavicular joint,
Acromioclavicular ligament

Coraco-acromial ligament

Acromion of scapula

Tendon of long head
of biceps brachii muscle

Spine of scapula

Glenoid labrum

Glenoid cavity
of scapula

Infraglenoid tubercle

Clavicle

Coracoclavicular ligament
– Conoid ligament
– Trapezoid ligament

Coracohumeral ligament

Coracoid process of scapula

〈Superior〉 glenohumeral ligament

Communication with subtendinous
bursa of subscapularis muscle

〈Middle and inferior〉
glenohumeral ligaments

Articular capsule
of glenohumeral joint

b

Acromion,
Acromioclavicular ligament

Deltoid muscle

Subdeltoid and subacromial bursae
(combined)

Articular capsule
of glenohumeral joint

Articular cavity
of glenohumeral joint

Tendon of long head
of biceps brachii muscle

Intertubercular tendon sheath

Body of humerus

Clavicle

Glenoid labrum

Glenoid cavity
of scapula

Articular cavity
of glenohumeral joint

Head of humerus

Glenoid labrum

〈Axillary recess〉
of glenohumeral joint

96 Right glenohumeral (= shoulder) joint (100%)
  a Shoulder joint socket and supra-articular ligaments,
     lateral aspect
  b Frontal section, ventral aspect

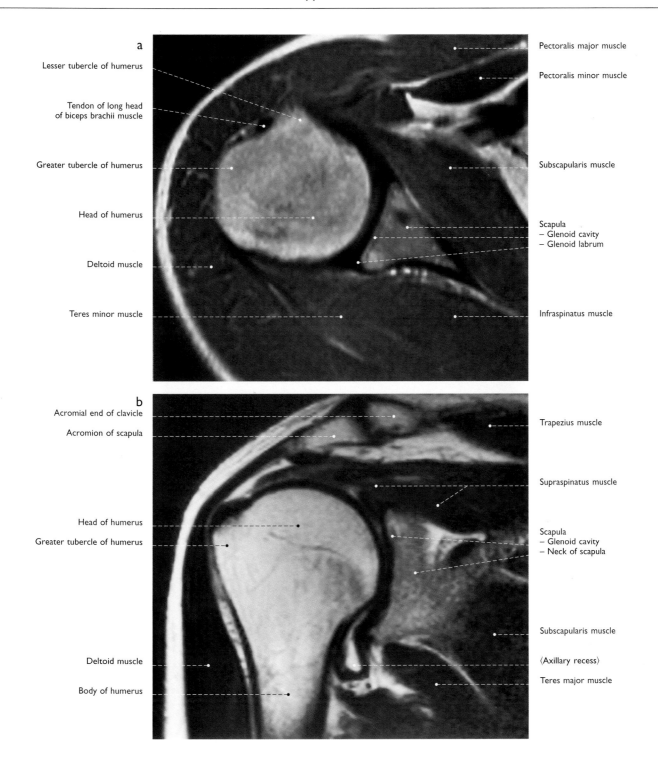

a
Lesser tubercle of humerus

Tendon of long head
of biceps brachii muscle

Greater tubercle of humerus

Head of humerus

Deltoid muscle

Teres minor muscle

Pectoralis major muscle

Pectoralis minor muscle

Subscapularis muscle

Scapula
– Glenoid cavity
– Glenoid labrum

Infraspinatus muscle

b
Acromial end of clavicle
Acromion of scapula

Head of humerus
Greater tubercle of humerus

Deltoid muscle

Body of humerus

Trapezius muscle

Supraspinatus muscle

Scapula
– Glenoid cavity
– Neck of scapula

Subscapularis muscle

⟨Axillary recess⟩

Teres major muscle

97 Right glenohumeral (= shoulder) joint (100%)

a Transverse magnetic resonance image (MRI, T$_2$-weighted),
   inferior aspect
b Coronal magnetic resonance image (MRI, T$_2$-weighted),
   ventral aspect

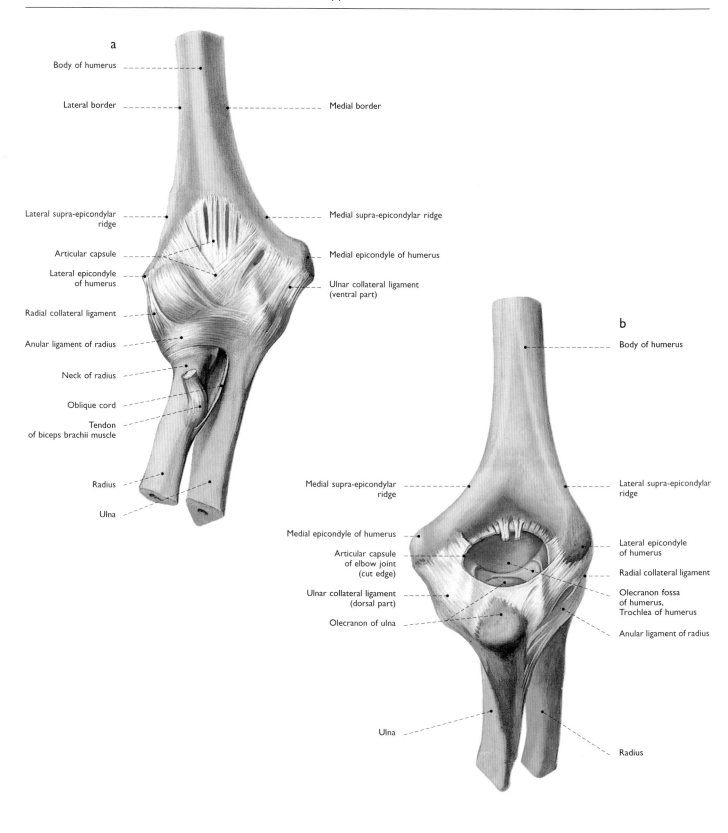

a

Body of humerus

Lateral border

Medial border

Lateral supra-epicondylar ridge

Medial supra-epicondylar ridge

Articular capsule

Medial epicondyle of humerus

Lateral epicondyle of humerus

Radial collateral ligament

Ulnar collateral ligament (ventral part)

Anular ligament of radius

Neck of radius

Oblique cord

Tendon of biceps brachii muscle

Radius

Ulna

b

Body of humerus

Medial supra-epicondylar ridge

Lateral supra-epicondylar ridge

Medial epicondyle of humerus

Lateral epicondyle of humerus

Articular capsule of elbow joint (cut edge)

Radial collateral ligament

Ulnar collateral ligament (dorsal part)

Olecranon fossa of humerus, Trochlea of humerus

Olecranon of ulna

Anular ligament of radius

Ulna

Radius

98   Right elbow joint (85%)
a   Ventral aspect
b   Dorsal aspect

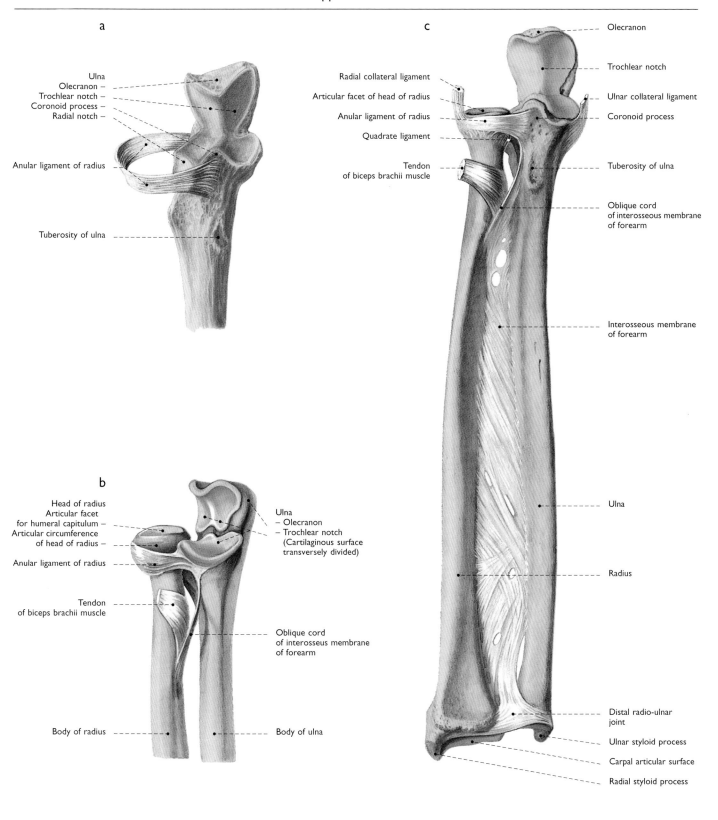

a

Ulna
Olecranon –
Trochlear notch –
Coronoid process –
Radial notch –

Anular ligament of radius –

Tuberosity of ulna

b

Head of radius
Articular facet
for humeral capitulum –
Articular circumference
of head of radius –

Anular ligament of radius –

Tendon
of biceps brachii muscle –

Body of radius

Ulna
– Olecranon
– Trochlear notch
(Cartilaginous surface
transversely divided)

Oblique cord
of interosseus membrane
of forearm

Body of ulna

c

Radial collateral ligament

Articular facet of head of radius

Anular ligament of radius

Quadrate ligament

Tendon
of biceps brachii muscle

Olecranon

Trochlear notch

Ulnar collateral ligament

Coronoid process

Tuberosity of ulna

Oblique cord
of interosseous membrane
of forearm

Interosseous membrane
of forearm

Ulna

Radius

Distal radio-ulnar
joint

Ulnar styloid process

Carpal articular surface

Radial styloid process

99   Radio-ulnar joints of the right forearm

a   Proximal end of ulna and anular ligament of radius (80%),
    ventral aspect
b   Proximal radio-ulnar joint (70%), ventral aspect
c   Forearm bones in supinated position (70%), ventral aspect

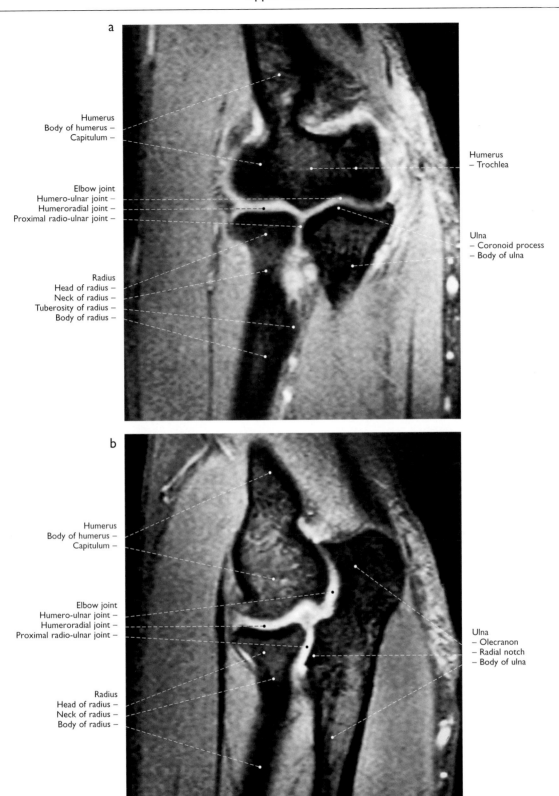

a

Humerus
Body of humerus –
Capitulum –

Humerus
– Trochlea

Elbow joint
Humero-ulnar joint –
Humeroradial joint –
Proximal radio-ulnar joint –

Ulna
– Coronoid process
– Body of ulna

Radius
Head of radius –
Neck of radius –
Tuberosity of radius –
Body of radius –

b

Humerus
Body of humerus –
Capitulum –

Elbow joint
Humero-ulnar joint –
Humeroradial joint –
Proximal radio-ulnar joint –

Ulna
– Olecranon
– Radial notch
– Body of ulna

Radius
Head of radius –
Neck of radius –
Body of radius –

100 Right elbow joint (100%)
Coronal magnetic resonance images (MRI, T$_2$-weighted)
a   through the ventral part
b   through the dorsal part
of the elbow joint, ventral aspect

a

b

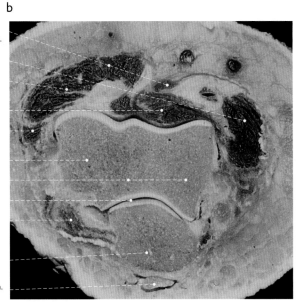

Brachioradialis muscle,
Tendon of biceps brachii m.

Pronator teres muscle

Extensor carpi radialis
longus muscle

Brachialis muscle

Extensor carpi radialis
brevis muscle

Capitulum of humerus

Trochlea of humerus

Humero-ulnar joint

Anconeus muscle

Olecranon of ulna

Tendon of triceps brachii m.

c

d

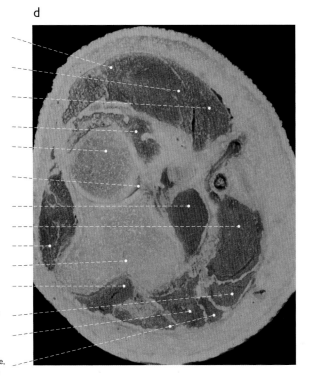

Extensor carpi radialis
brevis muscle

Extensor carpi radialis
longus muscle

Brachioradialis muscle

Supinator muscle

Head of radius

Proximal radio-ulnar
joint

Brachialis muscle

Pronator teres muscle

Anconeus muscle

Body of ulna

Flexor digitorum
profundus muscle

Flexor carpi radialis m.

Flexor digitorum
superficialis muscle

Flexor carpi ulnaris muscle,
Palmaris longus muscle

101 Right elbow joint (90%)

a, b Transverse sections through the distal arm
and the humero-ulnar joint
c, d Transverse sections through the proximal forearm
and the proximal radio-ulnar joint
a, c Magnetic resonance images (MRI, T$_2$-weighted),
distal aspect
b, d Anatomical sections, distal aspect
The pictures c and d are rotated by about 90°
in relation to a and b.

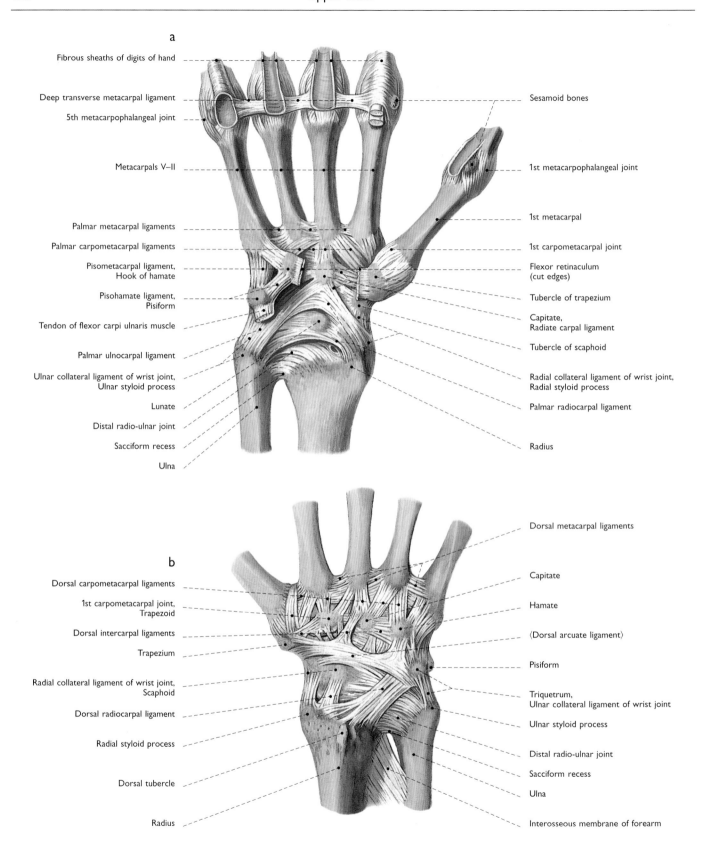

a

Fibrous sheaths of digits of hand

Deep transverse metacarpal ligament

5th metacarpophalangeal joint

Metacarpals V–II

Palmar metacarpal ligaments

Palmar carpometacarpal ligaments

Pisometacarpal ligament,
Hook of hamate

Pisohamate ligament,
Pisiform

Tendon of flexor carpi ulnaris muscle

Palmar ulnocarpal ligament

Ulnar collateral ligament of wrist joint,
Ulnar styloid process

Lunate

Distal radio-ulnar joint

Sacciform recess

Ulna

Sesamoid bones

1st metacarpophalangeal joint

1st metacarpal

1st carpometacarpal joint

Flexor retinaculum
(cut edges)

Tubercle of trapezium

Capitate,
Radiate carpal ligament

Tubercle of scaphoid

Radial collateral ligament of wrist joint,
Radial styloid process

Palmar radiocarpal ligament

Radius

b

Dorsal carpometacarpal ligaments

1st carpometacarpal joint,
Trapezoid

Dorsal intercarpal ligaments

Trapezium

Radial collateral ligament of wrist joint,
Scaphoid

Dorsal radiocarpal ligament

Radial styloid process

Dorsal tubercle

Radius

Dorsal metacarpal ligaments

Capitate

Hamate

⟨Dorsal arcuate ligament⟩

Pisiform

Triquetrum,
Ulnar collateral ligament of wrist joint

Ulnar styloid process

Distal radio-ulnar joint

Sacciform recess

Ulna

Interosseous membrane of forearm

102 Joints of the right hand (75%)
a Palmar aspect
b Dorsal aspect

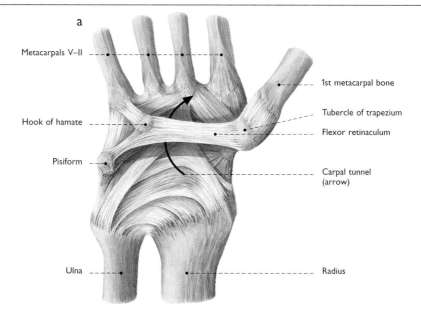

a

Metacarpals V–II

1st metacarpal bone

Hook of hamate

Tubercle of trapezium

Flexor retinaculum

Pisiform

Carpal tunnel
(arrow)

Ulna

Radius

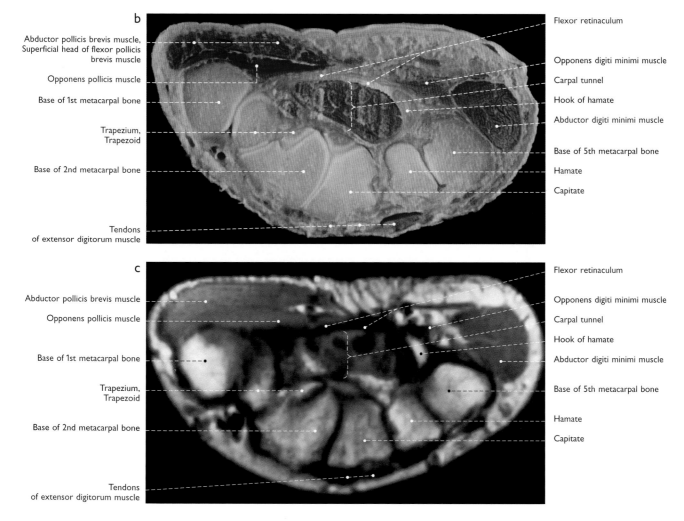

b

Abductor pollicis brevis muscle,
Superficial head of flexor pollicis
brevis muscle

Flexor retinaculum

Opponens pollicis muscle

Opponens digiti minimi muscle

Base of 1st metacarpal bone

Carpal tunnel

Hook of hamate

Trapezium,
Trapezoid

Abductor digiti minimi muscle

Base of 2nd metacarpal bone

Base of 5th metacarpal bone

Hamate

Capitate

Tendons
of extensor digitorum muscle

c

Abductor pollicis brevis muscle

Flexor retinaculum

Opponens pollicis muscle

Opponens digiti minimi muscle

Carpal tunnel

Base of 1st metacarpal bone

Hook of hamate

Abductor digiti minimi muscle

Trapezium,
Trapezoid

Base of 5th metacarpal bone

Base of 2nd metacarpal bone

Hamate

Capitate

Tendons
of extensor digitorum muscle

103 Carpal tunnel of the right hand

a   Palmar aspect (80%)
b   Anatomical section through the wrist and the carpal tunnel (130%),
    distal aspect
c   Transverse magnetic resonance image (MRI, T$_1$-weighted)
    of the wrist and the carpal tunnel (140%), distal aspect
b, c   Hand in full supination

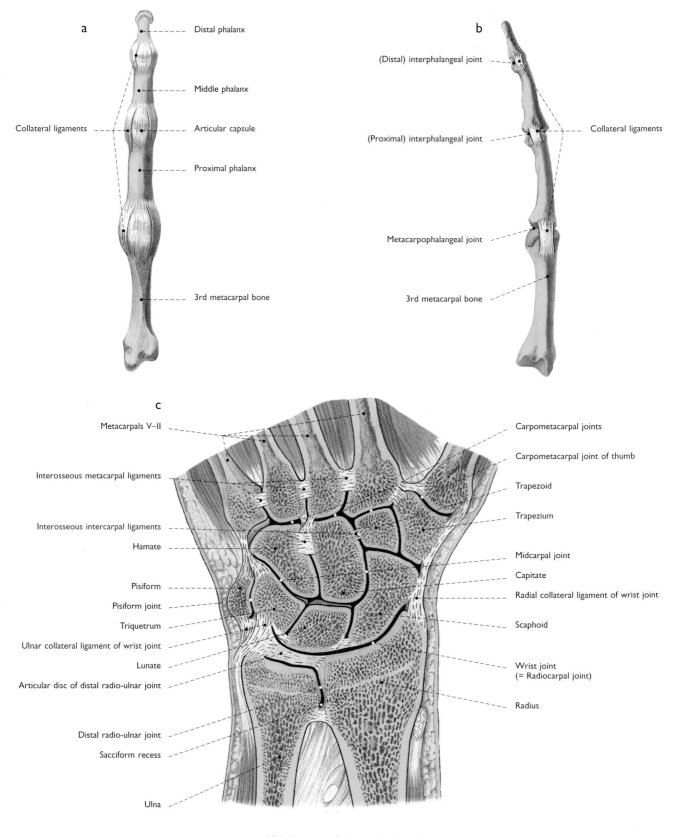

a

Distal phalanx

Middle phalanx

Collateral ligaments

Articular capsule

Proximal phalanx

3rd metacarpal bone

b

(Distal) interphalangeal joint

(Proximal) interphalangeal joint

Collateral ligaments

Metacarpophalangeal joint

3rd metacarpal bone

c

Metacarpals V–II

Interosseous metacarpal ligaments

Interosseous intercarpal ligaments

Hamate

Pisiform

Pisiform joint

Triquetrum

Ulnar collateral ligament of wrist joint

Lunate

Articular disc of distal radio-ulnar joint

Distal radio-ulnar joint

Sacciform recess

Ulna

Carpometacarpal joints

Carpometacarpal joint of thumb

Trapezoid

Trapezium

Midcarpal joint

Capitate

Radial collateral ligament of wrist joint

Scaphoid

Wrist joint
(= Radiocarpal joint)

Radius

104 Joints of the right hand
a, b Middle finger (60%)
   a Dorsal aspect
   b Lateral aspect
   c Radio-ulnar cut through the wrist (100%),
      palmar aspect

Upper Limb

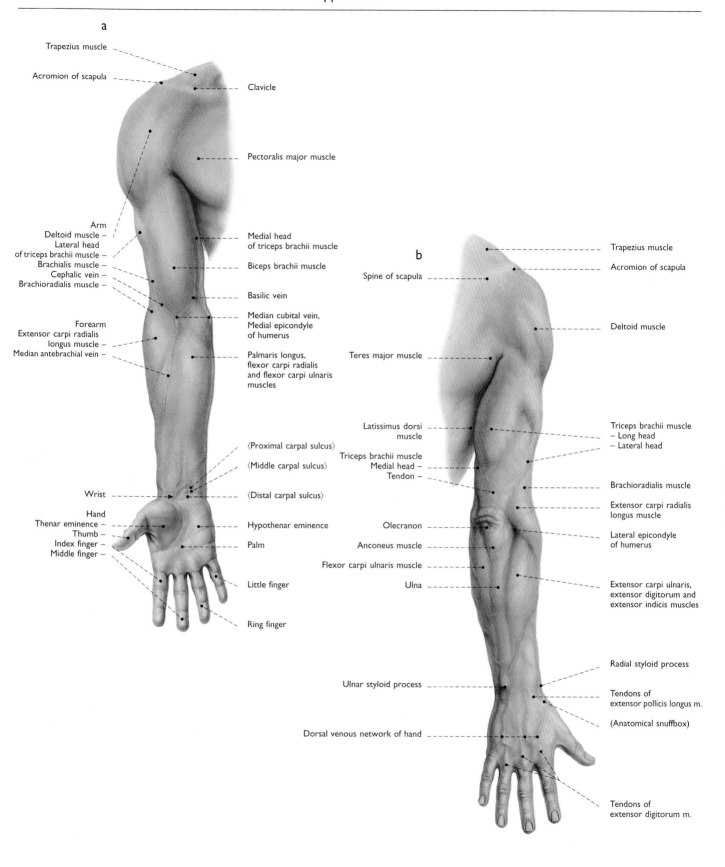

a

Trapezius muscle

Acromion of scapula

Clavicle

Pectoralis major muscle

Arm
Deltoid muscle –
Lateral head
of triceps brachii muscle –
Brachialis muscle –
Cephalic vein –
Brachioradialis muscle –

Medial head
of triceps brachii muscle

Biceps brachii muscle

Basilic vein

Median cubital vein,
Medial epicondyle
of humerus

Forearm
Extensor carpi radialis
longus muscle –
Median antebrachial vein –

Palmaris longus,
flexor carpi radialis
and flexor carpi ulnaris
muscles

⟨Proximal carpal sulcus⟩

⟨Middle carpal sulcus⟩

Wrist

⟨Distal carpal sulcus⟩

Hand
Thenar eminence –
Thumb –
Index finger –
Middle finger –

Hypothenar eminence

Palm

Little finger

Ring finger

b

Spine of scapula

Trapezius muscle

Acromion of scapula

Deltoid muscle

Teres major muscle

Latissimus dorsi
muscle

Triceps brachii muscle
Medial head –
Tendon –

Olecranon

Anconeus muscle

Flexor carpi ulnaris muscle

Ulna

Triceps brachii muscle
– Long head
– Lateral head

Brachioradialis muscle

Extensor carpi radialis
longus muscle

Lateral epicondyle
of humerus

Extensor carpi ulnaris,
extensor digitorum and
extensor indicis muscles

Ulnar styloid process

Dorsal venous network of hand

Radial styloid process

Tendons of
extensor pollicis longus m.

⟨Anatomical snuffbox⟩

Tendons of
extensor digitorum m.

105 Surface anatomy of the right upper limb (20%)
a Ventral aspect
b Dorsal aspect

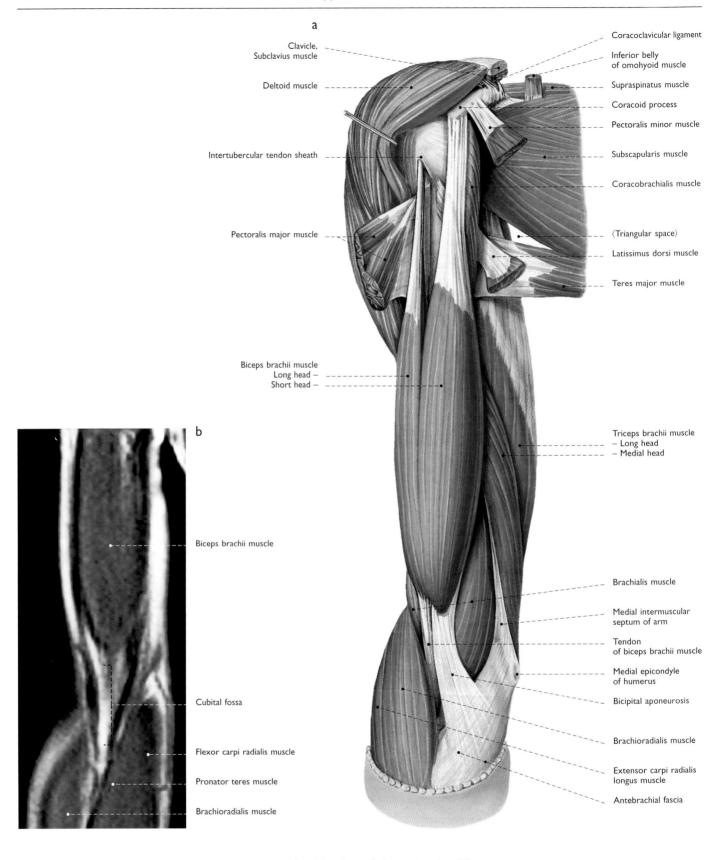

a

Clavicle,
Subclavius muscle

Deltoid muscle

Intertubercular tendon sheath

Pectoralis major muscle

Biceps brachii muscle
Long head –
Short head –

Coracoclavicular ligament

Inferior belly
of omohyoid muscle

Supraspinatus muscle

Coracoid process

Pectoralis minor muscle

Subscapularis muscle

Coracobrachialis muscle

⟨Triangular space⟩

Latissimus dorsi muscle

Teres major muscle

Triceps brachii muscle
– Long head
– Medial head

Brachialis muscle

Medial intermuscular
septum of arm

Tendon
of biceps brachii muscle

Medial epicondyle
of humerus

Bicipital aponeurosis

Brachioradialis muscle

Extensor carpi radialis
longus muscle

Antebrachial fascia

b

Biceps brachii muscle

Cubital fossa

Flexor carpi radialis muscle

Pronator teres muscle

Brachioradialis muscle

106 Muscles of the right shoulder
     and the right arm (50%)
   a Ventral aspect
   b Coronal magnetic resonance image
      of the anterior region of elbow (MRI, T$_1$-weighted)

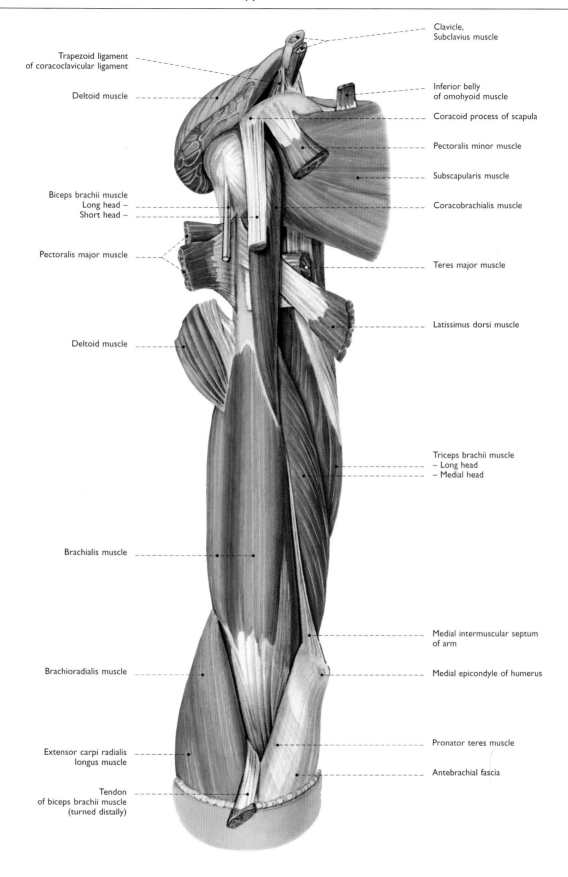

Clavicle,
Subclavius muscle

Trapezoid ligament
of coracoclavicular ligament

Deltoid muscle

Inferior belly
of omohyoid muscle

Coracoid process of scapula

Pectoralis minor muscle

Subscapularis muscle

Biceps brachii muscle
Long head –
Short head –

Coracobrachialis muscle

Pectoralis major muscle

Teres major muscle

Latissimus dorsi muscle

Deltoid muscle

Triceps brachii muscle
– Long head
– Medial head

Brachialis muscle

Medial intermuscular septum
of arm

Brachioradialis muscle

Medial epicondyle of humerus

Extensor carpi radialis
longus muscle

Pronator teres muscle

Antebrachial fascia

Tendon
of biceps brachii muscle
(turned distally)

**107　Muscles of the right shoulder
and the right arm** (50%)
The deltoid muscle was partially removed. Ventral aspect

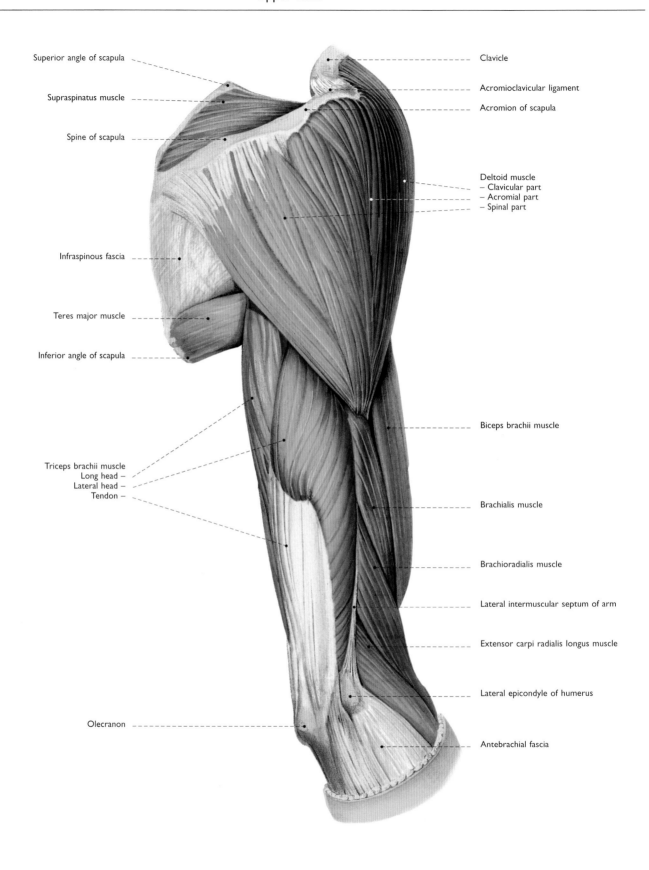

Superior angle of scapula

Supraspinatus muscle

Spine of scapula

Infraspinous fascia

Teres major muscle

Inferior angle of scapula

Triceps brachii muscle
Long head –
Lateral head –
Tendon –

Olecranon

Clavicle

Acromioclavicular ligament

Acromion of scapula

Deltoid muscle
– Clavicular part
– Acromial part
– Spinal part

Biceps brachii muscle

Brachialis muscle

Brachioradialis muscle

Lateral intermuscular septum of arm

Extensor carpi radialis longus muscle

Lateral epicondyle of humerus

Antebrachial fascia

108 Muscles of the right shoulder
and the right arm (50%)
Dorsolateral aspect

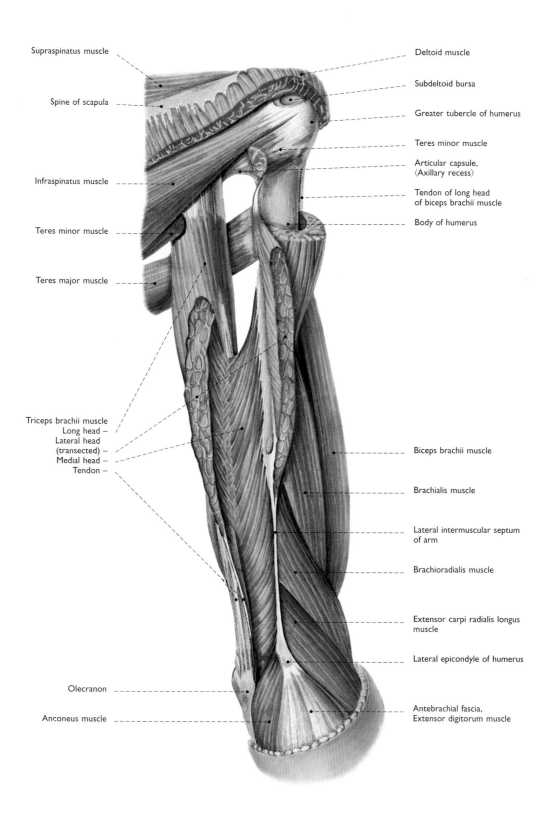

Supraspinatus muscle

Spine of scapula

Infraspinatus muscle

Teres minor muscle

Teres major muscle

Triceps brachii muscle
Long head –
Lateral head
(transected) –
Medial head –
Tendon –

Olecranon

Anconeus muscle

Deltoid muscle

Subdeltoid bursa

Greater tubercle of humerus

Teres minor muscle

Articular capsule,
(Axillary recess)

Tendon of long head
of biceps brachii muscle

Body of humerus

Biceps brachii muscle

Brachialis muscle

Lateral intermuscular septum
of arm

Brachioradialis muscle

Extensor carpi radialis longus
muscle

Lateral epicondyle of humerus

Antebrachial fascia,
Extensor digitorum muscle

**109 Muscles of the right shoulder
and the right arm** (50%)
The deltoid muscle was partially removed.
Dorsolateral aspect

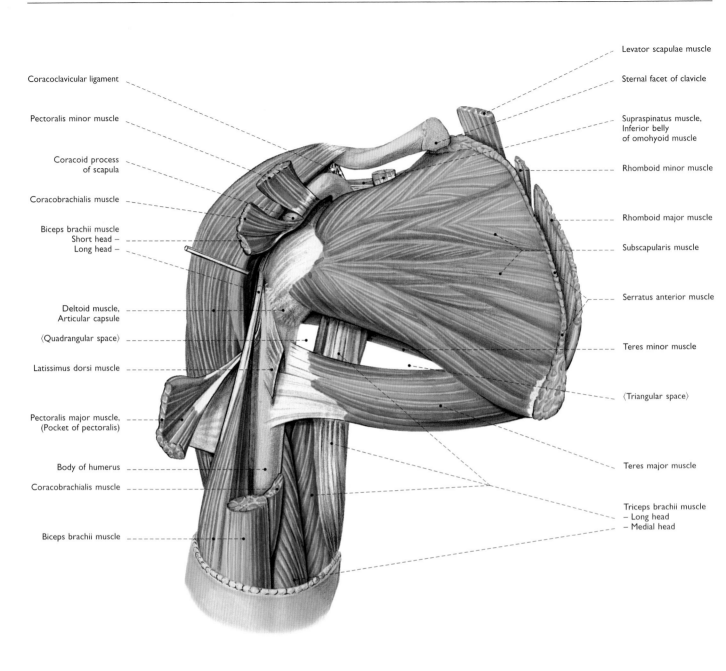

Coracoclavicular ligament

Pectoralis minor muscle

Coracoid process
of scapula

Coracobrachialis muscle

Biceps brachii muscle
Short head –
Long head –

Deltoid muscle,
Articular capsule

〈Quadrangular space〉

Latissimus dorsi muscle

Pectoralis major muscle,
(Pocket of pectoralis)

Body of humerus

Coracobrachialis muscle

Biceps brachii muscle

Levator scapulae muscle

Sternal facet of clavicle

Supraspinatus muscle,
Inferior belly
of omohyoid muscle

Rhomboid minor muscle

Rhomboid major muscle

Subscapularis muscle

Serratus anterior muscle

Teres minor muscle

〈Triangular space〉

Teres major muscle

Triceps brachii muscle
– Long head
– Medial head

**110 Muscles of the right shoulder
and the right arm** (60%)
Ventromedial aspect

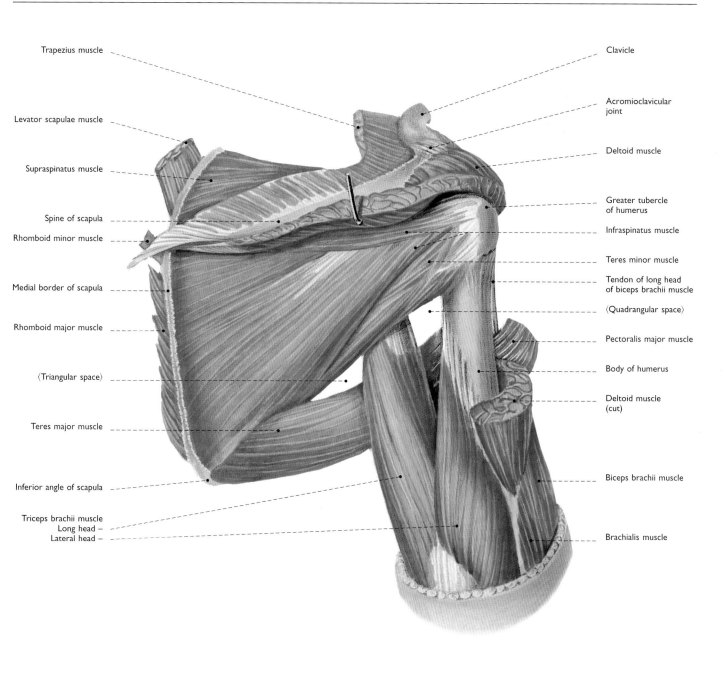

Trapezius muscle

Levator scapulae muscle

Supraspinatus muscle

Spine of scapula

Rhomboid minor muscle

Medial border of scapula

Rhomboid major muscle

⟨Triangular space⟩

Teres major muscle

Inferior angle of scapula

Triceps brachii muscle
Long head –
Lateral head –

Clavicle

Acromioclavicular
joint

Deltoid muscle

Greater tubercle
of humerus

Infraspinatus muscle

Teres minor muscle

Tendon of long head
of biceps brachii muscle

⟨Quadrangular space⟩

Pectoralis major muscle

Body of humerus

Deltoid muscle
(cut)

Biceps brachii muscle

Brachialis muscle

**111 Muscles of the right shoulder
and the right arm** (60%)
The deltoid muscle was partially removed.
Dorsal aspect

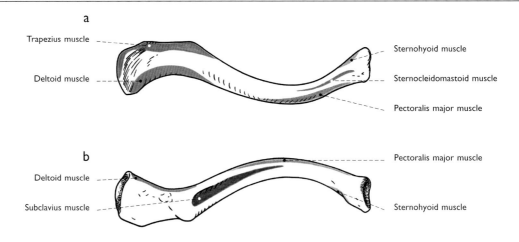

a

Trapezius muscle - Sternohyoid muscle

Deltoid muscle - Sternocleidomastoid muscle

- - - - - - - - - Pectoralis major muscle

b

- - - - - - - - - Pectoralis major muscle

Deltoid muscle - - - - - - - - - - - - -

Subclavius muscle - Sternohyoid muscle

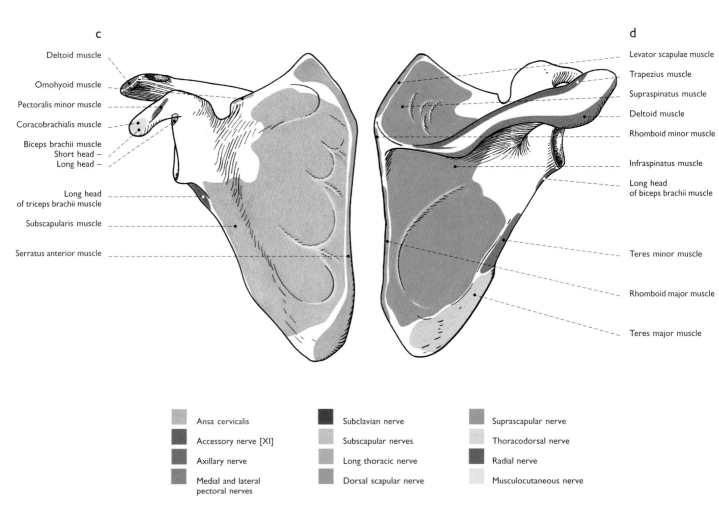

c

Deltoid muscle - - - - - - - - - -

Omohyoid muscle - - - - - - - - - -

Pectoralis minor muscle - - - - - - - - - -

Coracobrachialis muscle - - - - - - - - - -

Biceps brachii muscle
Short head –
Long head –

Long head - - - - - - - - - -
of triceps brachii muscle

Subscapularis muscle - - - - - - - - - -

Serratus anterior muscle - - - - - - - - - -

d

Levator scapulae muscle

Trapezius muscle

Supraspinatus muscle

Deltoid muscle

Rhomboid minor muscle

Infraspinatus muscle

Long head
of biceps brachii muscle

Teres minor muscle

Rhomboid major muscle

Teres major muscle

Ansa cervicalis

Accessory nerve [XI]

Axillary nerve

Medial and lateral
pectoral nerves

Subclavian nerve

Subscapular nerves

Long thoracic nerve

Dorsal scapular nerve

Suprascapular nerve

Thoracodorsal nerve

Radial nerve

Musculocutaneous nerve

112 Muscle attachments to the right pectoral girdle
The colors indicate the innervation of the muscles
attaching to the
a superior surface of the clavicle
b inferior surface of the clavicle
c costal surface of the scapula
d posterior surface of the scapula.

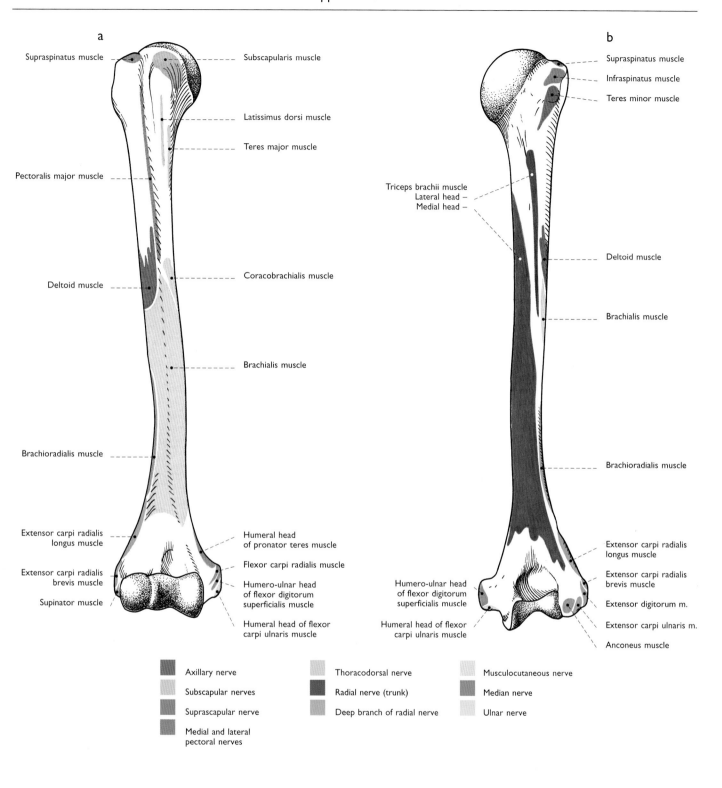

a

Supraspinatus muscle

Subscapularis muscle

Latissimus dorsi muscle

Teres major muscle

Pectoralis major muscle

Deltoid muscle

Coracobrachialis muscle

Brachialis muscle

Brachioradialis muscle

Extensor carpi radialis longus muscle

Extensor carpi radialis brevis muscle

Supinator muscle

Humeral head of pronator teres muscle

Flexor carpi radialis muscle

Humero-ulnar head of flexor digitorum superficialis muscle

Humeral head of flexor carpi ulnaris muscle

b

Supraspinatus muscle

Infraspinatus muscle

Teres minor muscle

Triceps brachii muscle
Lateral head —
Medial head —

Deltoid muscle

Brachialis muscle

Brachioradialis muscle

Extensor carpi radialis longus muscle

Extensor carpi radialis brevis muscle

Extensor digitorum m.

Extensor carpi ulnaris m.

Anconeus muscle

Humero-ulnar head of flexor digitorum superficialis muscle

Humeral head of flexor carpi ulnaris muscle

Axillary nerve

Subscapular nerves

Suprascapular nerve

Medial and lateral pectoral nerves

Thoracodorsal nerve

Radial nerve (trunk)

Deep branch of radial nerve

Musculocutaneous nerve

Median nerve

Ulnar nerve

113 Muscle attachments to the right humerus
The colors indicate the innervation of the muscles attaching to the
a ventral surface
b dorsal surface.

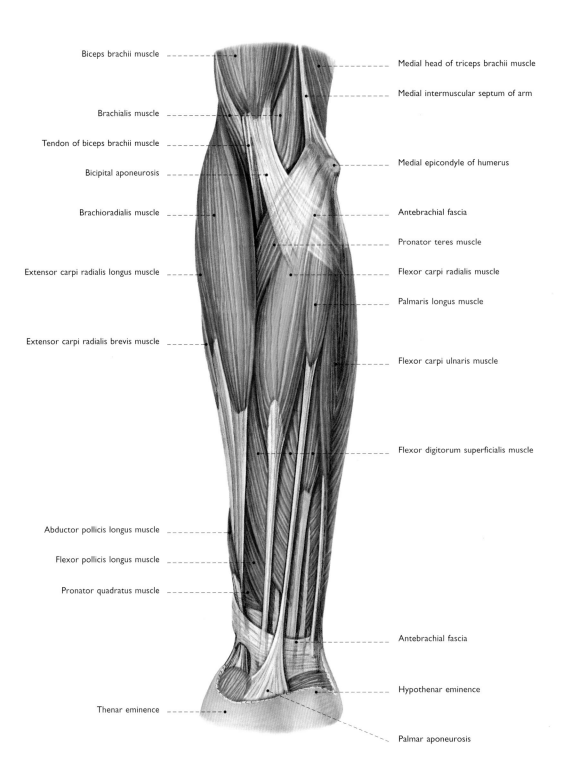

Biceps brachii muscle

Brachialis muscle

Tendon of biceps brachii muscle

Bicipital aponeurosis

Brachioradialis muscle

Extensor carpi radialis longus muscle

Extensor carpi radialis brevis muscle

Abductor pollicis longus muscle

Flexor pollicis longus muscle

Pronator quadratus muscle

Thenar eminence

Medial head of triceps brachii muscle

Medial intermuscular septum of arm

Medial epicondyle of humerus

Antebrachial fascia

Pronator teres muscle

Flexor carpi radialis muscle

Palmaris longus muscle

Flexor carpi ulnaris muscle

Flexor digitorum superficialis muscle

Antebrachial fascia

Hypothenar eminence

Palmar aponeurosis

114 Muscles of the right forearm (50%)
Superficial layer, ventral aspect

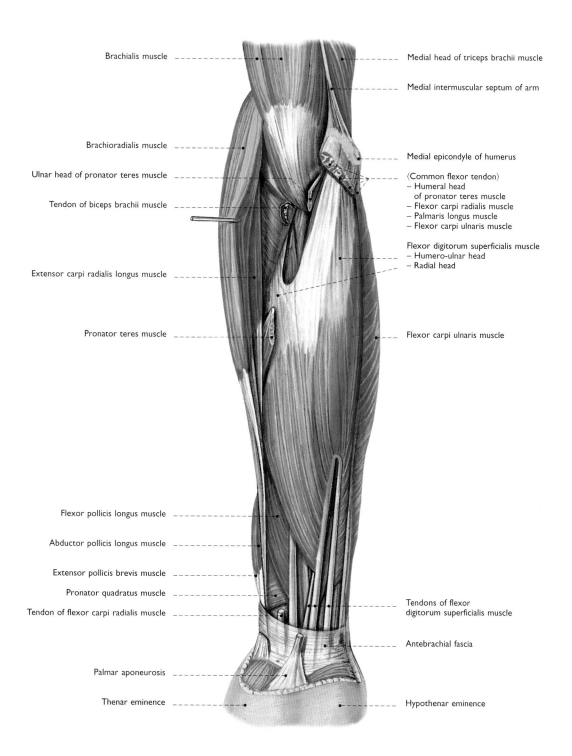

Brachialis muscle

Brachioradialis muscle

Ulnar head of pronator teres muscle

Tendon of biceps brachii muscle

Extensor carpi radialis longus muscle

Pronator teres muscle

Flexor pollicis longus muscle

Abductor pollicis longus muscle

Extensor pollicis brevis muscle

Pronator quadratus muscle

Tendon of flexor carpi radialis muscle

Palmar aponeurosis

Thenar eminence

Medial head of triceps brachii muscle

Medial intermuscular septum of arm

Medial epicondyle of humerus

⟨Common flexor tendon⟩
– Humeral head
  of pronator teres muscle
– Flexor carpi radialis muscle
– Palmaris longus muscle
– Flexor carpi ulnaris muscle

Flexor digitorum superficialis muscle
– Humero-ulnar head
– Radial head

Flexor carpi ulnaris muscle

Tendons of flexor
digitorum superficialis muscle

Antebrachial fascia

Hypothenar eminence

115 Muscles of the right forearm (50%)
Superficial layer. Some superficial forearm flexors were removed.
Ventral aspect

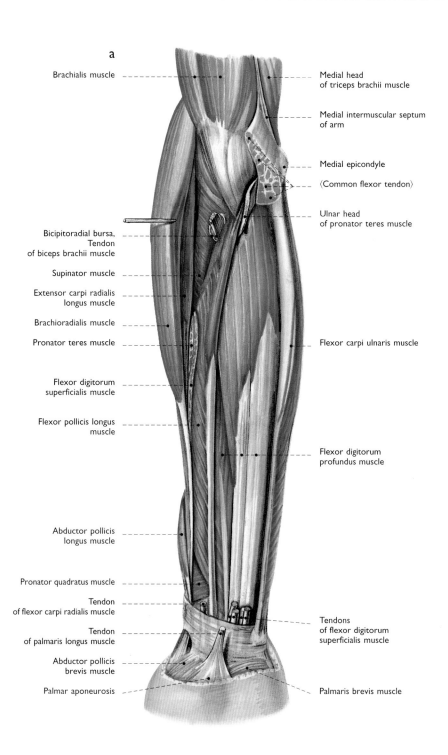

a

Brachialis muscle

Medial head
of triceps brachii muscle

Medial intermuscular septum
of arm

Medial epicondyle

⟨Common flexor tendon⟩

Ulnar head
of pronator teres muscle

Bicipitoradial bursa,
Tendon
of biceps brachii muscle

Supinator muscle

Extensor carpi radialis
longus muscle

Brachioradialis muscle

Pronator teres muscle

Flexor carpi ulnaris muscle

Flexor digitorum
superficialis muscle

Flexor pollicis longus
muscle

Flexor digitorum
profundus muscle

Abductor pollicis
longus muscle

Pronator quadratus muscle

Tendon
of flexor carpi radialis muscle

Tendon
of palmaris longus muscle

Abductor pollicis
brevis muscle

Palmar aponeurosis

Tendons
of flexor digitorum
superficialis muscle

Palmaris brevis muscle

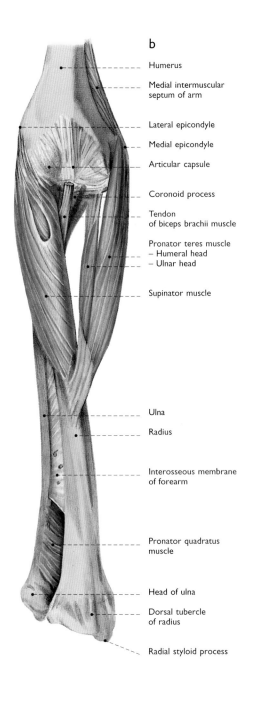

b

Humerus

Medial intermuscular
septum of arm

Lateral epicondyle

Medial epicondyle

Articular capsule

Coronoid process

Tendon
of biceps brachii muscle

Pronator teres muscle
– Humeral head
– Ulnar head

Supinator muscle

Ulna

Radius

Interosseous membrane
of forearm

Pronator quadratus
muscle

Head of ulna

Dorsal tubercle
of radius

Radial styloid process

116 Muscles of the right forearm (50%)

Ventral aspect
a Deep layer
b Supinator and pronator muscles in pronated position
   of the forearm

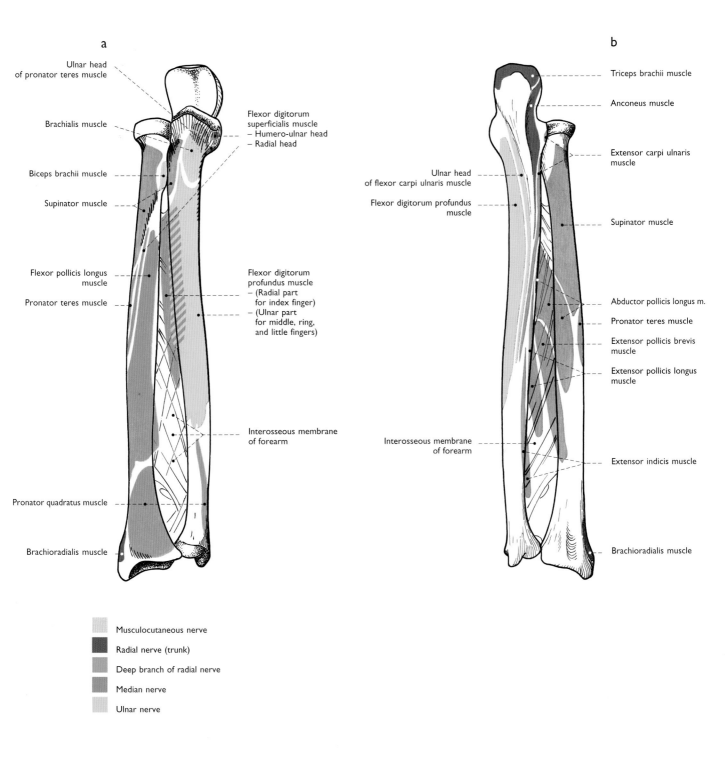

a

Ulnar head
of pronator teres muscle

Brachialis muscle

Biceps brachii muscle

Supinator muscle

Flexor pollicis longus
muscle

Pronator teres muscle

Pronator quadratus muscle

Brachioradialis muscle

Flexor digitorum
superficialis muscle
– Humero-ulnar head
– Radial head

Flexor digitorum
profundus muscle
– (Radial part
for index finger)
– (Ulnar part
for middle, ring,
and little fingers)

Interosseous membrane
of forearm

b

Ulnar head
of flexor carpi ulnaris muscle

Flexor digitorum profundus
muscle

Interosseous membrane
of forearm

Triceps brachii muscle

Anconeus muscle

Extensor carpi ulnaris
muscle

Supinator muscle

Abductor pollicis longus m.

Pronator teres muscle

Extensor pollicis brevis
muscle

Extensor pollicis longus
muscle

Extensor indicis muscle

Brachioradialis muscle

Musculocutaneous nerve

Radial nerve (trunk)

Deep branch of radial nerve

Median nerve

Ulnar nerve

117 Muscle attachments to the radius,
ulna, and interosseous membrane
of the right forearm

The colors indicate the innervation of the muscles
attaching to the
a ventral surface
b dorsal surface
of the forearm.

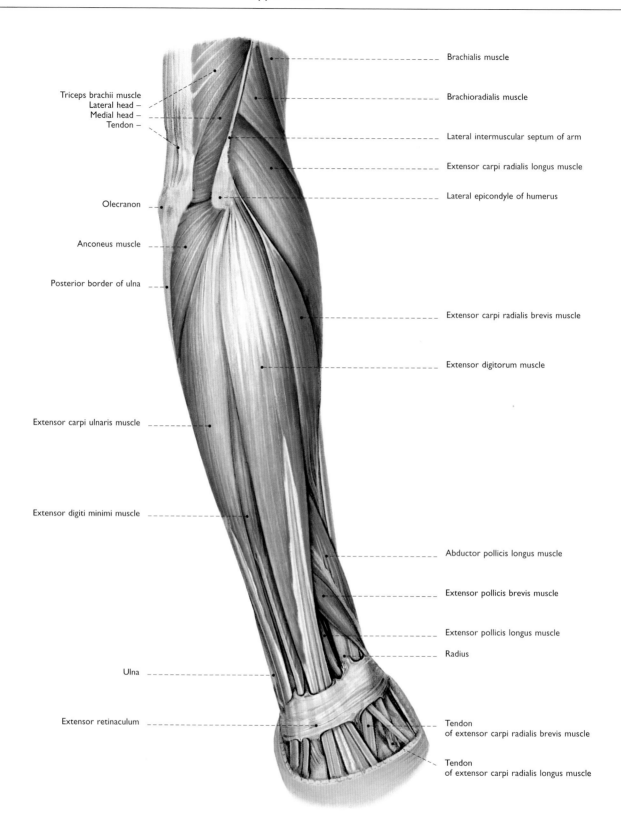

Brachialis muscle

Triceps brachii muscle
Lateral head –
Medial head –
Tendon –

Brachioradialis muscle

Lateral intermuscular septum of arm

Extensor carpi radialis longus muscle

Olecranon

Lateral epicondyle of humerus

Anconeus muscle

Posterior border of ulna

Extensor carpi radialis brevis muscle

Extensor digitorum muscle

Extensor carpi ulnaris muscle

Extensor digiti minimi muscle

Abductor pollicis longus muscle

Extensor pollicis brevis muscle

Extensor pollicis longus muscle

Radius

Ulna

Extensor retinaculum

Tendon
of extensor carpi radialis brevis muscle

Tendon
of extensor carpi radialis longus muscle

118 Muscles of the right forearm (50%)
Superficial layer. The forearm is slightly pronated.
Dorsolateral aspect

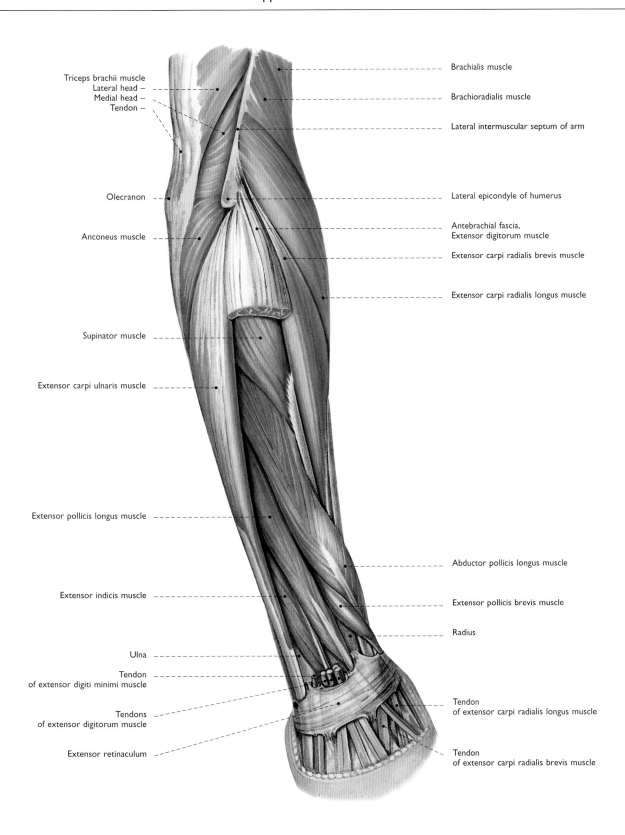

Triceps brachii muscle
Lateral head –
Medial head –
Tendon –

Olecranon

Anconeus muscle

Supinator muscle

Extensor carpi ulnaris muscle

Extensor pollicis longus muscle

Extensor indicis muscle

Ulna

Tendon
of extensor digiti minimi muscle

Tendons
of extensor digitorum muscle

Extensor retinaculum

Brachialis muscle

Brachioradialis muscle

Lateral intermuscular septum of arm

Lateral epicondyle of humerus

Antebrachial fascia,
Extensor digitorum muscle

Extensor carpi radialis brevis muscle

Extensor carpi radialis longus muscle

Abductor pollicis longus muscle

Extensor pollicis brevis muscle

Radius

Tendon
of extensor carpi radialis longus muscle

Tendon
of extensor carpi radialis brevis muscle

119   Muscles of the right forearm (50%)
Deep layer. The forearm is slightly pronated.
Dorsolateral aspect

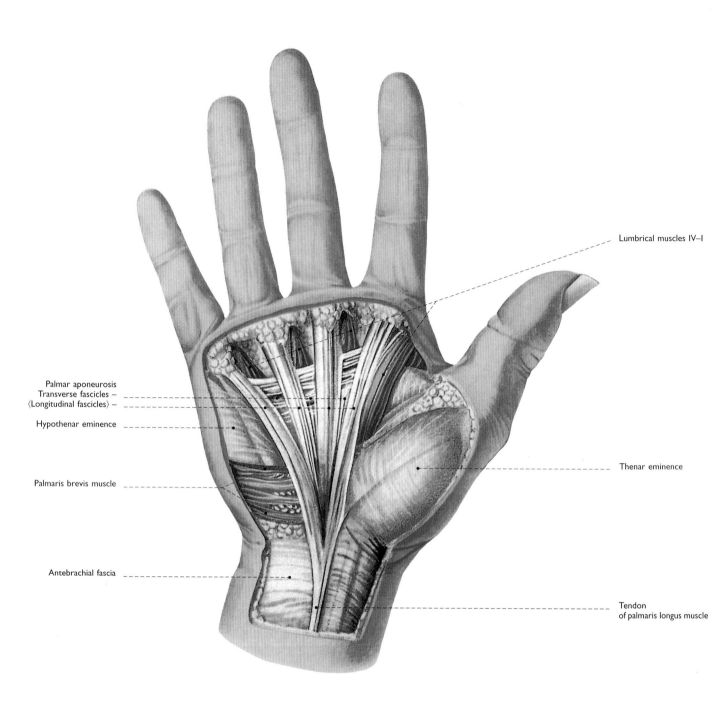

Lumbrical muscles IV–I

Palmar aponeurosis
Transverse fascicles –
⟨Longitudinal fascicles⟩ –

Hypothenar eminence

Thenar eminence

Palmaris brevis muscle

Antebrachial fascia

Tendon
of palmaris longus muscle

120 Palmar aponeurosis of the right hand (75%)
Palmar aspect

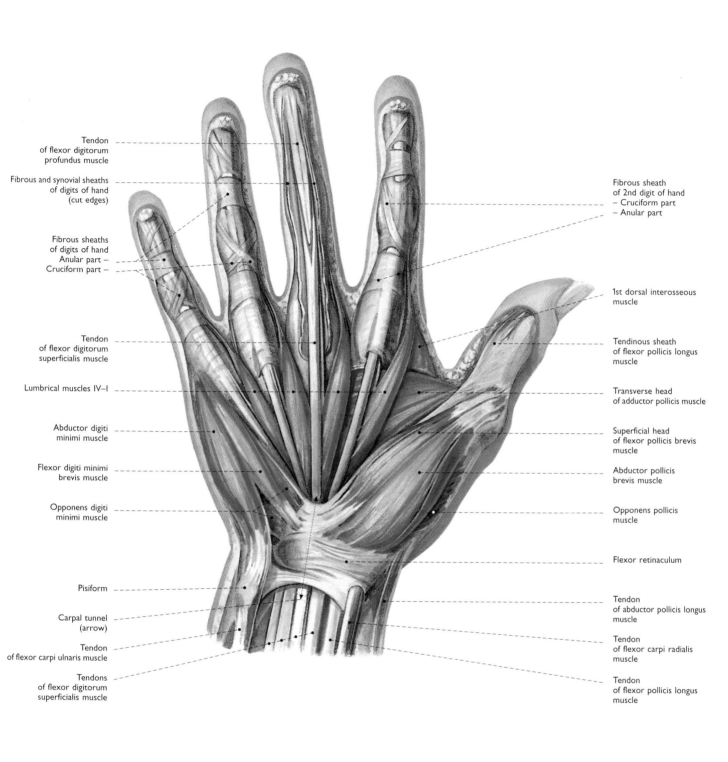

Tendon
of flexor digitorum
profundus muscle

Fibrous and synovial sheaths
of digits of hand
(cut edges)

Fibrous sheaths
of digits of hand
Anular part –
Cruciform part –

Tendon
of flexor digitorum
superficialis muscle

Lumbrical muscles IV–I

Abductor digiti
minimi muscle

Flexor digiti minimi
brevis muscle

Opponens digiti
minimi muscle

Pisiform

Carpal tunnel
(arrow)

Tendon
of flexor carpi ulnaris muscle

Tendons
of flexor digitorum
superficialis muscle

Fibrous sheath
of 2nd digit of hand
– Cruciform part
– Anular part

1st dorsal interosseous
muscle

Tendinous sheath
of flexor pollicis longus
muscle

Transverse head
of adductor pollicis muscle

Superficial head
of flexor pollicis brevis
muscle

Abductor pollicis
brevis muscle

Opponens pollicis
muscle

Flexor retinaculum

Tendon
of abductor pollicis longus
muscle

Tendon
of flexor carpi radialis
muscle

Tendon
of flexor pollicis longus
muscle

121 Muscles of the right hand (75%)
Superficial layer. The palmar aponeurosis was removed.
Palmar aspect

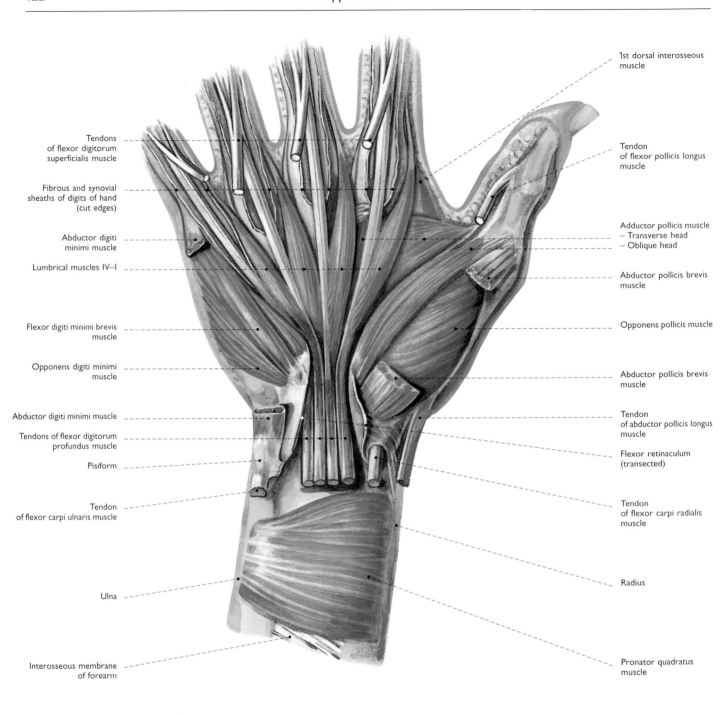

Tendons
of flexor digitorum
superficialis muscle

Fibrous and synovial
sheaths of digits of hand
(cut edges)

Abductor digiti
minimi muscle

Lumbrical muscles IV–I

Flexor digiti minimi brevis
muscle

Opponens digiti minimi
muscle

Abductor digiti minimi muscle

Tendons of flexor digitorum
profundus muscle

Pisiform

Tendon
of flexor carpi ulnaris muscle

Ulna

Interosseous membrane
of forearm

1st dorsal interosseous
muscle

Tendon
of flexor pollicis longus
muscle

Adductor pollicis muscle
– Transverse head
– Oblique head

Abductor pollicis brevis
muscle

Opponens pollicis muscle

Abductor pollicis brevis
muscle

Tendon
of abductor pollicis longus
muscle

Flexor retinaculum
(transected)

Tendon
of flexor carpi radialis
muscle

Radius

Pronator quadratus
muscle

122 Muscles of the right hand (75%)
Superficial layer. The flexor superficialis muscle
was removed and the carpal tunnel opened.
Palmar aspect

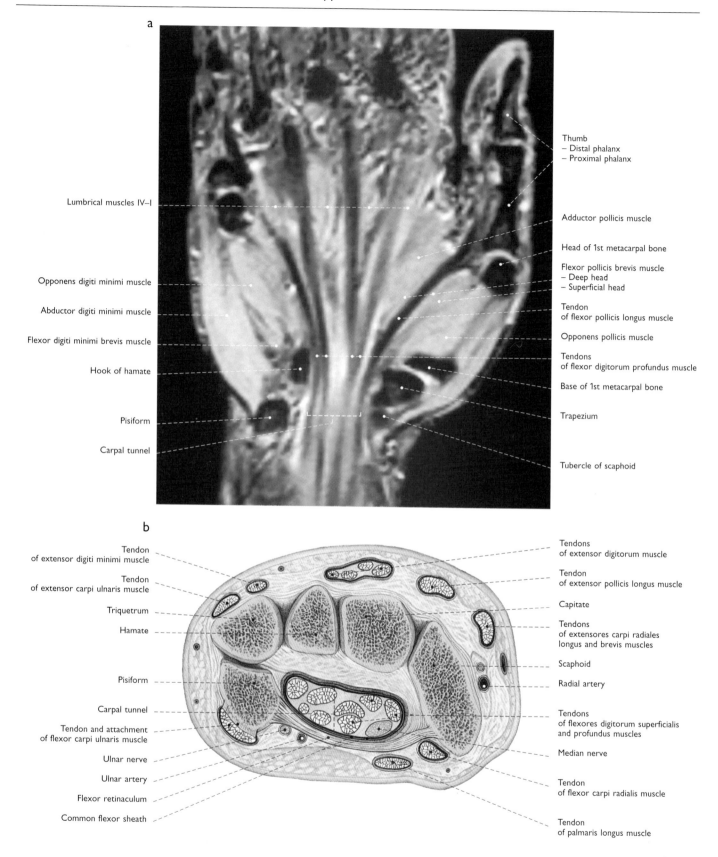

a

Thumb
– Distal phalanx
– Proximal phalanx

Lumbrical muscles IV–I

Adductor pollicis muscle

Head of 1st metacarpal bone

Flexor pollicis brevis muscle
– Deep head
– Superficial head

Opponens digiti minimi muscle

Tendon
of flexor pollicis longus muscle

Abductor digiti minimi muscle

Opponens pollicis muscle

Flexor digiti minimi brevis muscle

Tendons
of flexor digitorum profundus muscle

Hook of hamate

Base of 1st metacarpal bone

Trapezium

Pisiform

Carpal tunnel

Tubercle of scaphoid

b

Tendon
of extensor digiti minimi muscle

Tendons
of extensor digitorum muscle

Tendon
of extensor carpi ulnaris muscle

Tendon
of extensor pollicis longus muscle

Triquetrum

Capitate

Hamate

Tendons
of extensores carpi radiales
longus and brevis muscles

Pisiform

Scaphoid

Radial artery

Carpal tunnel

Tendon and attachment
of flexor carpi ulnaris muscle

Tendons
of flexores digitorum superficialis
and profundus muscles

Ulnar nerve

Median nerve

Ulnar artery

Flexor retinaculum

Tendon
of flexor carpi radialis muscle

Common flexor sheath

Tendon
of palmaris longus muscle

123 Muscles of the right hand

a Radio-ulnar (coronal) magnetic resonance image
(MRI, T$_2$-weighted) (100%)
b Transverse section through the wrist and the carpal tunnel (140%),
hand in pronated position, distal aspect

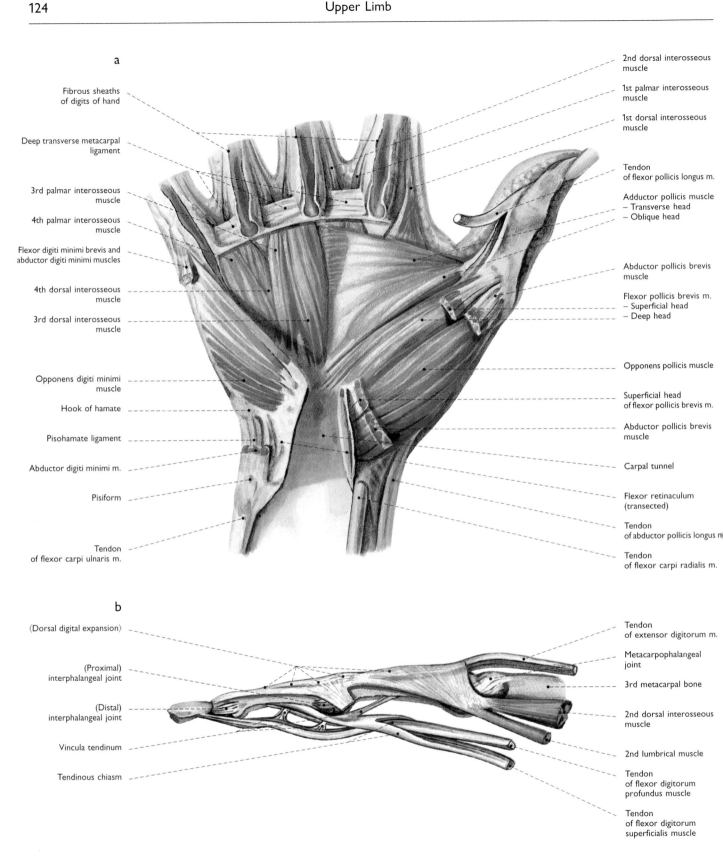

a

Fibrous sheaths
of digits of hand

Deep transverse metacarpal
ligament

3rd palmar interosseous
muscle

4th palmar interosseous
muscle

Flexor digiti minimi brevis and
abductor digiti minimi muscles

4th dorsal interosseous
muscle

3rd dorsal interosseous
muscle

Opponens digiti minimi
muscle

Hook of hamate

Pisohamate ligament

Abductor digiti minimi m.

Pisiform

Tendon
of flexor carpi ulnaris m.

2nd dorsal interosseous
muscle

1st palmar interosseous
muscle

1st dorsal interosseous
muscle

Tendon
of flexor pollicis longus m.

Adductor pollicis muscle
– Transverse head
– Oblique head

Abductor pollicis brevis
muscle

Flexor pollicis brevis m.
– Superficial head
– Deep head

Opponens pollicis muscle

Superficial head
of flexor pollicis brevis m.

Abductor pollicis brevis
muscle

Carpal tunnel

Flexor retinaculum
(transected)

Tendon
of abductor pollicis longus m

Tendon
of flexor carpi radialis m.

b

⟨Dorsal digital expansion⟩

(Proximal)
interphalangeal joint

(Distal)
interphalangeal joint

Vincula tendinum

Tendinous chiasm

Tendon
of extensor digitorum m.

Metacarpophalangeal
joint

3rd metacarpal bone

2nd dorsal interosseous
muscle

2nd lumbrical muscle

Tendon
of flexor digitorum
profundus muscle

Tendon
of flexor digitorum
superficialis muscle

124 Muscles of the right hand (75%)
a Deep layer, palmar aspect
b Middle finger with the dorsal digital expansion,
  radial aspect

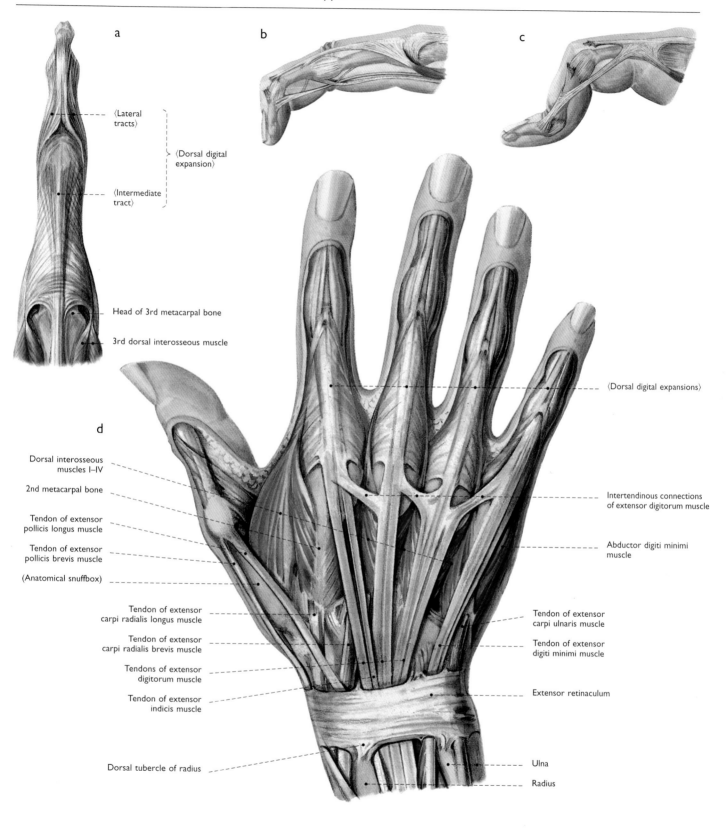

a

⟨Lateral tracts⟩

⟨Dorsal digital expansion⟩

⟨Intermediate tract⟩

Head of 3rd metacarpal bone

3rd dorsal interosseous muscle

b

c

⟨Dorsal digital expansions⟩

d

Dorsal interosseous muscles I–IV

2nd metacarpal bone

Tendon of extensor pollicis longus muscle

Tendon of extensor pollicis brevis muscle

(Anatomical snuffbox)

Tendon of extensor carpi radialis longus muscle

Tendon of extensor carpi radialis brevis muscle

Tendons of extensor digitorum muscle

Tendon of extensor indicis muscle

Dorsal tubercle of radius

Intertendinous connections of extensor digitorum muscle

Abductor digiti minimi muscle

Tendon of extensor carpi ulnaris muscle

Tendon of extensor digiti minimi muscle

Extensor retinaculum

Ulna

Radius

125   Muscles of the right hand

a   Muscles of the dorsum and dorsal digital expansion of the middle finger (75%), dorsal aspect

b, c   Ruptures of the dorsal digital expansion above the proximal (b) and distal (c) interphalangeal joints (50%)

d   Muscles of the dorsum of hand (75%), dorsal aspect

a

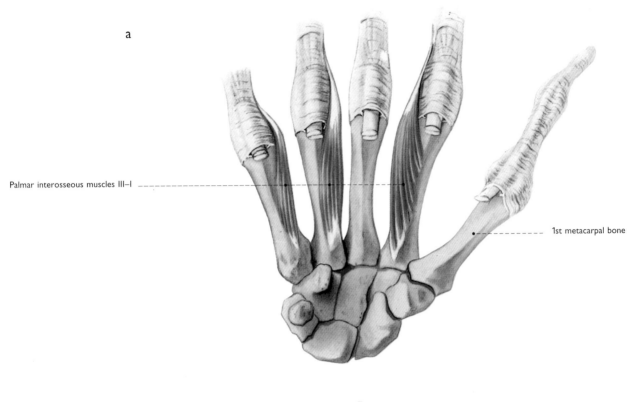

Palmar interosseous muscles III–I

1st metacarpal bone

b

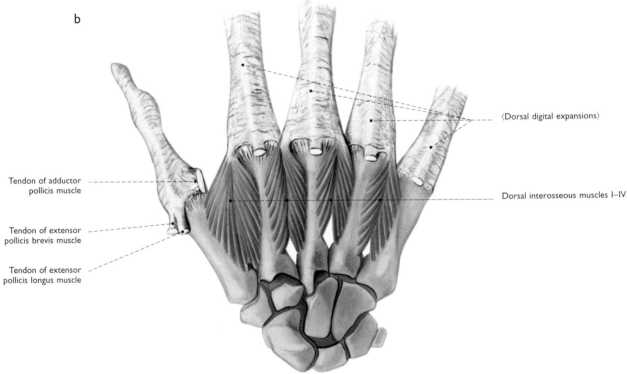

(Dorsal digital expansions)

Tendon of adductor
pollicis muscle

Dorsal interosseous muscles I–IV

Tendon of extensor
pollicis brevis muscle

Tendon of extensor
pollicis longus muscle

126 Interosseous muscles of the right hand (75%)
    a Palmar interosseous muscles, palmar aspect
    b Dorsal interosseous muscles, dorsal aspect

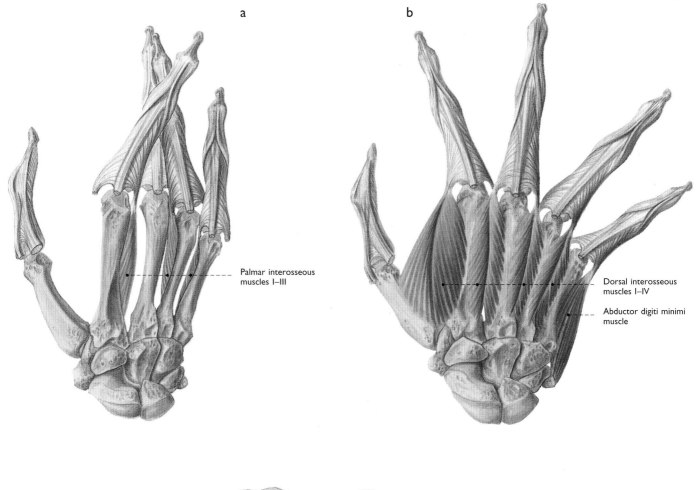

a

b

Palmar interosseous
muscles I–III

Dorsal interosseous
muscles I–IV

Abductor digiti minimi
muscle

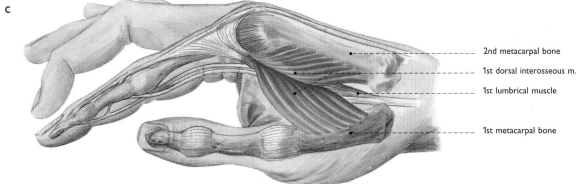

c

2nd metacarpal bone

1st dorsal interosseous m.

1st lumbrical muscle

1st metacarpal bone

**127 Interosseous and lumbrical muscles
of the right hand** (60%)

a Function of the palmar interosseous muscles, dorsal aspect
b Function of the dorsal interosseous muscles, dorsal aspect
c Function of the first lumbrical and first dorsal interosseous muscles,
   radial aspect

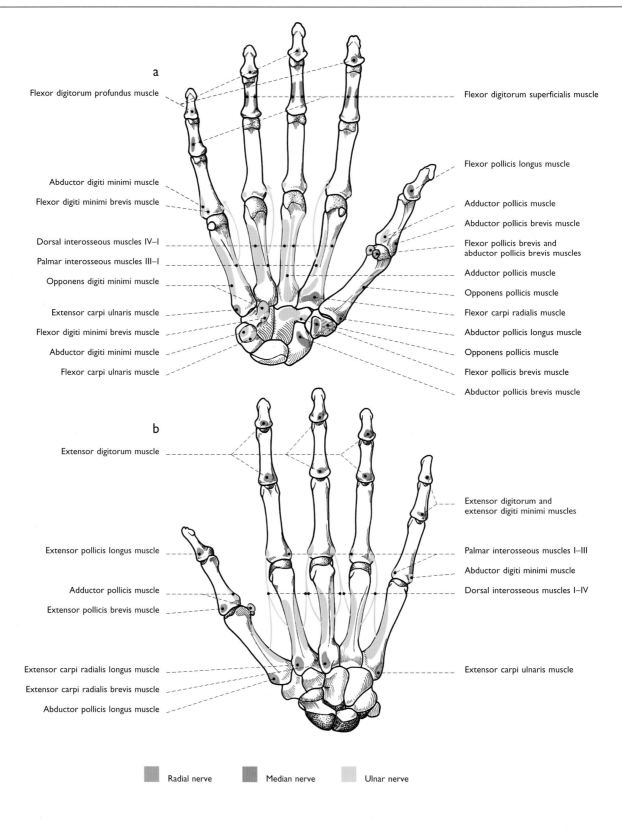

a

Flexor digitorum profundus muscle

Flexor digitorum superficialis muscle

Flexor pollicis longus muscle

Abductor digiti minimi muscle

Flexor digiti minimi brevis muscle

Adductor pollicis muscle

Abductor pollicis brevis muscle

Dorsal interosseous muscles IV–I

Palmar interosseous muscles III–I

Flexor pollicis brevis and
abductor pollicis brevis muscles

Opponens digiti minimi muscle

Adductor pollicis muscle

Opponens pollicis muscle

Extensor carpi ulnaris muscle

Flexor carpi radialis muscle

Flexor digiti minimi brevis muscle

Abductor pollicis longus muscle

Abductor digiti minimi muscle

Opponens pollicis muscle

Flexor carpi ulnaris muscle

Flexor pollicis brevis muscle

Abductor pollicis brevis muscle

b

Extensor digitorum muscle

Extensor digitorum and
extensor digiti minimi muscles

Extensor pollicis longus muscle

Palmar interosseous muscles I–III

Abductor digiti minimi muscle

Adductor pollicis muscle

Dorsal interosseous muscles I–IV

Extensor pollicis brevis muscle

Extensor carpi radialis longus muscle

Extensor carpi ulnaris muscle

Extensor carpi radialis brevis muscle

Abductor pollicis longus muscle

Radial nerve   Median nerve   Ulnar nerve

**128 Muscle attachments to the bones
of the right hand**
The colors indicate the innervation of the muscles
attaching to the
a palmar surface
b dorsal surface.

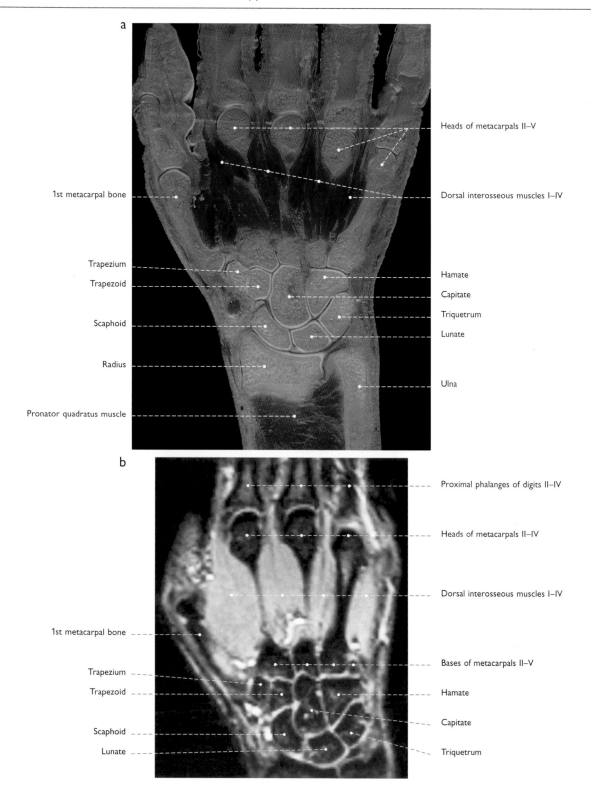

a

Heads of metacarpals II–V

Dorsal interosseous muscles I–IV

1st metacarpal bone

Trapezium
Trapezoid

Scaphoid

Radius

Pronator quadratus muscle

Hamate
Capitate
Triquetrum
Lunate

Ulna

b

Proximal phalanges of digits II–IV

Heads of metacarpals II–IV

Dorsal interosseous muscles I–IV

1st metacarpal bone

Trapezium
Trapezoid

Scaphoid
Lunate

Bases of metacarpals II–V

Hamate

Capitate

Triquetrum

**129 Dorsal interosseous muscles
       of the right hand** (75%)

a Anatomical radio-ulnar section, dorsal aspect
b Radio-ulnar (coronal) magnetic resonance image
   (MRI, T$_2$-weighted) of the wrist and the metacarpus

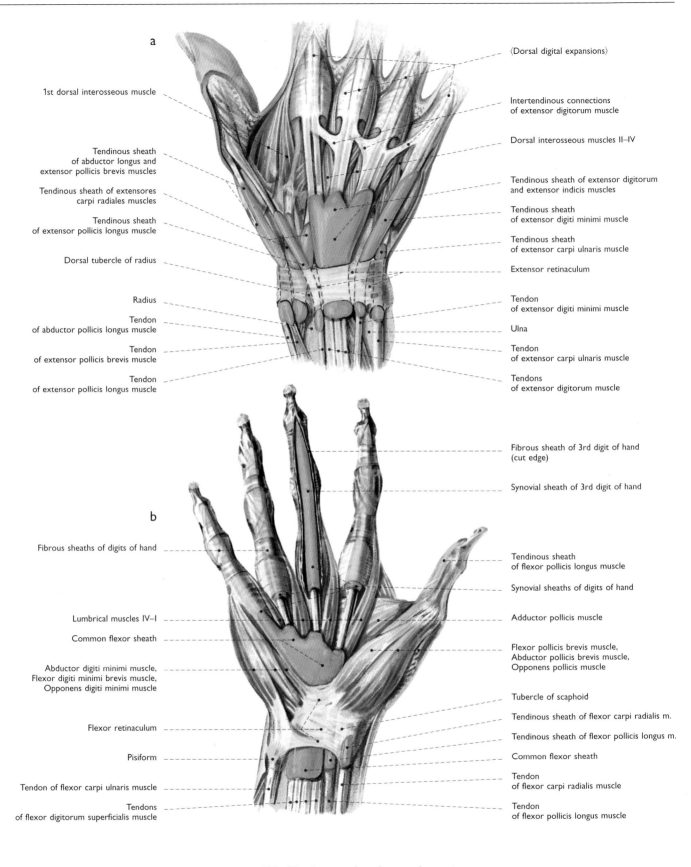

a

1st dorsal interosseous muscle

Tendinous sheath
of abductor longus and
extensor pollicis brevis muscles

Tendinous sheath of extensores
carpi radiales muscles

Tendinous sheath
of extensor pollicis longus muscle

Dorsal tubercle of radius

Radius

Tendon
of abductor pollicis longus muscle

Tendon
of extensor pollicis brevis muscle

Tendon
of extensor pollicis longus muscle

⟨Dorsal digital expansions⟩

Intertendinous connections
of extensor digitorum muscle

Dorsal interosseous muscles II–IV

Tendinous sheath of extensor digitorum
and extensor indicis muscles

Tendinous sheath
of extensor digiti minimi muscle

Tendinous sheath
of extensor carpi ulnaris muscle

Extensor retinaculum

Tendon
of extensor digiti minimi muscle

Ulna

Tendon
of extensor carpi ulnaris muscle

Tendons
of extensor digitorum muscle

b

Fibrous sheaths of digits of hand

Lumbrical muscles IV–I

Common flexor sheath

Abductor digiti minimi muscle,
Flexor digiti minimi brevis muscle,
Opponens digiti minimi muscle

Flexor retinaculum

Pisiform

Tendon of flexor carpi ulnaris muscle

Tendons
of flexor digitorum superficialis muscle

Fibrous sheath of 3rd digit of hand
(cut edge)

Synovial sheath of 3rd digit of hand

Tendinous sheath
of flexor pollicis longus muscle

Synovial sheaths of digits of hand

Adductor pollicis muscle

Flexor pollicis brevis muscle,
Abductor pollicis brevis muscle,
Opponens pollicis muscle

Tubercle of scaphoid

Tendinous sheath of flexor carpi radialis m.

Tendinous sheath of flexor pollicis longus m.

Common flexor sheath

Tendon
of flexor carpi radialis muscle

Tendon
of flexor pollicis longus muscle

130 Tendinous sheaths on the wrist
and the fingers of the right hand (50%)
a Dorsal aspect
b Palmar aspect

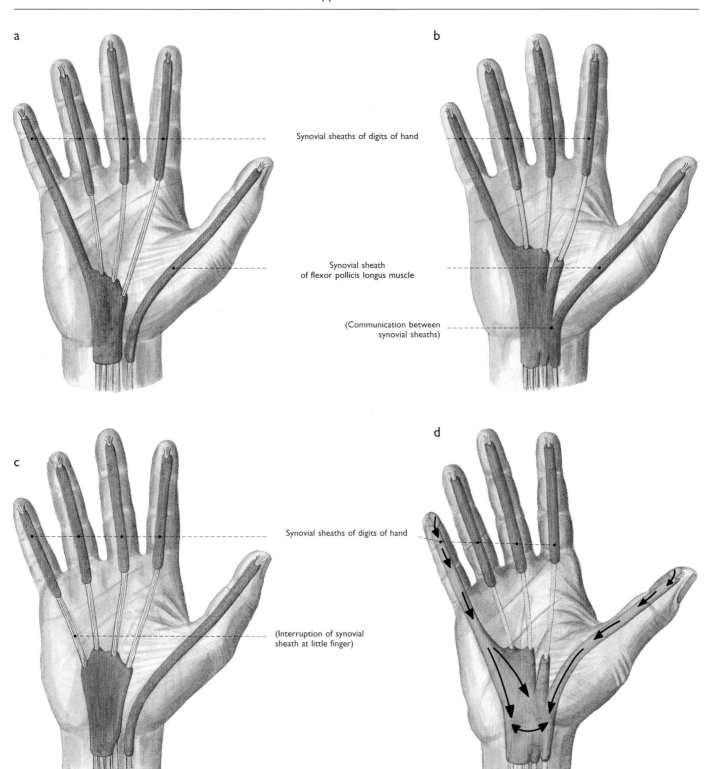

a

b

Synovial sheaths of digits of hand

Synovial sheath
of flexor pollicis longus muscle

(Communication between
synovial sheaths)

d

c

Synovial sheaths of digits of hand

(Interruption of synovial
sheath at little finger)

**131 Tendinous sheaths on the wrist
and the fingers of the right hand** (40%)

Palmar aspect
a Usual arrangement
b Most common variation
c Other common variation
d V-phlegmona following an abscess at the distal phalanx
   of the thumb or the little finger

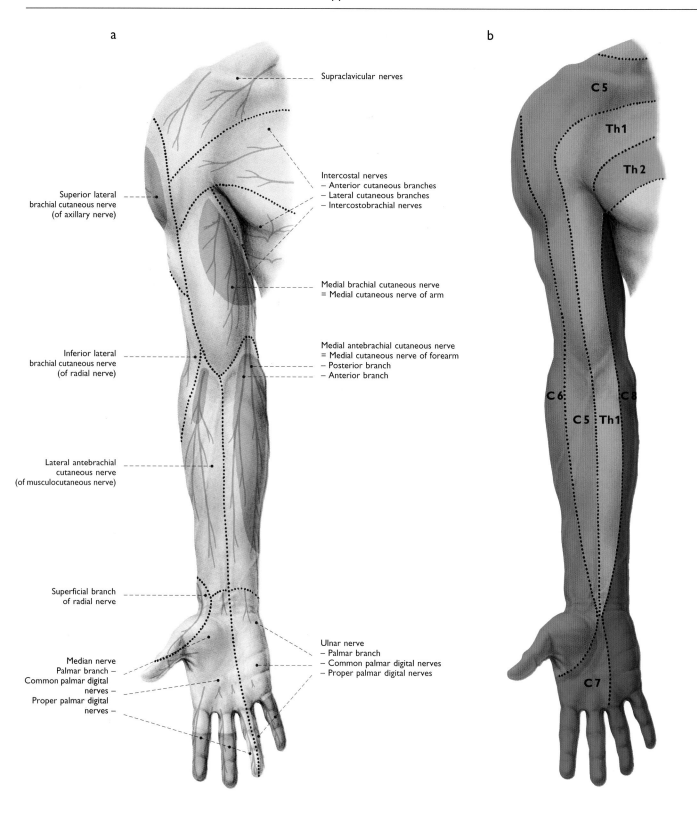

a

Supraclavicular nerves

Intercostal nerves
– Anterior cutaneous branches
– Lateral cutaneous branches
– Intercostobrachial nerves

Superior lateral
brachial cutaneous nerve
(of axillary nerve)

Medial brachial cutaneous nerve
= Medial cutaneous nerve of arm

Medial antebrachial cutaneous nerve
= Medial cutaneous nerve of forearm
– Posterior branch
– Anterior branch

Inferior lateral
brachial cutaneous nerve
(of radial nerve)

Lateral antebrachial
cutaneous nerve
(of musculocutaneous nerve)

Superficial branch
of radial nerve

Median nerve
Palmar branch –
Common palmar digital
nerves –
Proper palmar digital
nerves –

Ulnar nerve
– Palmar branch
– Common palmar digital nerves
– Proper palmar digital nerves

b

C 5

Th 1

Th 2

C 6

C 8

C 5 Th 1

C 7

**132 Cutaneous and segmental innervation
of the right upper limb** (25%)

Schematic representations, ventral aspect
a Cutaneous nerves and areas of distribution,
the autonomic areas of the different nerves
are given in a darker gray.
b Segmental innervation (dermatomes)

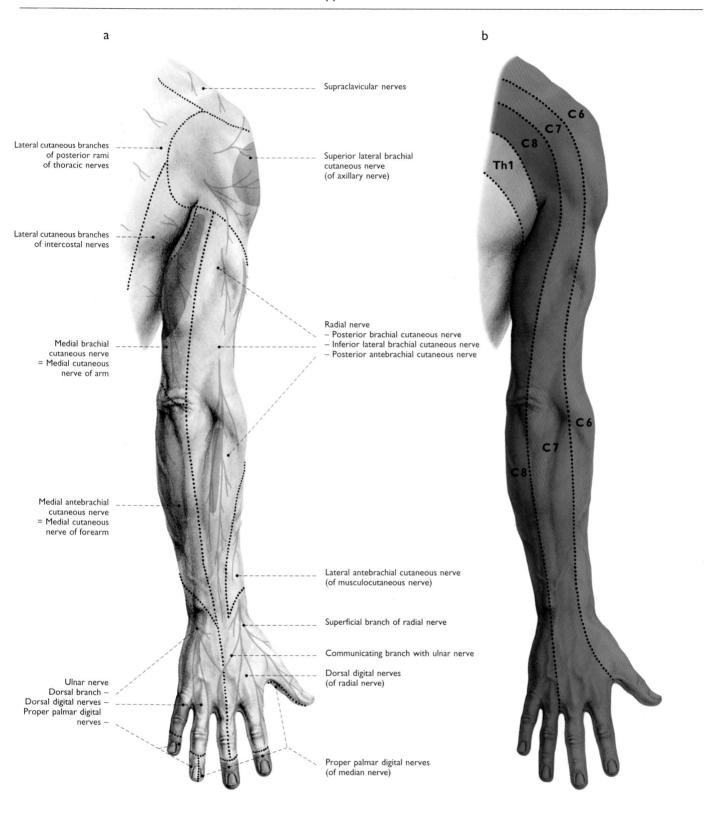

a

Supraclavicular nerves

Lateral cutaneous branches
of posterior rami
of thoracic nerves

Superior lateral brachial
cutaneous nerve
(of axillary nerve)

Lateral cutaneous branches
of intercostal nerves

Radial nerve
– Posterior brachial cutaneous nerve
– Inferior lateral brachial cutaneous nerve
– Posterior antebrachial cutaneous nerve

Medial brachial
cutaneous nerve
= Medial cutaneous
nerve of arm

Medial antebrachial
cutaneous nerve
= Medial cutaneous
nerve of forearm

Lateral antebrachial cutaneous nerve
(of musculocutaneous nerve)

Superficial branch of radial nerve

Communicating branch with ulnar nerve

Dorsal digital nerves
(of radial nerve)

Ulnar nerve
Dorsal branch –
Dorsal digital nerves –
Proper palmar digital
nerves –

Proper palmar digital nerves
(of median nerve)

b

C 6
C 7
C 8
Th1

C 6
C 7
C 8

**133 Cutaneous and segmental innervation
of the right upper limb** (25%)
Schematic representations, dorsal aspect
a Cutaneous nerves and areas of distribution,
   the autonomic areas of the different nerves
   are given in a darker gray.
b Segmental innervation (dermatomes)

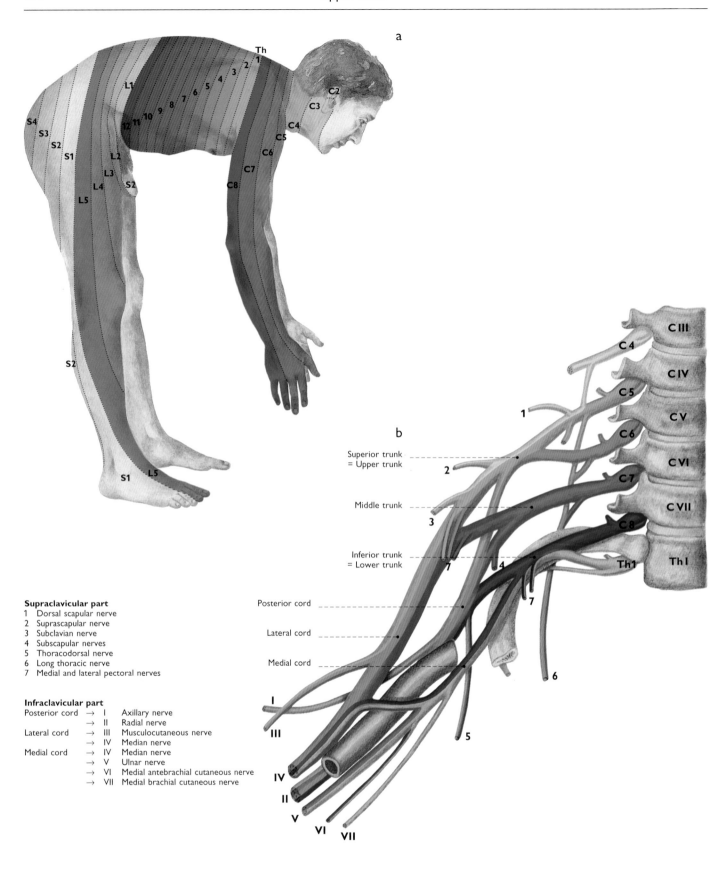

Supraclavicular part

1   Dorsal scapular nerve
2   Suprascapular nerve
3   Subclavian nerve
4   Subscapular nerves
5   Thoracodorsal nerve
6   Long thoracic nerve
7   Medial and lateral pectoral nerves

Infraclavicular part

Posterior cord	→	I	Axillary nerve
	→	II	Radial nerve
Lateral cord	→	III	Musculocutaneous nerve
	→	IV	Median nerve
Medial cord	→	IV	Median nerve
	→	V	Ulnar nerve
	→	VI	Medial antebrachial cutaneous nerve
	→	VII	Medial brachial cutaneous nerve

134   Segmental innervation and brachial plexus

a   Segmental innervation (dermatomes) of the upper limb, trunk, and lower limb (according to von Lanz and Wachsmuth, 1959)

b   Plan of the brachial plexus

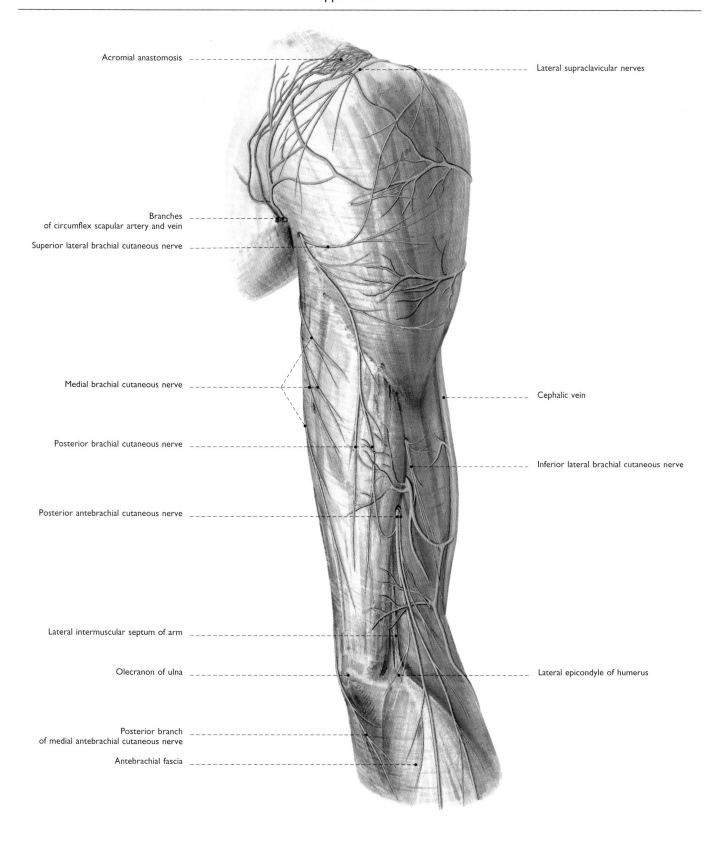

Acromial anastomosis

Lateral supraclavicular nerves

Branches of circumflex scapular artery and vein

Superior lateral brachial cutaneous nerve

Medial brachial cutaneous nerve

Cephalic vein

Posterior brachial cutaneous nerve

Inferior lateral brachial cutaneous nerve

Posterior antebrachial cutaneous nerve

Lateral intermuscular septum of arm

Olecranon of ulna

Lateral epicondyle of humerus

Posterior branch of medial antebrachial cutaneous nerve

Antebrachial fascia

135 Subcutaneous veins and nerves of the right shoulder and the right arm (50%)
In this case the inferior lateral brachial cutaneous nerve originates from the axillary nerve. Dorsolateral aspect

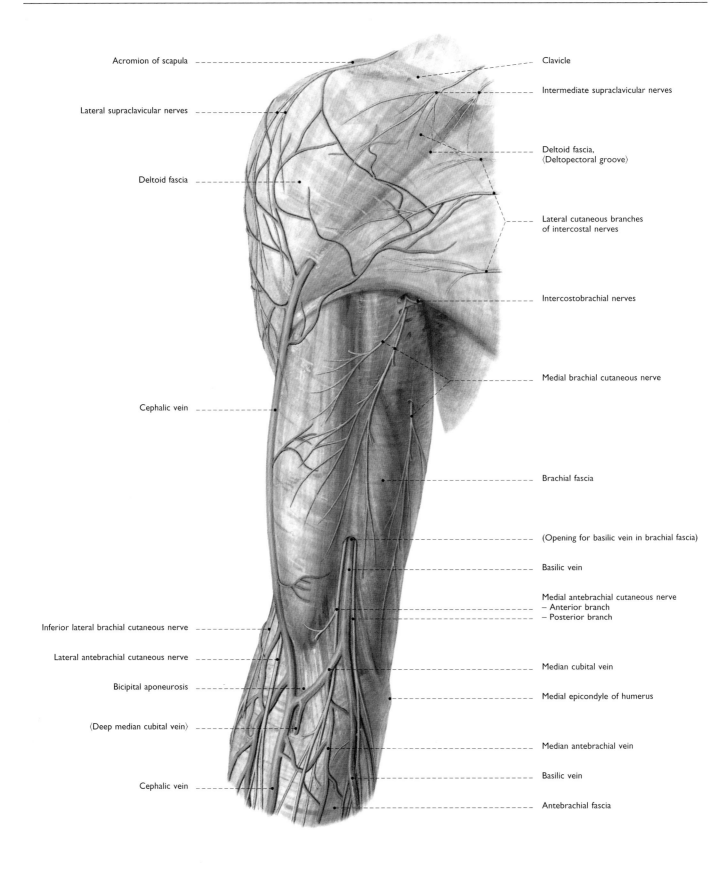

Acromion of scapula

Lateral supraclavicular nerves

Deltoid fascia

Cephalic vein

Inferior lateral brachial cutaneous nerve

Lateral antebrachial cutaneous nerve

Bicipital aponeurosis

⟨Deep median cubital vein⟩

Cephalic vein

Clavicle

Intermediate supraclavicular nerves

Deltoid fascia,
⟨Deltopectoral groove⟩

Lateral cutaneous branches
of intercostal nerves

Intercostobrachial nerves

Medial brachial cutaneous nerve

Brachial fascia

⟨Opening for basilic vein in brachial fascia⟩

Basilic vein

Medial antebrachial cutaneous nerve
– Anterior branch
– Posterior branch

Median cubital vein

Medial epicondyle of humerus

Median antebrachial vein

Basilic vein

Antebrachial fascia

**136 Subcutaneous veins and nerves of the
right shoulder and the right arm** (50%)
Ventral aspect

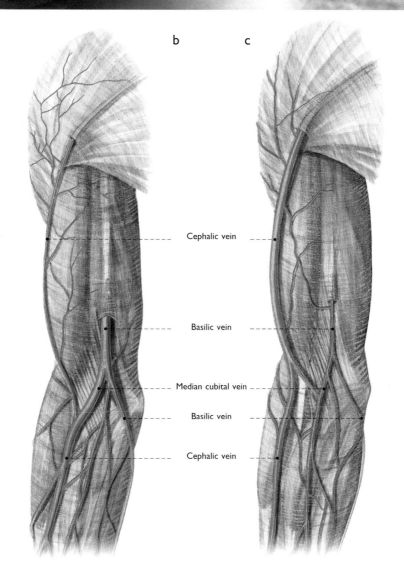

a

Cephalic vein

Head of humerus

Scapula

Brachial veins
(with valves)

Thoraco-acromial vein

Clavicle

Subclavian vein

Brachiocephalic vein

Axillary vein

b   **c**

Cephalic vein

Basilic vein

Median cubital vein

Basilic vein

Cephalic vein

**137 Subcutaneous veins of the right shoulder,
the right arm and forearm**

a   Phlebogram of the veins of the arm
and the axilla (50%)

b, c   Common variations of the subcutaneous veins
of the arm and the anterior region of elbow (30%), ventral aspect

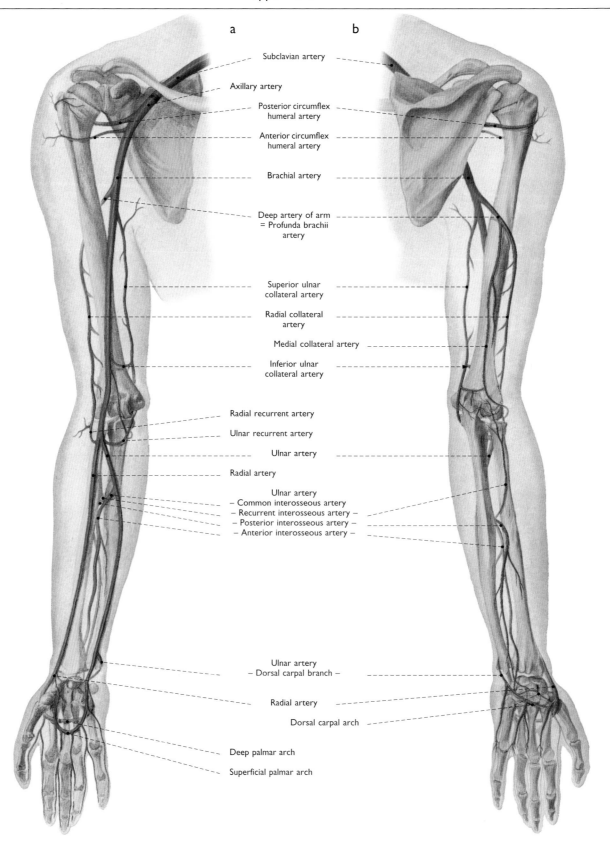

a

b

Subclavian artery

Axillary artery

Posterior circumflex
humeral artery

Anterior circumflex
humeral artery

Brachial artery

Deep artery of arm
= Profunda brachii
artery

Superior ulnar
collateral artery

Radial collateral
artery

Medial collateral artery

Inferior ulnar
collateral artery

Radial recurrent artery

Ulnar recurrent artery

Ulnar artery

Radial artery

Ulnar artery
– Common interosseous artery
– Recurrent interosseous artery –
– Posterior interosseous artery –
– Anterior interosseous artery –

Ulnar artery
– Dorsal carpal branch –

Radial artery

Dorsal carpal arch

Deep palmar arch

Superficial palmar arch

138 Arteries of the right upper limb (30%)
Schematic representations
a   Ventral aspect
b   Dorsal aspect

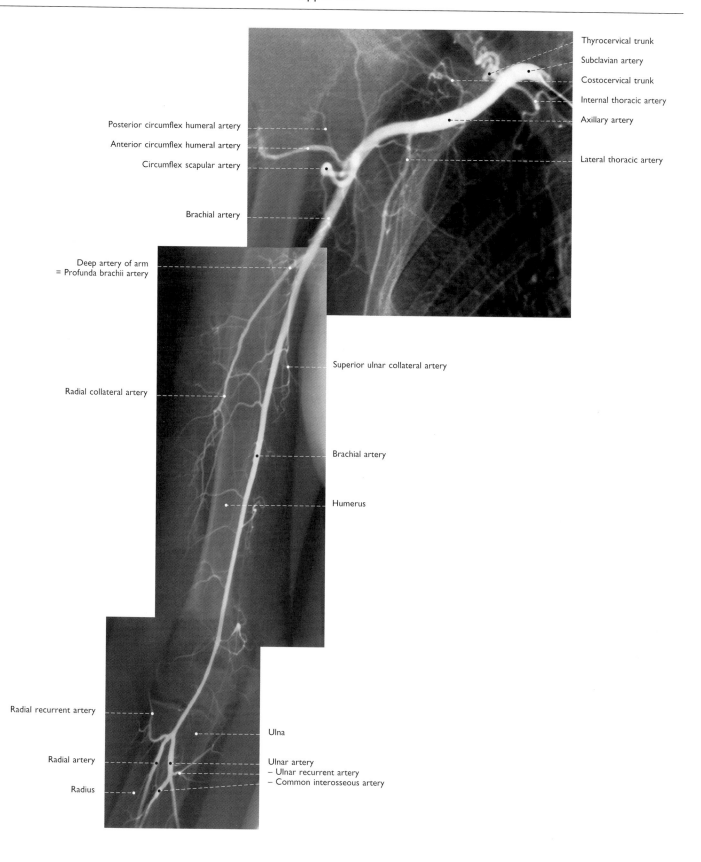

Thyrocervical trunk
Subclavian artery
Costocervical trunk
Internal thoracic artery
Axillary artery

Lateral thoracic artery

Posterior circumflex humeral artery
Anterior circumflex humeral artery
Circumflex scapular artery

Brachial artery

Deep artery of arm
= Profunda brachii artery

Superior ulnar collateral artery

Radial collateral artery

Brachial artery

Humerus

Radial recurrent artery

Ulna

Radial artery

Ulnar artery
– Ulnar recurrent artery
– Common interosseous artery

Radius

139 Arteries of the right upper limb (50%)
Arteriogram of the arteries of the upper limb
(subclavian, axillary, brachial, radial, and ulnar arteries)

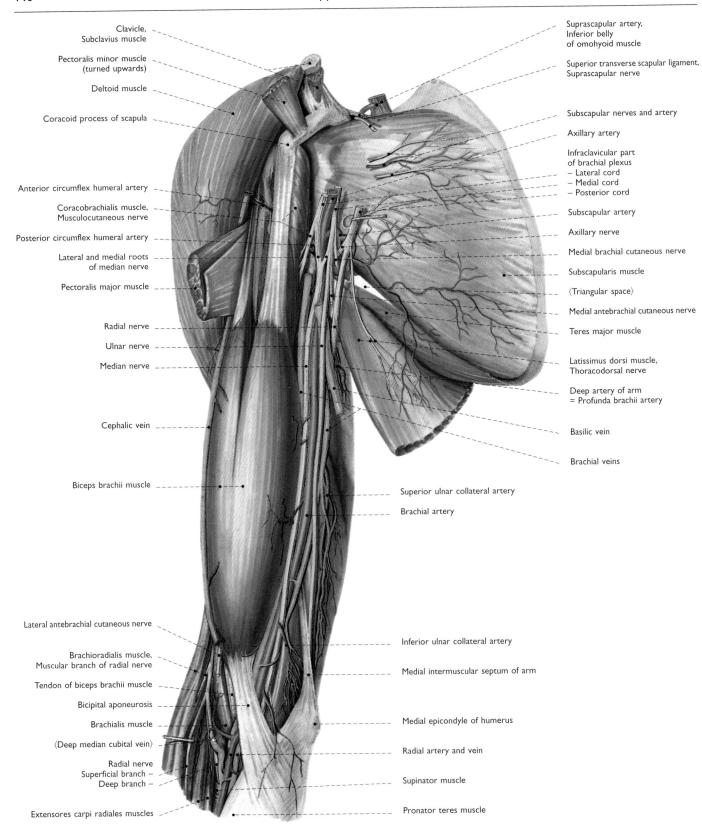

Clavicle, Subclavius muscle

Pectoralis minor muscle (turned upwards)

Deltoid muscle

Coracoid process of scapula

Anterior circumflex humeral artery

Coracobrachialis muscle, Musculocutaneous nerve

Posterior circumflex humeral artery

Lateral and medial roots of median nerve

Pectoralis major muscle

Radial nerve

Ulnar nerve

Median nerve

Cephalic vein

Biceps brachii muscle

Lateral antebrachial cutaneous nerve

Brachioradialis muscle, Muscular branch of radial nerve

Tendon of biceps brachii muscle

Bicipital aponeurosis

Brachialis muscle

⟨Deep median cubital vein⟩

Radial nerve
Superficial branch –
Deep branch –

Extensores carpi radiales muscles

Suprascapular artery, Inferior belly of omohyoid muscle

Superior transverse scapular ligament, Suprascapular nerve

Subscapular nerves and artery

Axillary artery

Infraclavicular part of brachial plexus
– Lateral cord
– Medial cord
– Posterior cord

Subscapular artery

Axillary nerve

Medial brachial cutaneous nerve

Subscapularis muscle

⟨Triangular space⟩

Medial antebrachial cutaneous nerve

Teres major muscle

Latissimus dorsi muscle, Thoracodorsal nerve

Deep artery of arm = Profunda brachii artery

Basilic vein

Brachial veins

Superior ulnar collateral artery

Brachial artery

Inferior ulnar collateral artery

Medial intermuscular septum of arm

Medial epicondyle of humerus

Radial artery and vein

Supinator muscle

Pronator teres muscle

140 Blood vessels and nerves
of the right shoulder, the arm,
and the anterior region of elbow (50%)
Ventral aspect

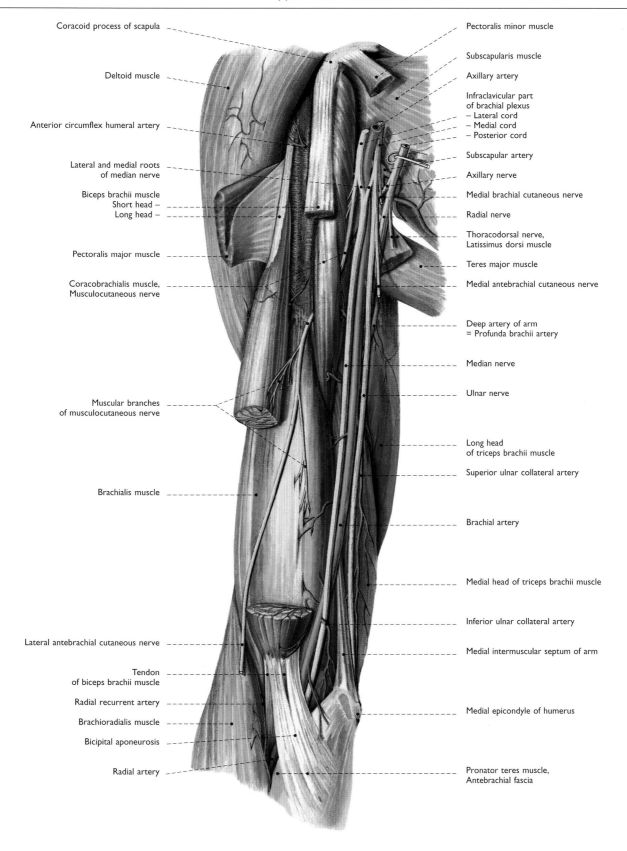

Coracoid process of scapula

Deltoid muscle

Anterior circumflex humeral artery

Lateral and medial roots of median nerve

Biceps brachii muscle
Short head –
Long head –

Pectoralis major muscle

Coracobrachialis muscle, Musculocutaneous nerve

Muscular branches of musculocutaneous nerve

Brachialis muscle

Lateral antebrachial cutaneous nerve

Tendon of biceps brachii muscle

Radial recurrent artery

Brachioradialis muscle

Bicipital aponeurosis

Radial artery

Pectoralis minor muscle

Subscapularis muscle

Axillary artery

Infraclavicular part of brachial plexus
– Lateral cord
– Medial cord
– Posterior cord

Subscapular artery

Axillary nerve

Medial brachial cutaneous nerve

Radial nerve

Thoracodorsal nerve, Latissimus dorsi muscle

Teres major muscle

Medial antebrachial cutaneous nerve

Deep artery of arm = Profunda brachii artery

Median nerve

Ulnar nerve

Long head of triceps brachii muscle

Superior ulnar collateral artery

Brachial artery

Medial head of triceps brachii muscle

Inferior ulnar collateral artery

Medial intermuscular septum of arm

Medial epicondyle of humerus

Pronator teres muscle, Antebrachial fascia

141 Arteries and nerves of the right arm and the anterior region of elbow (50%)
The biceps brachii muscle was partially removed.
Ventral aspect

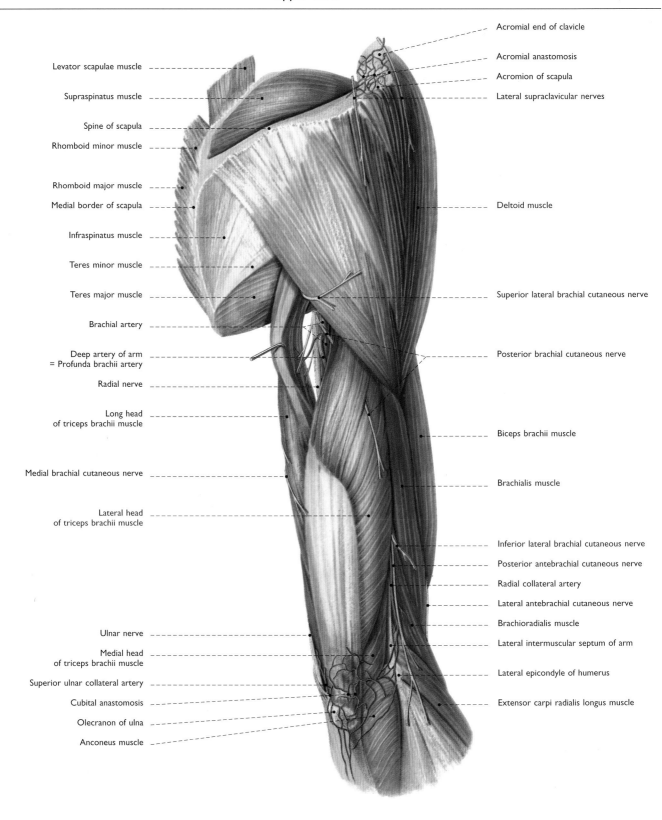

Levator scapulae muscle

Supraspinatus muscle

Spine of scapula

Rhomboid minor muscle

Rhomboid major muscle

Medial border of scapula

Infraspinatus muscle

Teres minor muscle

Teres major muscle

Brachial artery

Deep artery of arm
= Profunda brachii artery

Radial nerve

Long head
of triceps brachii muscle

Medial brachial cutaneous nerve

Lateral head
of triceps brachii muscle

Ulnar nerve

Medial head
of triceps brachii muscle

Superior ulnar collateral artery

Cubital anastomosis

Olecranon of ulna

Anconeus muscle

Acromial end of clavicle

Acromial anastomosis

Acromion of scapula

Lateral supraclavicular nerves

Deltoid muscle

Superior lateral brachial cutaneous nerve

Posterior brachial cutaneous nerve

Biceps brachii muscle

Brachialis muscle

Inferior lateral brachial cutaneous nerve

Posterior antebrachial cutaneous nerve

Radial collateral artery

Lateral antebrachial cutaneous nerve

Brachioradialis muscle

Lateral intermuscular septum of arm

Lateral epicondyle of humerus

Extensor carpi radialis longus muscle

**142 Arteries and nerves of the right shoulder,
the right arm, and the posterior region of elbow** (50%)
Dorsolateral aspect

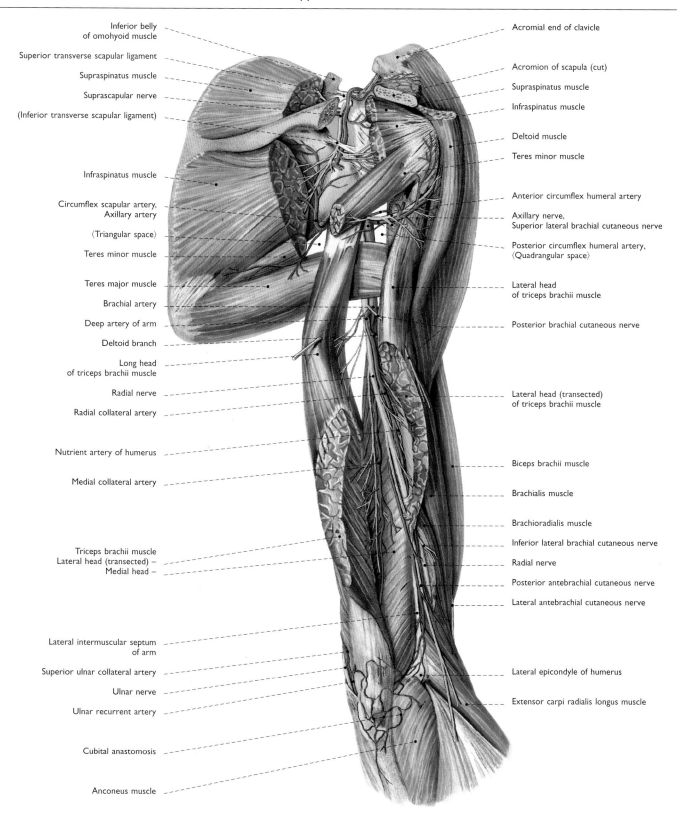

Inferior belly of omohyoid muscle

Superior transverse scapular ligament

Supraspinatus muscle

Suprascapular nerve

(Inferior transverse scapular ligament)

Infraspinatus muscle

Circumflex scapular artery, Axillary artery

⟨Triangular space⟩

Teres minor muscle

Teres major muscle

Brachial artery

Deep artery of arm

Deltoid branch

Long head of triceps brachii muscle

Radial nerve

Radial collateral artery

Nutrient artery of humerus

Medial collateral artery

Triceps brachii muscle
Lateral head (transected) —
Medial head —

Lateral intermuscular septum of arm

Superior ulnar collateral artery

Ulnar nerve

Ulnar recurrent artery

Cubital anastomosis

Anconeus muscle

Acromial end of clavicle

Acromion of scapula (cut)

Supraspinatus muscle

Infraspinatus muscle

Deltoid muscle

Teres minor muscle

Anterior circumflex humeral artery

Axillary nerve,
Superior lateral brachial cutaneous nerve

Posterior circumflex humeral artery,
⟨Quadrangular space⟩

Lateral head
of triceps brachii muscle

Posterior brachial cutaneous nerve

Lateral head (transected)
of triceps brachii muscle

Biceps brachii muscle

Brachialis muscle

Brachioradialis muscle

Inferior lateral brachial cutaneous nerve

Radial nerve

Posterior antebrachial cutaneous nerve

Lateral antebrachial cutaneous nerve

Lateral epicondyle of humerus

Extensor carpi radialis longus muscle

**143 Arteries and nerves of the right shoulder,
the right arm, and the posterior region of elbow** (50%)

The lateral head of the triceps brachii muscle was divided,
the radial nerve channel opened. Dorsolateral aspect

a

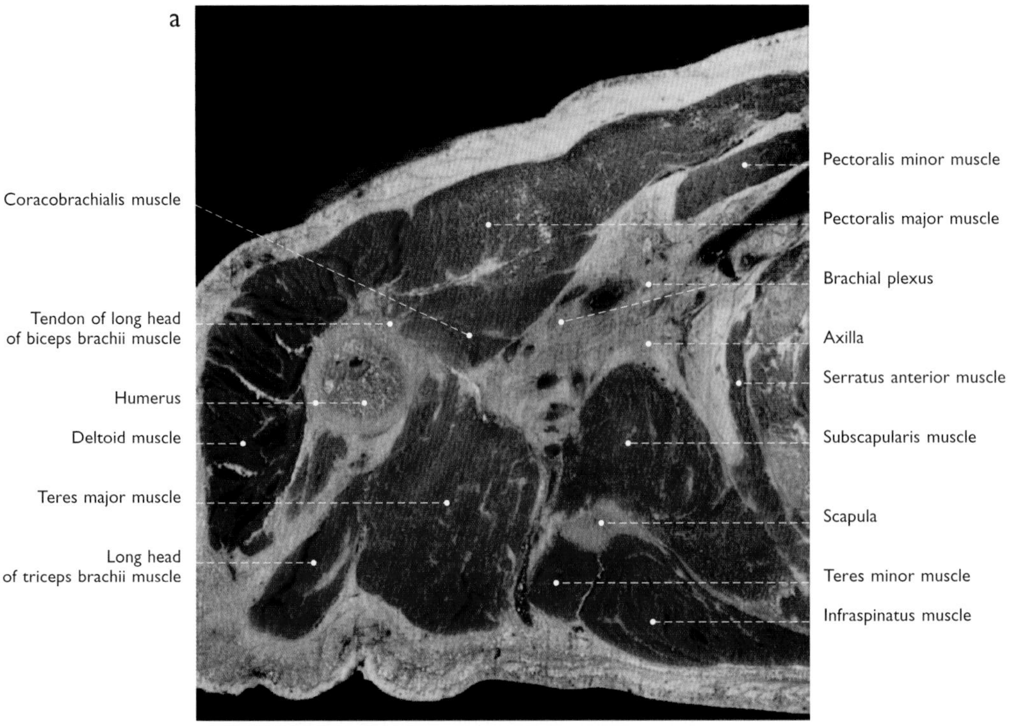

Coracobrachialis muscle

Tendon of long head
of biceps brachii muscle

Humerus

Deltoid muscle

Teres major muscle

Long head
of triceps brachii muscle

Pectoralis minor muscle

Pectoralis major muscle

Brachial plexus

Axilla

Serratus anterior muscle

Subscapularis muscle

Scapula

Teres minor muscle

Infraspinatus muscle

b

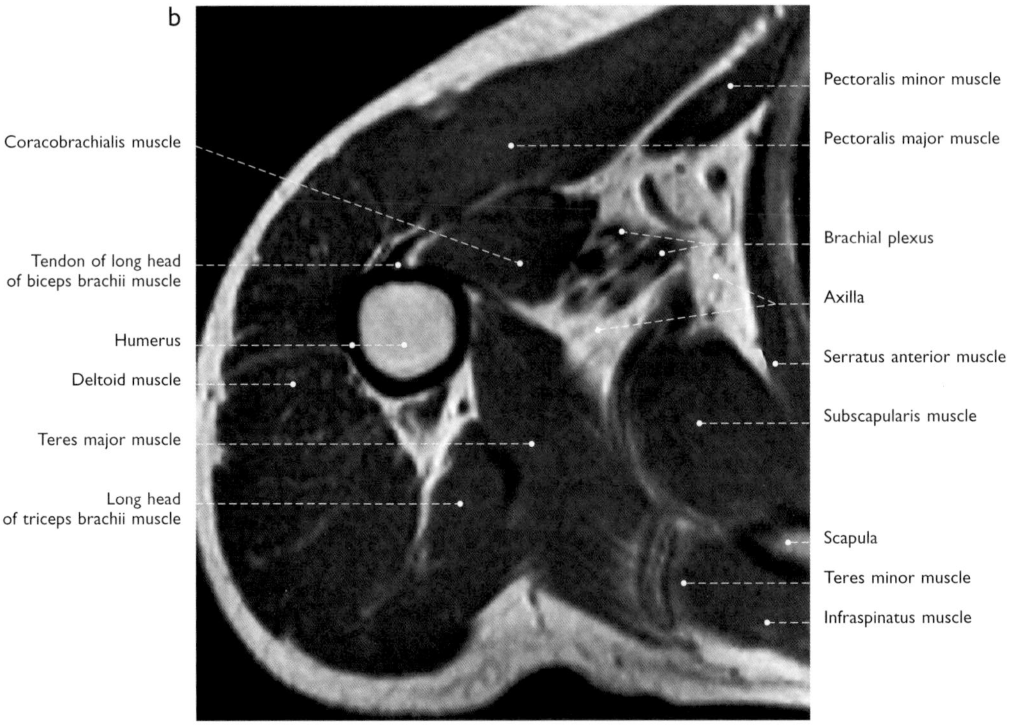

Coracobrachialis muscle

Tendon of long head
of biceps brachii muscle

Humerus

Deltoid muscle

Teres major muscle

Long head
of triceps brachii muscle

Pectoralis minor muscle

Pectoralis major muscle

Brachial plexus

Axilla

Serratus anterior muscle

Subscapularis muscle

Scapula

Teres minor muscle

Infraspinatus muscle

144 Right arm (80%)

Transverse sections through the proximal arm
at the level of the shoulder and the axilla, distal aspect
a Anatomical section
b Magnetic resonance image (MRI, T$_1$-weighted)

a

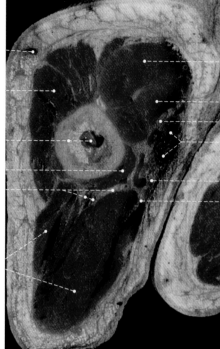

Cephalic vein

Deltoid muscle

Body of humerus

Triceps brachii muscle
Medial head –

Radial nerve,
Deep artery and vein of arm

Triceps brachii muscle
Lateral head –
Long head –

Biceps brachii muscle

Coracobrachialis muscle

Musculocutaneous nerve

Brachial artery and vein

Median nerve

Ulnar nerve

b

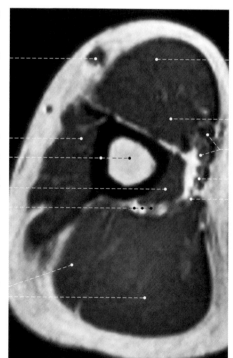

Cephalic vein

Deltoid muscle

Body of humerus

Triceps brachii muscle
Medial head –

Deep artery and vein of arm,
Radial nerve

Triceps brachii muscle
Lateral head –
Long head –

Biceps brachii muscle

Coracobrachialis muscle

Brachial artery and vein

Median nerve

Ulnar nerve

145 Right arm (80%)

Transverse sections through the proximal third
of the arm, distal aspect

a   Anatomical section
b   Magnetic resonance image (MRI, T$_1$-weighted)

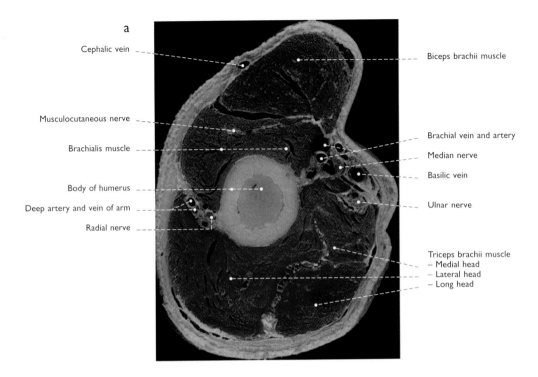

a

Cephalic vein

Musculocutaneous nerve

Brachialis muscle

Body of humerus

Deep artery and vein of arm

Radial nerve

Biceps brachii muscle

Brachial vein and artery

Median nerve

Basilic vein

Ulnar nerve

Triceps brachii muscle
– Medial head
– Lateral head
– Long head

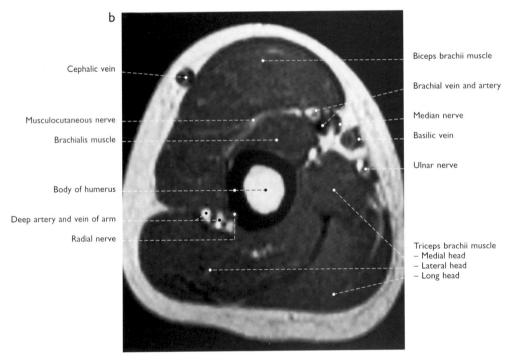

b

Cephalic vein

Musculocutaneous nerve

Brachialis muscle

Body of humerus

Deep artery and vein of arm

Radial nerve

Biceps brachii muscle

Brachial vein and artery

Median nerve

Basilic vein

Ulnar nerve

Triceps brachii muscle
– Medial head
– Lateral head
– Long head

146 Right arm (100%)

Transverse sections through the middle third
of the arm, distal aspect
a Anatomical section
b Magnetic resonance image (MRI, T$_1$-weighted)

a

Tendon
of biceps brachii muscle

Brachioradialis muscle

Radial nerve

Extensor carpi radialis longus muscle

Humerus

Triceps brachii muscle

Cephalic vein

Biceps brachii muscle

Brachial vein and artery

Median nerve

Brachialis muscle

Basilic vein

Pronator teres muscle

Ulnar nerve

Tendon
of triceps brachii muscle

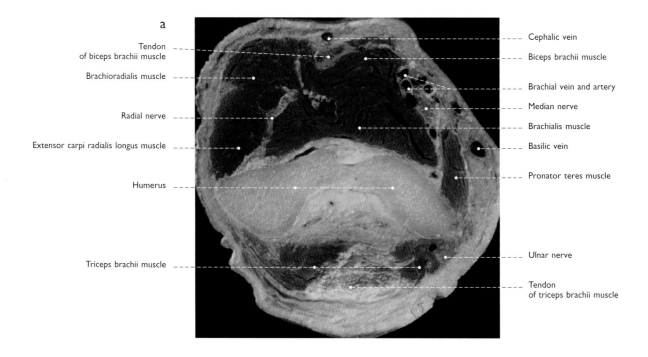

b

Cephalic vein

Tendon
of biceps brachii muscle

Brachioradialis muscle

Radial nerve

Extensor carpi radialis longus muscle

Triceps brachii muscle

Brachial vein and artery

Median nerve

Basilic vein

Brachialis muscle

Humerus

Ulnar nerve

Tendon
of triceps brachii muscle

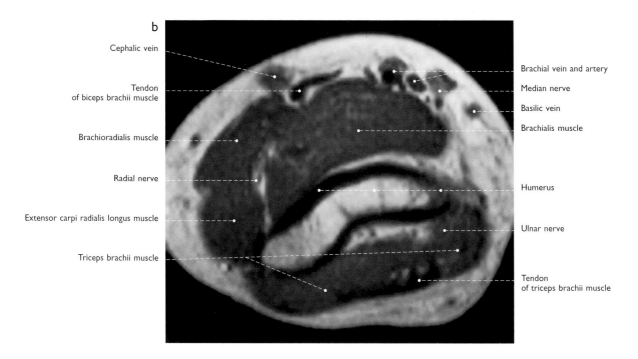

147 Right arm (100%)

Transverse sections through the distal third
of the arm just above the elbow joint,
distal aspect
a Anatomical section
b Magnetic resonance image (MRI, T$_1$-weighted)

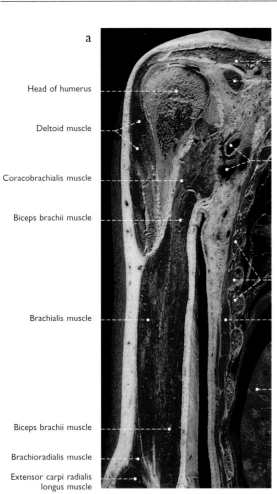

a

Head of humerus

Deltoid muscle

Coracobrachialis muscle

Biceps brachii muscle

Brachialis muscle

Biceps brachii muscle

Brachioradialis muscle

Extensor carpi radialis
longus muscle

Supraspinatus muscle

Coracoid process of scapula

Axillary artery and vein

Ribs

Serratus anterior muscle

Liver

b

Trapezius muscle

Spine of scapula

Infraspinatus muscle

Teres minor muscle

Deltoid muscle

Teres major muscle

Scapula

Triceps brachii muscle
Long head –
Lateral head –
Medial head –

Serratus anterior muscle

Latissimus dorsi muscle

Olecranon fossa

Lateral and medial
epicondyles of humerus

148 Right arm (35%)

Coronal anatomical sections
a   through the ventral part (flexor compartment)
b   through the dorsal part (extensor compartment) of the arm,
    ventral aspect

a

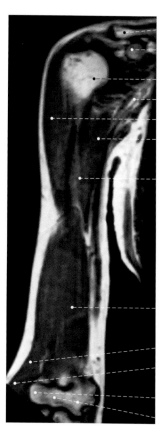

Clavicle

Coracoid process of scapula

Head of humerus

Axillary fossa

Deltoid muscle

Coracobrachialis muscle

Biceps brachii muscle

b

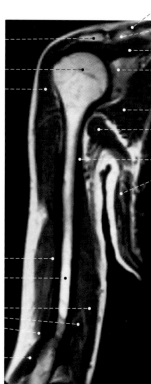

Acromion of scapula

Head of humerus

Deltoid muscle

Brachialis muscle

Brachioradialis muscle

Extensor carpi radialis
longus muscle

Capitulum of humerus

Trochlea of humerus

Clavicle

Trapezius muscle

Supraspinatus muscle

Scapula

Subscapularis muscle

Teres major muscle

Coracobrachialis muscle

Latissimus dorsi muscle

Brachialis muscle

Body of humerus

Triceps brachii muscle
Long head –
Medial head –
Lateral head –

Brachioradialis muscle

Capitulum of humerus

Olecranon of ulna

c

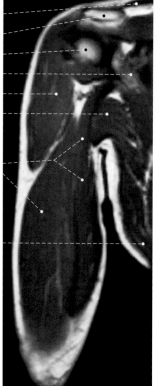

Trapezius muscle

Acromion of scapula

Head of humerus

Scapula

Deltoid muscle

Teres major muscle

Triceps brachii muscle
Long head –
Lateral head –

Latissimus dorsi muscle

149 Right arm (30%)

Coronal magnetic resonance images (MRI, T_1-weighted)
a through the ventral part (flexor compartment)
b through the middle part
c through the dorsal part (extensor compartment) of the arm,
ventral aspect

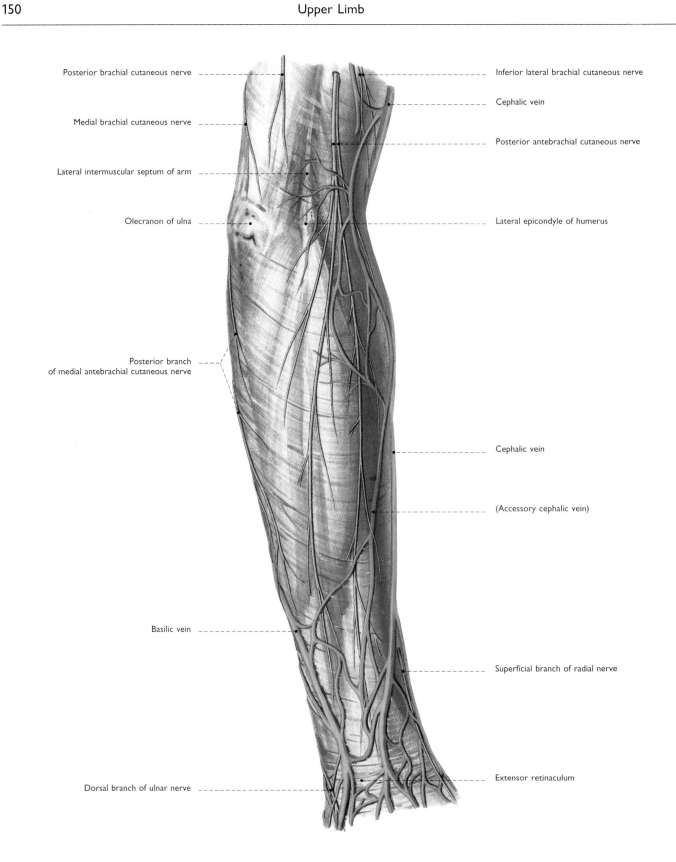

Posterior brachial cutaneous nerve

Medial brachial cutaneous nerve

Lateral intermuscular septum of arm

Olecranon of ulna

Posterior branch
of medial antebrachial cutaneous nerve

Basilic vein

Dorsal branch of ulnar nerve

Inferior lateral brachial cutaneous nerve

Cephalic vein

Posterior antebrachial cutaneous nerve

Lateral epicondyle of humerus

Cephalic vein

(Accessory cephalic vein)

Superficial branch of radial nerve

Extensor retinaculum

**150 Subcutaneous veins and nerves
of the posterior (extensor) region
of the right forearm** (50%)
Dorsolateral aspect

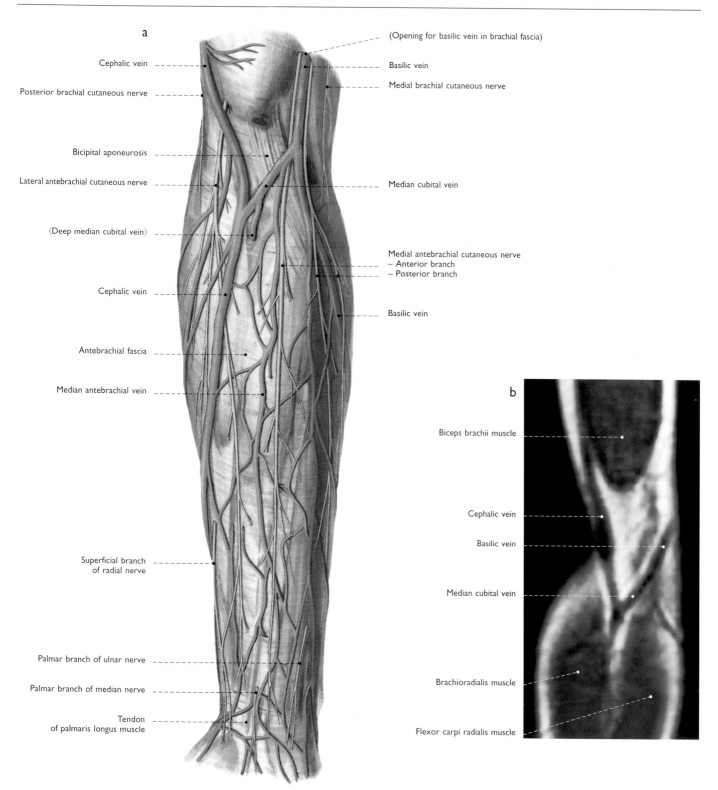

a

Cephalic vein

Posterior brachial cutaneous nerve

Bicipital aponeurosis

Lateral antebrachial cutaneous nerve

⟨Deep median cubital vein⟩

Cephalic vein

Antebrachial fascia

Median antebrachial vein

Superficial branch of radial nerve

Palmar branch of ulnar nerve

Palmar branch of median nerve

Tendon of palmaris longus muscle

(Opening for basilic vein in brachial fascia)

Basilic vein

Medial brachial cutaneous nerve

Median cubital vein

Medial antebrachial cutaneous nerve
– Anterior branch
– Posterior branch

Basilic vein

b

Biceps brachii muscle

Cephalic vein

Basilic vein

Median cubital vein

Brachioradialis muscle

Flexor carpi radialis muscle

151 Subcutaneous veins and nerves
of the anterior region of elbow
and the anterior (flexor) region
of the right forearm (50%)
a   Ventral aspect
b   Coronal magnetic resonance image (MRI, T_1-weighted)

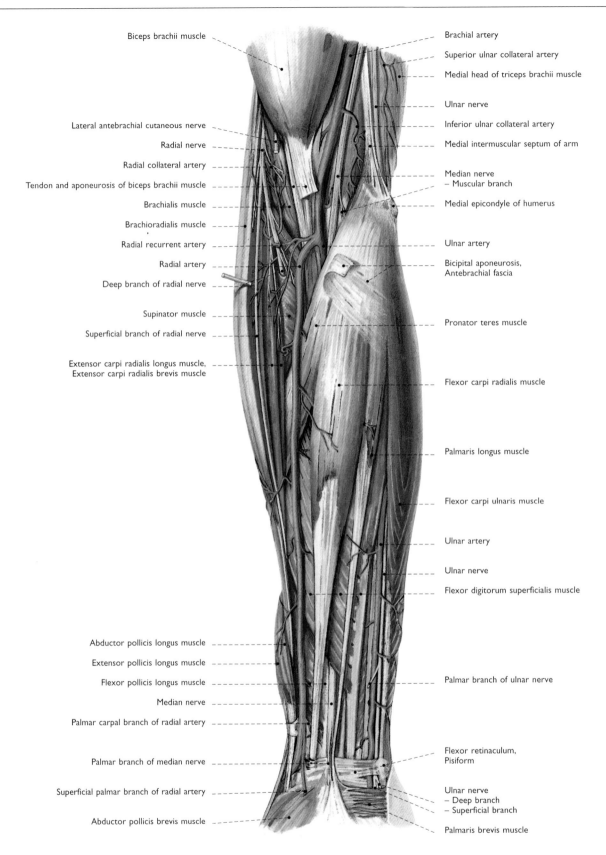

Biceps brachii muscle

Lateral antebrachial cutaneous nerve

Radial nerve

Radial collateral artery

Tendon and aponeurosis of biceps brachii muscle

Brachialis muscle

Brachioradialis muscle

Radial recurrent artery

Radial artery

Deep branch of radial nerve

Supinator muscle

Superficial branch of radial nerve

Extensor carpi radialis longus muscle,
Extensor carpi radialis brevis muscle

Abductor pollicis longus muscle

Extensor pollicis longus muscle

Flexor pollicis longus muscle

Median nerve

Palmar carpal branch of radial artery

Palmar branch of median nerve

Superficial palmar branch of radial artery

Abductor pollicis brevis muscle

Brachial artery

Superior ulnar collateral artery

Medial head of triceps brachii muscle

Ulnar nerve

Inferior ulnar collateral artery

Medial intermuscular septum of arm

Median nerve
– Muscular branch

Medial epicondyle of humerus

Ulnar artery

Bicipital aponeurosis,
Antebrachial fascia

Pronator teres muscle

Flexor carpi radialis muscle

Palmaris longus muscle

Flexor carpi ulnaris muscle

Ulnar artery

Ulnar nerve

Flexor digitorum superficialis muscle

Palmar branch of ulnar nerve

Flexor retinaculum,
Pisiform

Ulnar nerve
– Deep branch
– Superficial branch

Palmaris brevis muscle

152 Arteries and nerves of the right forearm (50%)
Ventral aspect

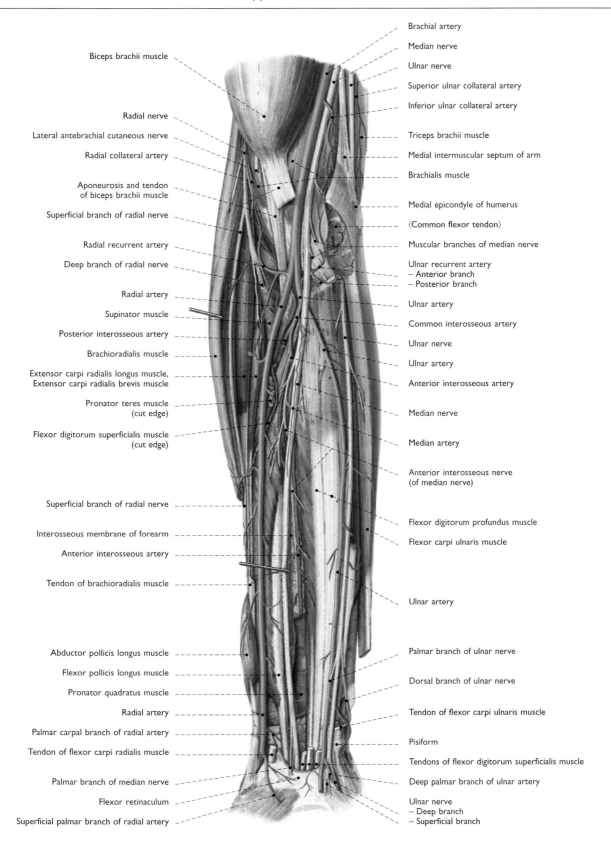

Biceps brachii muscle

Radial nerve

Lateral antebrachial cutaneous nerve

Radial collateral artery

Aponeurosis and tendon
of biceps brachii muscle

Superficial branch of radial nerve

Radial recurrent artery

Deep branch of radial nerve

Radial artery

Supinator muscle

Posterior interosseous artery

Brachioradialis muscle

Extensor carpi radialis longus muscle,
Extensor carpi radialis brevis muscle

Pronator teres muscle
(cut edge)

Flexor digitorum superficialis muscle
(cut edge)

Superficial branch of radial nerve

Interosseous membrane of forearm

Anterior interosseous artery

Tendon of brachioradialis muscle

Abductor pollicis longus muscle

Flexor pollicis longus muscle

Pronator quadratus muscle

Radial artery

Palmar carpal branch of radial artery

Tendon of flexor carpi radialis muscle

Palmar branch of median nerve

Flexor retinaculum

Superficial palmar branch of radial artery

Brachial artery

Median nerve

Ulnar nerve

Superior ulnar collateral artery

Inferior ulnar collateral artery

Triceps brachii muscle

Medial intermuscular septum of arm

Brachialis muscle

Medial epicondyle of humerus

⟨Common flexor tendon⟩

Muscular branches of median nerve

Ulnar recurrent artery
– Anterior branch
– Posterior branch

Ulnar artery

Common interosseous artery

Ulnar nerve

Ulnar artery

Anterior interosseous artery

Median nerve

Median artery

Anterior interosseous nerve
(of median nerve)

Flexor digitorum profundus muscle

Flexor carpi ulnaris muscle

Ulnar artery

Palmar branch of ulnar nerve

Dorsal branch of ulnar nerve

Tendon of flexor carpi ulnaris muscle

Pisiform

Tendons of flexor digitorum superficialis muscle

Deep palmar branch of ulnar artery

Ulnar nerve
– Deep branch
– Superficial branch

153 Arteries and nerves of the right forearm (50%)
The superficial muscles were removed.
Ventral aspect

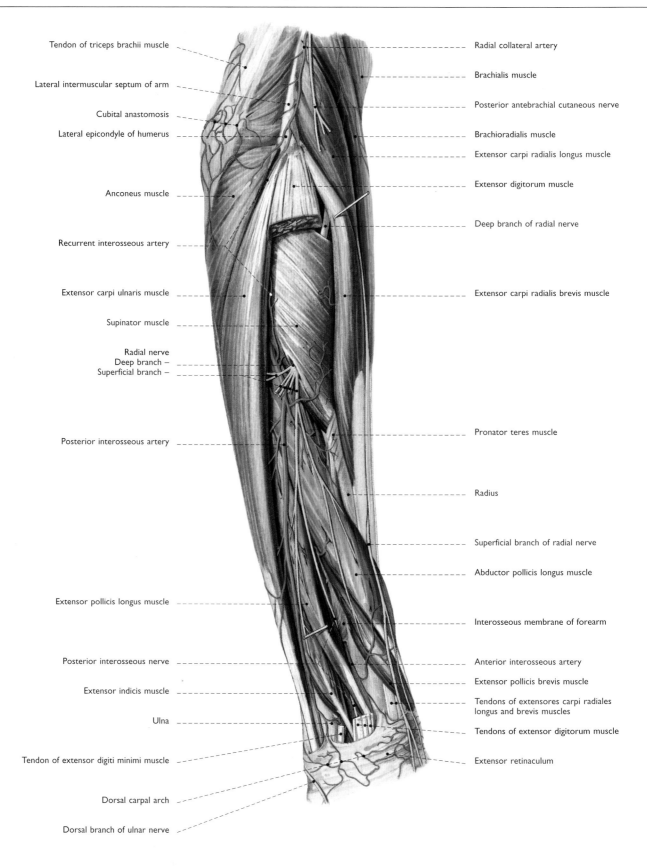

Tendon of triceps brachii muscle

Lateral intermuscular septum of arm

Cubital anastomosis

Lateral epicondyle of humerus

Anconeus muscle

Recurrent interosseous artery

Extensor carpi ulnaris muscle

Supinator muscle

Radial nerve
Deep branch —
Superficial branch —

Posterior interosseous artery

Extensor pollicis longus muscle

Posterior interosseous nerve

Extensor indicis muscle

Ulna

Tendon of extensor digiti minimi muscle

Dorsal carpal arch

Dorsal branch of ulnar nerve

Radial collateral artery

Brachialis muscle

Posterior antebrachial cutaneous nerve

Brachioradialis muscle

Extensor carpi radialis longus muscle

Extensor digitorum muscle

Deep branch of radial nerve

Extensor carpi radialis brevis muscle

Pronator teres muscle

Radius

Superficial branch of radial nerve

Abductor pollicis longus muscle

Interosseous membrane of forearm

Anterior interosseous artery

Extensor pollicis brevis muscle

Tendons of extensores carpi radiales
longus and brevis muscles

Tendons of extensor digitorum muscle

Extensor retinaculum

154 Arteries and nerves of the right forearm (50%)
The superficial muscles were partially removed.
Dorsolateral aspect

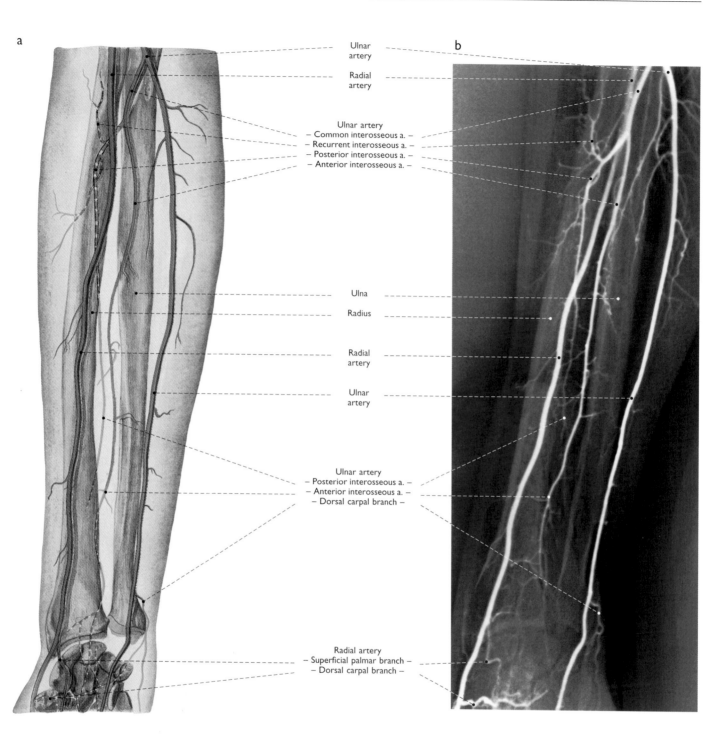

a

Ulnar
artery

Radial
artery

Ulnar artery
– Common interosseous a. –
– Recurrent interosseous a. –
– Posterior interosseous a. –
– Anterior interosseous a. –

b

Ulna

Radius

Radial
artery

Ulnar
artery

Ulnar artery
– Posterior interosseous a. –
– Anterior interosseous a. –
– Dorsal carpal branch –

Radial artery
– Superficial palmar branch –
– Dorsal carpal branch –

155 Arteries of the right forearm (60%)
Ventral aspect
a Schematic representation
b Arteriogram

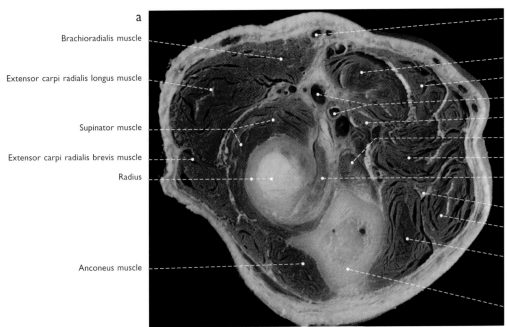

a

Brachioradialis muscle

Extensor carpi radialis longus muscle

Supinator muscle

Extensor carpi radialis brevis muscle

Radius

Anconeus muscle

Cephalic vein

Pronator teres muscle

Flexor carpi radialis muscle

Brachial vein and artery

Median nerve

Brachialis muscle

Flexor digitorum superficialis muscle

Tendon of biceps brachii muscle

Ulnar nerve

Flexor carpi ulnaris muscle

Flexor digitorum profundus muscle

Ulna

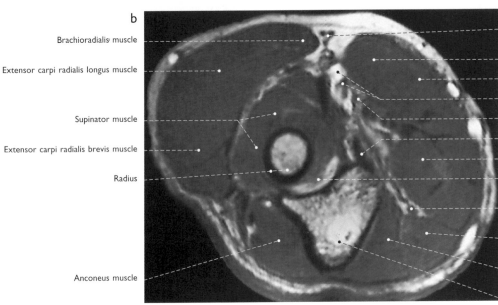

b

Brachioradialis muscle

Extensor carpi radialis longus muscle

Supinator muscle

Extensor carpi radialis brevis muscle

Radius

Anconeus muscle

Cephalic vein

Pronator teres muscle

Flexor carpi radialis muscle

Brachial vein and artery

Median nerve

Brachialis muscle

Flexor digitorum superficialis muscle

Tendon of biceps brachii muscle

Ulnar nerve

Flexor carpi ulnaris muscle

Flexor digitorum profundus muscle

Ulna

156 Right forearm (110%)

Transverse sections through the proximal forearm
just below the elbow joint, distal aspect
a Anatomical section
b Magnetic resonance image (MRI, T$_1$-weighted)

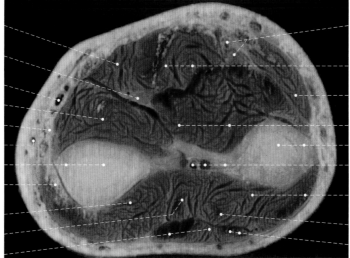

a

Flexor carpi radialis muscle

Median nerve

Radial artery

Flexor pollicis longus muscle

Superficial branch of radial nerve

Cephalic vein

Radius

Extensores carpi radiales
longus and brevis muscles

Extensor pollicis brevis muscle

Abductor pollicis longus muscle

Extensor digitorum muscle,
Extensor digiti minimi muscle

Ulnar artery and nerve

Flexor digitorum superficialis muscle

Flexor carpi ulnaris muscle

Flexor digitorum profundus muscle

Ulna

Anterior interosseous artery and vein,
Interosseous membrane of forearm

Extensor indicis muscle,
Extensor carpi ulnaris muscle

Extensor pollicis longus muscle

Deep branch of radial nerve,
Posterior interosseous artery

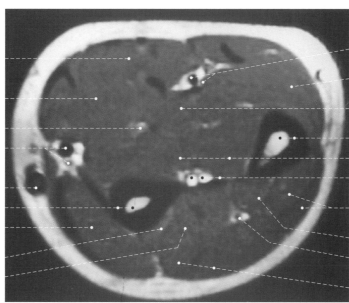

b

Flexor carpi radialis muscle

Flexor pollicis longus muscle

Median nerve

Radial artery,
Superficial branch of radial nerve

Cephalic vein

Radius

Extensores carpi radiales
longus and brevis muscles

Extensor pollicis brevis muscle

Abductor pollicis longus muscle

Ulnar artery and nerve

Flexor carpi ulnaris muscle

Flexor digitorum superficialis muscle

Ulna

Flexor digitorum profundus muscle

Anterior interosseous artery and vein,
Interosseous membrane of forearm

Extensor indicis muscle,
Extensor carpi ulnaris muscle

Extensor pollicis longus muscle

Deep branch of radial nerve,
Posterior interosseous artery

Extensor digitorum muscle,
Extensor digiti minimi muscle

157 Right forearm (110%)

Transverse sections through the proximal third
of the forearm in supinated position, distal aspect
a Anatomical section
b Magnetic resonance image (MRI, T$_1$-weighted)

a

Tendon
of flexor carpi radialis muscle

Median nerve

Flexor pollicis longus muscle

Radial artery

Tendon
of extensor carpi radialis longus muscle

Radius

Interosseous membrane of forearm

Abductor pollicis longus muscle

Extensor pollicis brevis muscle

Flexor digitorum superficialis muscle

Ulnar artery and nerve

Flexor carpi ulnaris muscle

Flexor digitorum profundus muscle

Pronator quadratus muscle

Ulna

Extensor indicis muscle

Extensor pollicis longus muscle,
Extensor carpi ulnaris muscle

Extensor digitorum muscle,
Extensor digiti minimi muscle

b

Tendon
of flexor carpi radialis muscle

Median nerve

Radial artery

Flexor pollicis longus muscle

Tendon
of extensor carpi radialis longus muscle

Radius

Extensor pollicis longus muscle

Abductor pollicis longus muscle,
Extensor pollicis brevis muscle

Flexor digitorum superficialis muscle

Ulnar artery and nerve

Flexor carpi ulnaris muscle

Flexor digitorum profundus muscle

Pronator quadratus muscle

Ulna

Extensor carpi ulnaris muscle

Extensor indicis muscle

Extensor digitorum muscle,
Extensor digiti minimi muscle

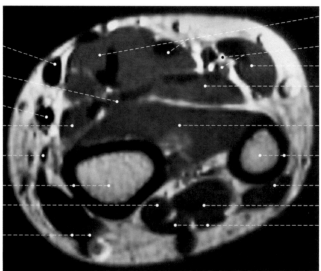

158 Right forearm (120%)

Transverse sections through the distal third
of the forearm in supinated position, distal aspect

a   Anatomical section

b   Magnetic resonance image (MRI, T$_1$-weighted)

a

Tendons
of flexor carpi radialis and
flexor pollicis longus muscles

Radial artery

Tendons
of abductor pollicis longus and
extensor pollicis brevis muscles

Scaphoid

Radial styloid process

Tendon
of extensor carpi radialis longus muscle

Tendon
of extensor carpi radialis brevis muscle

Tendons
of extensor indicis and
extensor digitorum muscles

Median nerve

Tendons
of flexor digitorum superficialis muscle

Ulnar nerve and artery

Tendons
of flexor digitorum profundus muscle

Lunate

Triquetrum

Tendon
of extensor carpi ulnaris muscle

Tendon
of extensor digiti minimi muscle

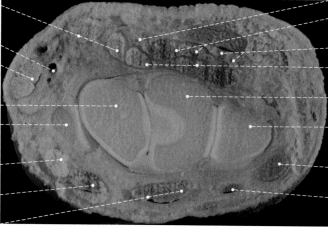

b

Tendons
of flexor carpi radialis and
flexor pollicis longus muscles

Radial artery

Tendons
of abductor pollicis longus and
extensor pollicis brevis muscles

Scaphoid

Radial styloid process

Tendon
of extensor carpi radialis longus muscle

Tendon
of extensor carpi radialis brevis muscle

Tendons
of extensor indicis and
extensor digitorum muscles

Median nerve

Tendons
of flexor digitorum superficialis muscle

Ulnar nerve and artery

Tendons
of flexor digitorum profundus muscle

Lunate

Triquetrum

Tendon
of extensor carpi ulnaris muscle

Tendon
of extensor digiti minimi muscle

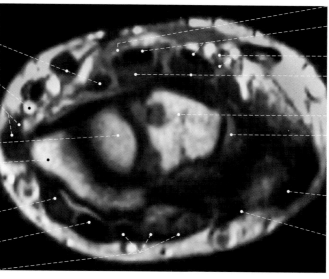

159   Right forearm (120%)

Transverse sections through the distal forearm
at the level of the wrist joint. Forearm and hand
in supinated position, distal aspect

a   Anatomical section
b   Magnetic resonance image (MRI, T$_1$-weighted)

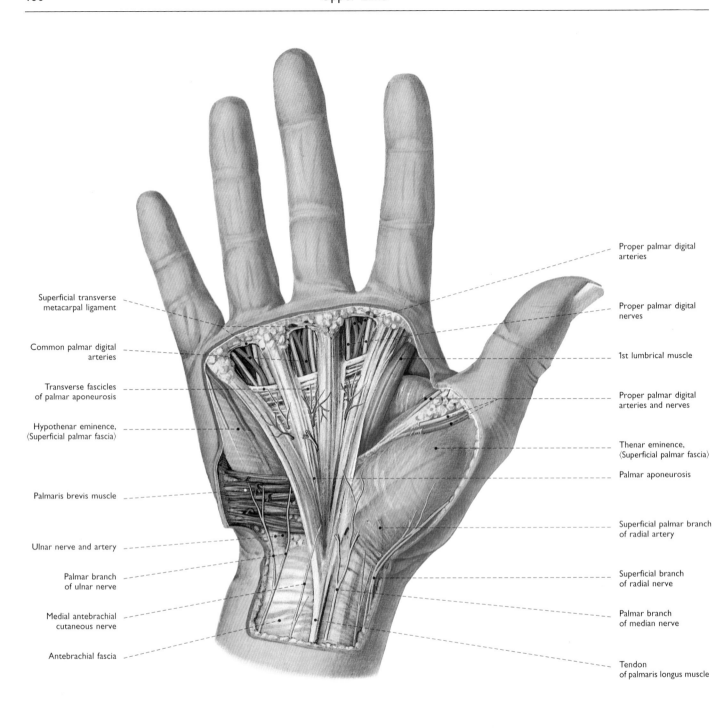

Superficial transverse
metacarpal ligament

Common palmar digital
arteries

Transverse fascicles
of palmar aponeurosis

Hypothenar eminence,
(Superficial palmar fascia)

Palmaris brevis muscle

Ulnar nerve and artery

Palmar branch
of ulnar nerve

Medial antebrachial
cutaneous nerve

Antebrachial fascia

Proper palmar digital
arteries

Proper palmar digital
nerves

1st lumbrical muscle

Proper palmar digital
arteries and nerves

Thenar eminence,
(Superficial palmar fascia)

Palmar aponeurosis

Superficial palmar branch
of radial artery

Superficial branch
of radial nerve

Palmar branch
of median nerve

Tendon
of palmaris longus muscle

**160 Arteries and nerves
of the palm of the right hand** (75%)
Palmar aspect

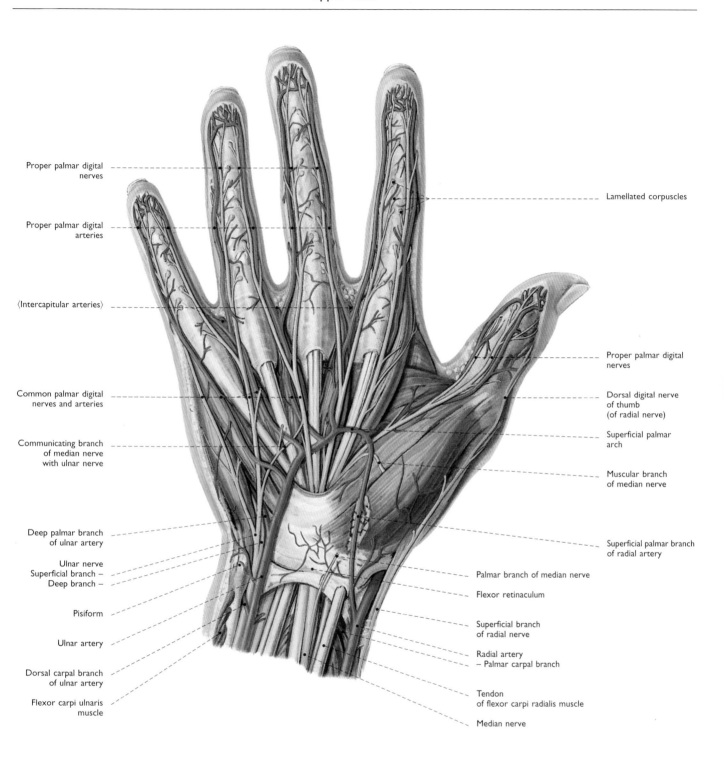

Proper palmar digital nerves

Proper palmar digital arteries

⟨Intercapitular arteries⟩

Common palmar digital nerves and arteries

Communicating branch of median nerve with ulnar nerve

Deep palmar branch of ulnar artery

Ulnar nerve
Superficial branch –
Deep branch –

Pisiform

Ulnar artery

Dorsal carpal branch of ulnar artery

Flexor carpi ulnaris muscle

Lamellated corpuscles

Proper palmar digital nerves

Dorsal digital nerve of thumb (of radial nerve)

Superficial palmar arch

Muscular branch of median nerve

Superficial palmar branch of radial artery

Palmar branch of median nerve

Flexor retinaculum

Superficial branch of radial nerve

Radial artery
– Palmar carpal branch

Tendon of flexor carpi radialis muscle

Median nerve

161 Arteries and nerves of the palm of the right hand (75%)
The palmar aponeurosis was removed.
Palmar aspect

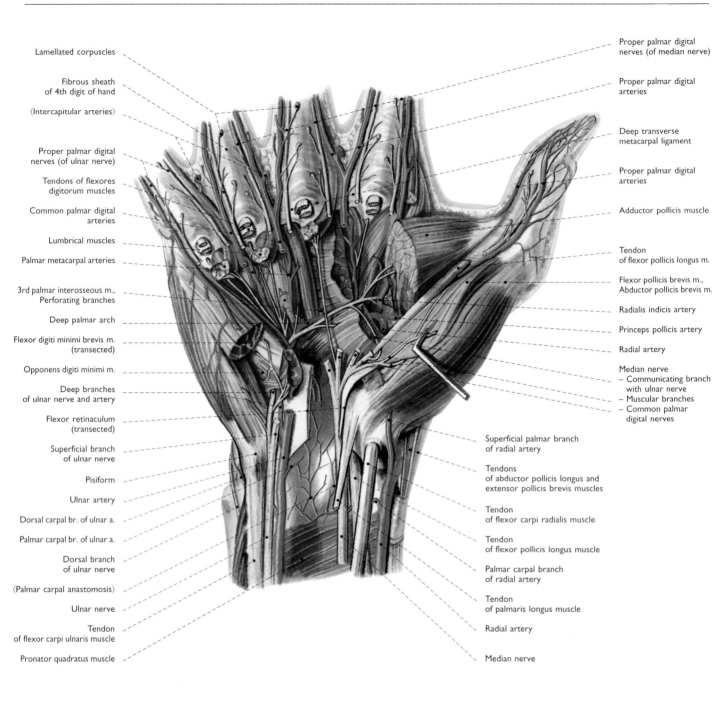

Lamellated corpuscles

Fibrous sheath
of 4th digit of hand

⟨Intercapitular arteries⟩

Proper palmar digital
nerves (of ulnar nerve)

Tendons of flexores
digitorum muscles

Common palmar digital
arteries

Lumbrical muscles

Palmar metacarpal arteries

3rd palmar interosseous m.,
Perforating branches

Deep palmar arch

Flexor digiti minimi brevis m.
(transected)

Opponens digiti minimi m.

Deep branches
of ulnar nerve and artery

Flexor retinaculum
(transected)

Superficial branch
of ulnar nerve

Pisiform

Ulnar artery

Dorsal carpal br. of ulnar a.

Palmar carpal br. of ulnar a.

Dorsal branch
of ulnar nerve

⟨Palmar carpal anastomosis⟩

Ulnar nerve

Tendon
of flexor carpi ulnaris muscle

Pronator quadratus muscle

Proper palmar digital
nerves (of median nerve)

Proper palmar digital
arteries

Deep transverse
metacarpal ligament

Proper palmar digital
arteries

Adductor pollicis muscle

Tendon
of flexor pollicis longus m.

Flexor pollicis brevis m.,
Abductor pollicis brevis m.

Radialis indicis artery

Princeps pollicis artery

Radial artery

Median nerve
– Communicating branch
  with ulnar nerve
– Muscular branches
– Common palmar
  digital nerves

Superficial palmar branch
of radial artery

Tendons
of abductor pollicis longus and
extensor pollicis brevis muscles

Tendon
of flexor carpi radialis muscle

Tendon
of flexor pollicis longus muscle

Palmar carpal branch
of radial artery

Tendon
of palmaris longus muscle

Radial artery

Median nerve

**162 Arteries and nerves
of the palm of the right hand** (75%)
The palmar aponeurosis and the flexor muscles
of the fingers were removed. Palmar aspect

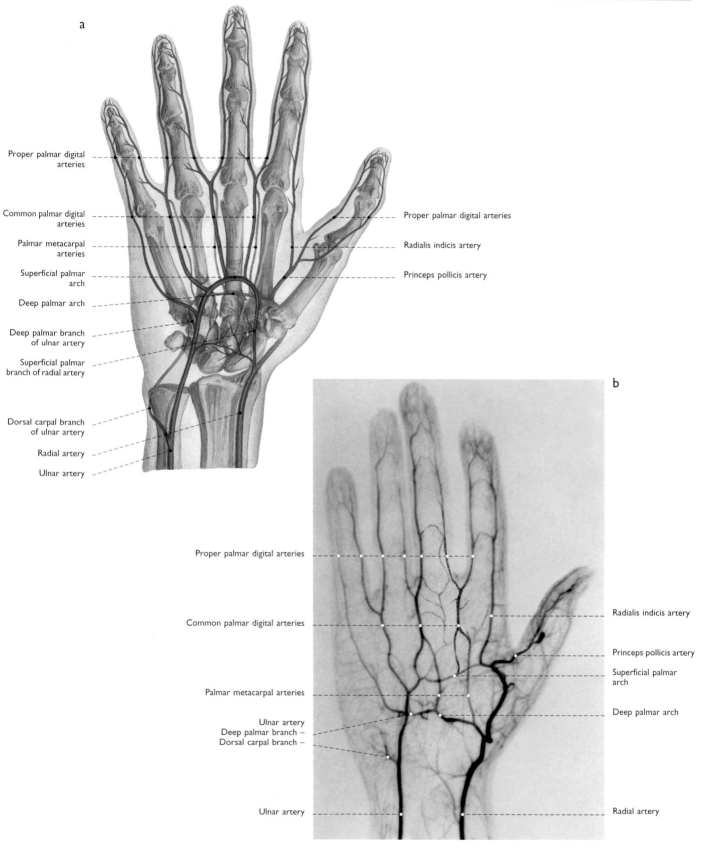

a

Proper palmar digital arteries

Common palmar digital arteries

Palmar metacarpal arteries

Superficial palmar arch

Deep palmar arch

Deep palmar branch of ulnar artery

Superficial palmar branch of radial artery

Dorsal carpal branch of ulnar artery

Radial artery

Ulnar artery

Proper palmar digital arteries

Radialis indicis artery

Princeps pollicis artery

b

Proper palmar digital arteries

Common palmar digital arteries

Palmar metacarpal arteries

Ulnar artery
Deep palmar branch –
Dorsal carpal branch –

Ulnar artery

Radialis indicis artery

Princeps pollicis artery

Superficial palmar arch

Deep palmar arch

Radial artery

163 Arteries of the right hand (50%)

Palmar aspect
a Schematic representation
b Arteriogram

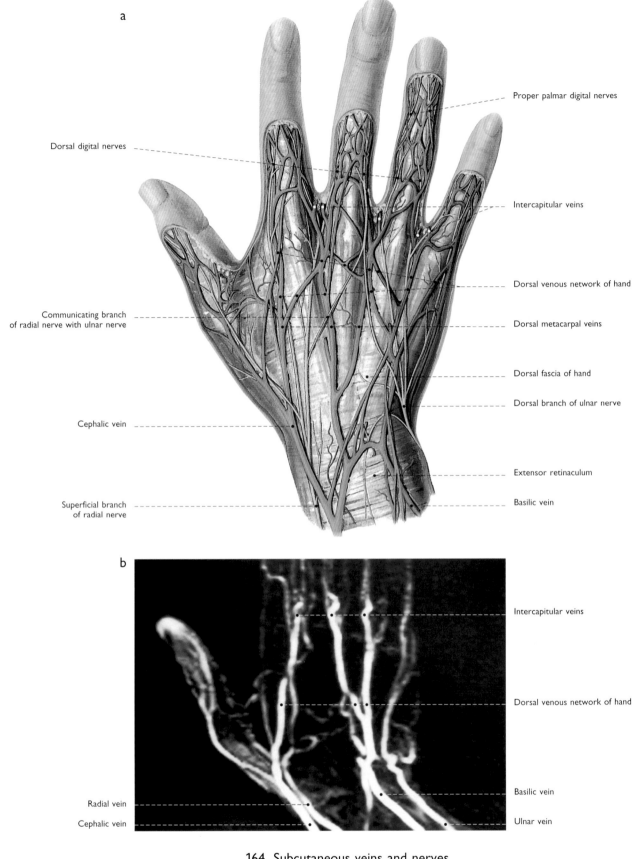

a

Proper palmar digital nerves

Dorsal digital nerves

Intercapitular veins

Dorsal venous network of hand

Communicating branch
of radial nerve with ulnar nerve

Dorsal metacarpal veins

Dorsal fascia of hand

Dorsal branch of ulnar nerve

Cephalic vein

Extensor retinaculum

Superficial branch
of radial nerve

Basilic vein

b

Intercapitular veins

Dorsal venous network of hand

Basilic vein

Radial vein

Cephalic vein

Ulnar vein

**164 Subcutaneous veins and nerves
of the dorsum of the right hand** (60%)
a   Dorsal aspect
b   Magnetic resonance angiogram (MRA)

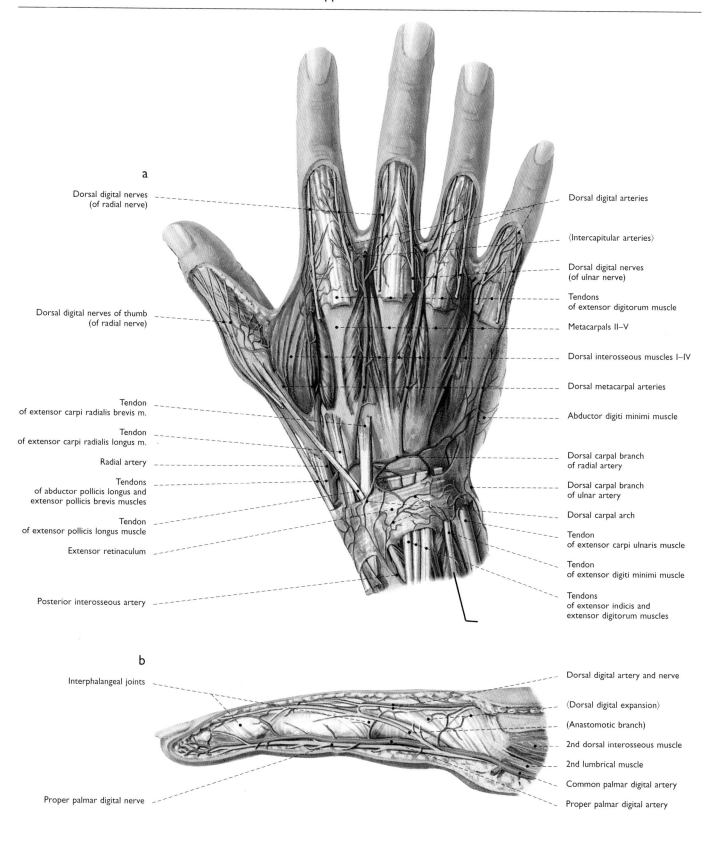

a

Dorsal digital nerves
(of radial nerve)

Dorsal digital nerves of thumb
(of radial nerve)

Tendon
of extensor carpi radialis brevis m.

Tendon
of extensor carpi radialis longus m.

Radial artery

Tendons
of abductor pollicis longus and
extensor pollicis brevis muscles

Tendon
of extensor pollicis longus muscle

Extensor retinaculum

Posterior interosseous artery

Dorsal digital arteries

〈Intercapitular arteries〉

Dorsal digital nerves
(of ulnar nerve)

Tendons
of extensor digitorum muscle

Metacarpals II–V

Dorsal interosseous muscles I–IV

Dorsal metacarpal arteries

Abductor digiti minimi muscle

Dorsal carpal branch
of radial artery

Dorsal carpal branch
of ulnar artery

Dorsal carpal arch

Tendon
of extensor carpi ulnaris muscle

Tendon
of extensor digiti minimi muscle

Tendons
of extensor indicis and
extensor digitorum muscles

b

Interphalangeal joints

Proper palmar digital nerve

Dorsal digital artery and nerve

〈Dorsal digital expansion〉

(Anastomotic branch)

2nd dorsal interosseous muscle

2nd lumbrical muscle

Common palmar digital artery

Proper palmar digital artery

**165 Arteries and nerves of the dorsum
of the right hand and the fingers**

a The extensor tendons to the fingers were removed.
Dorsal aspect of the dorsum of hand (60%)

b Middle finger (90%), radial aspect

a

Superficial head
of flexor pollicis brevis m.

Abductor pollicis brevis m.

Opponens pollicis muscle

Tendon
of flexor pollicis longus m.

1st metacarpal bone

Adductor pollicis muscle

Princeps pollicis artery

1st dorsal interosseous
muscle

2nd metacarpal bone

2nd dorsal interosseous
muscle

Palmar aponeurosis

Palmaris brevis muscle

Flexor retinaculum

Flexor digiti minimi brevis m

Opponens digiti minimi m.

Abductor digiti minimi
muscle

Carpal tunnel with
tendons of flexores
digitorum superficialis
and profundus muscles

5th metacarpal bone

4th dorsal interosseous
muscle

b

Superficial head
of flexor pollicis brevis m.

Opponens pollicis muscle

Abductor pollicis brevis m.

Tendon
of flexor pollicis longus m.

Adductor pollicis muscle

1st metacarpal bone

Princeps pollicis artery

1st dorsal interosseous m.

2nd metacarpal bone

Palmar aponeurosis

Flexor digiti minimi brevis m

Opponens digiti minimi m.

Abductor digiti minimi m.

Carpal tunnel with
tendons of flexores
digitorum superficialis
and profundus muscles

4th and 5th metacarpals

2nd and 3rd dorsal
interosseous muscles

166 Right hand (150%)

Transverse sections through the proximal metacarpus,
hand in full supination, distal aspect

a Anatomical section
b Magnetic resonance image (MRI, T$_1$-weighted)

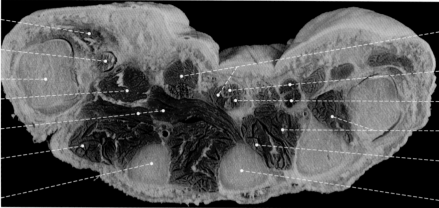

a

Superficial head
of flexor pollicis brevis muscle

Tendon
of flexor pollicis longus muscle

1st metacarpal bone

Deep head
of flexor pollicis brevis muscle

Adductor pollicis muscle

1st dorsal interosseous muscle

2nd metacarpal bone

1st and 2nd lumbrical muscles

Tendons (II and III)
of flexor digitorum superficialis m.

Tendons (II and III)
of flexor digitorum profundus m.

2nd and 3rd palmar interosseous
muscles

3rd dorsal interosseous muscle

3rd metacarpal bone

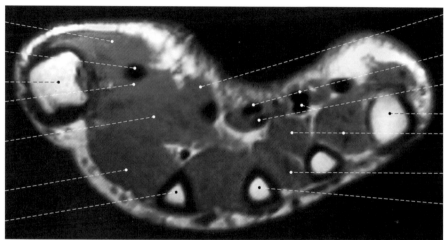

b

Superficial head
of flexor pollicis brevis muscle

Tendon
of flexor pollicis longus muscle

1st metacarpal bone

Deep head
of flexor pollicis brevis muscle

Adductor pollicis muscle

1st dorsal interosseous muscle

2nd metacarpal bone

1st lumbrical muscle

Tendons (II and III)
of flexor digitorum superficialis m.

Tendons (II and III)
of flexor digitorum profundus m.

5th metacarpal bone

2nd and 3rd palmar interosseous
muscles

3rd dorsal interosseous muscle

3rd metacarpal bone

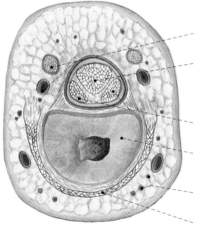

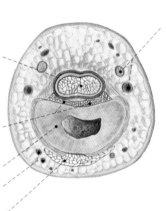

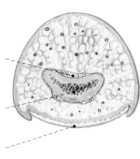

c   d   e

Proper palmar digital
nerve and artery

Tendon
of flexor digitorum
profundus muscle

Flexor digitorum
superficialis muscle
– Tendon
Insertion of tendon –

Proximal phalanx

Middle phalanx

Dorsal digital
artery and nerve

⟨Dorsal digital
expansion⟩

Proper palmar digital
nerve and artery

Insertion of tendon
of flexor digitorum
profundus muscle

Distal phalanx

Nail

167 Right hand

Hand in full supination

a, b Transverse sections through the middle part
      of the metacarpus (130%), distal aspect
   a Anatomical section
   b Magnetic resonance image (MRI, T$_1$-weighted)
c–e Transverse sections through
   c the proximal phalanx
   d the middle phalanx
   e the distal phalanx
      of the middle finger (230%), distal aspect

Lower Limb

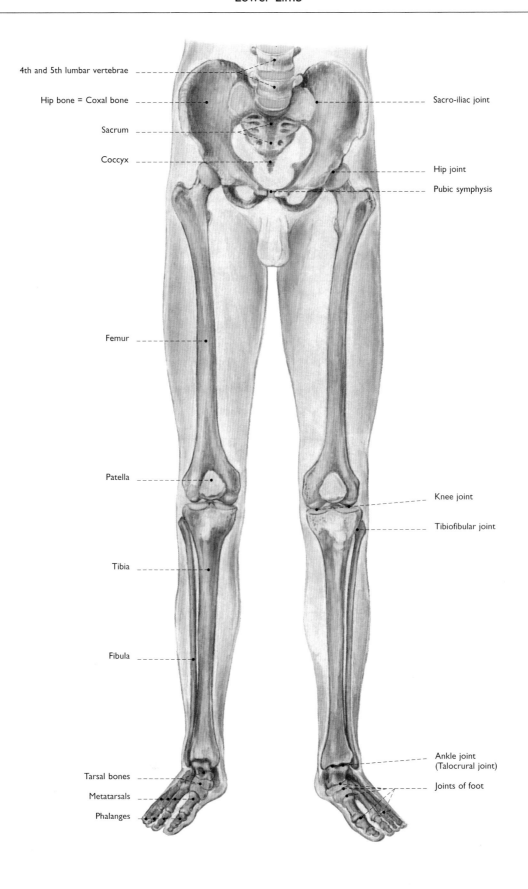

4th and 5th lumbar vertebrae

Hip bone = Coxal bone

Sacrum

Coccyx

Sacro-iliac joint

Hip joint

Pubic symphysis

Femur

Patella

Knee joint

Tibiofibular joint

Tibia

Fibula

Ankle joint
(Talocrural joint)

Tarsal bones

Joints of foot

Metatarsals

Phalanges

170 Lower limb (20%)
Ventral aspect

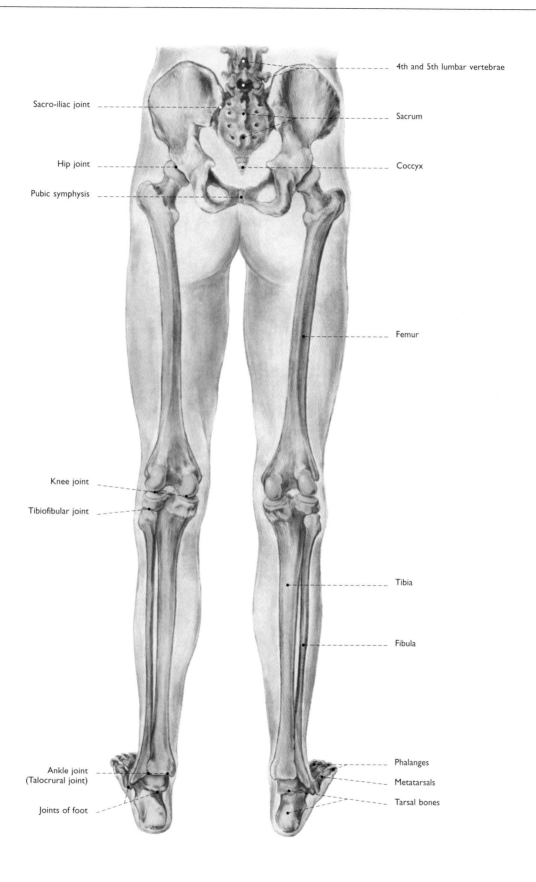

4th and 5th lumbar vertebrae

Sacro-iliac joint

Sacrum

Hip joint

Coccyx

Pubic symphysis

Femur

Knee joint

Tibiofibular joint

Tibia

Fibula

Phalanges

Ankle joint
(Talocrural joint)

Metatarsals

Tarsal bones

Joints of foot

171 Lower limb (20%)
Dorsal aspect

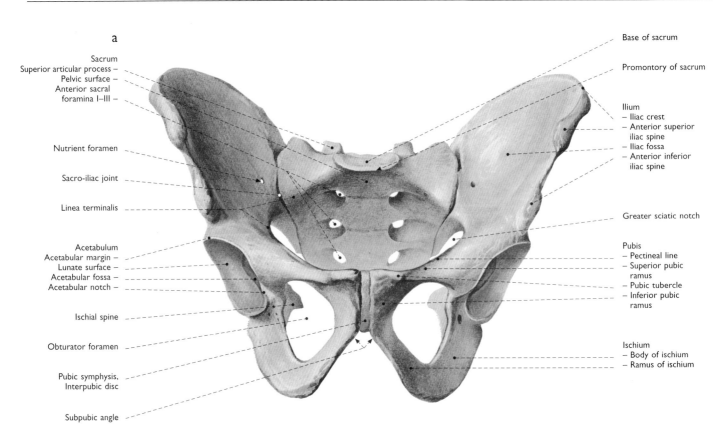

a

Sacrum
Superior articular process –
Pelvic surface –
Anterior sacral
foramina I–III –

Nutrient foramen

Sacro-iliac joint

Linea terminalis

Acetabulum
Acetabular margin –
Lunate surface –
Acetabular fossa –
Acetabular notch –

Ischial spine

Obturator foramen

Pubic symphysis,
Interpubic disc

Subpubic angle

Base of sacrum

Promontory of sacrum

Ilium
– Iliac crest
– Anterior superior
iliac spine
– Iliac fossa
– Anterior inferior
iliac spine

Greater sciatic notch

Pubis
– Pectineal line
– Superior pubic
ramus
– Pubic tubercle
– Inferior pubic
ramus

Ischium
– Body of ischium
– Ramus of ischium

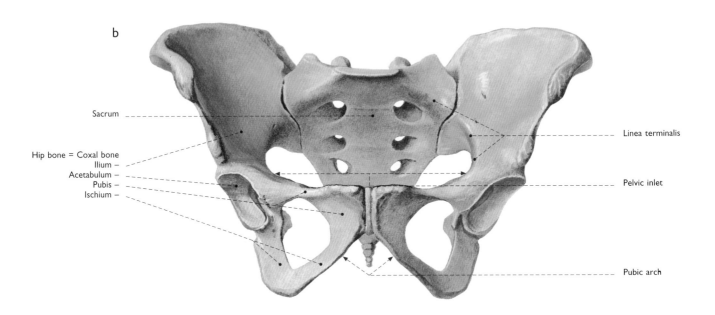

b

Sacrum

Hip bone = Coxal bone
Ilium –
Acetabulum –
Pubis –
Ischium –

Linea terminalis

Pelvic inlet

Pubic arch

172 Pelvic girdle (40%)
Ventral aspect
a Male pelvis
b Female pelvis

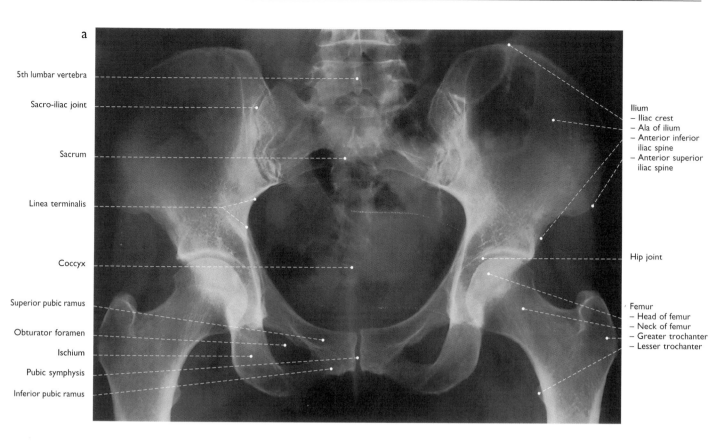

a

5th lumbar vertebra

Sacro-iliac joint

Sacrum

Linea terminalis

Coccyx

Superior pubic ramus

Obturator foramen

Ischium

Pubic symphysis

Inferior pubic ramus

Ilium
– Iliac crest
– Ala of ilium
– Anterior inferior iliac spine
– Anterior superior iliac spine

Hip joint

Femur
– Head of femur
– Neck of femur
– Greater trochanter
– Lesser trochanter

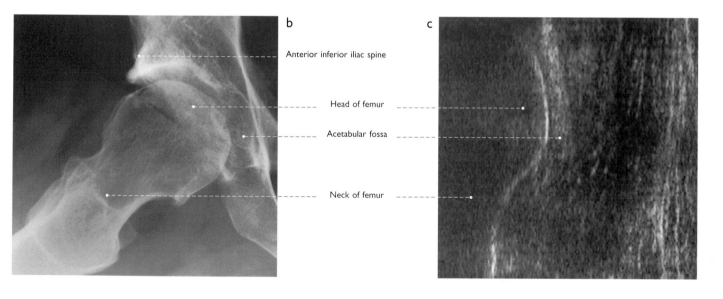

b

Anterior inferior iliac spine

Head of femur

Acetabular fossa

Neck of femur

c

173 Pelvic girdle and proximal
      thigh bones (= femora)
   a Anteroposterior radiograph (50%)
   b Anteroposterior radiograph of the right hip joint,
      the femur in abduction (65%)
   c Ultrasonic image of the right hip joint

a

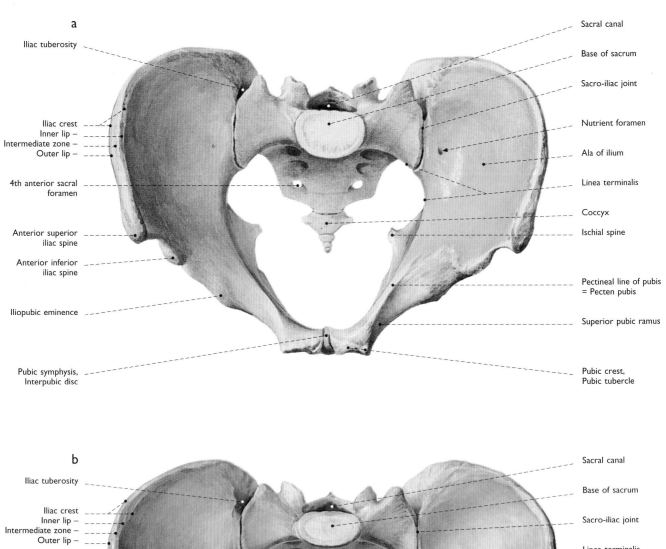

Iliac tuberosity

Iliac crest
Inner lip –
Intermediate zone –
Outer lip –

4th anterior sacral
foramen

Anterior superior
iliac spine

Anterior inferior
iliac spine

Iliopubic eminence

Pubic symphysis,
Interpubic disc

Sacral canal

Base of sacrum

Sacro-iliac joint

Nutrient foramen

Ala of ilium

Linea terminalis

Coccyx

Ischial spine

Pectineal line of pubis
= Pecten pubis

Superior pubic ramus

Pubic crest,
Pubic tubercle

b

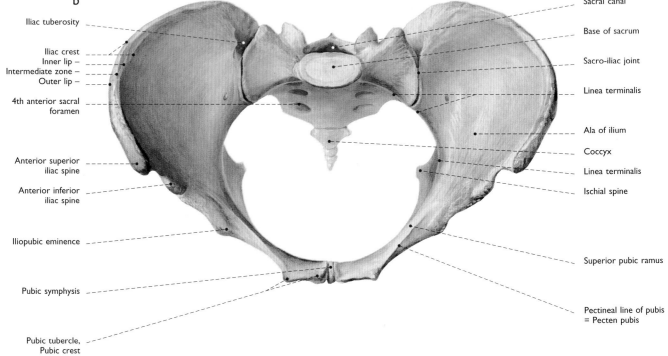

Iliac tuberosity

Iliac crest
Inner lip –
Intermediate zone –
Outer lip –

4th anterior sacral
foramen

Anterior superior
iliac spine

Anterior inferior
iliac spine

Iliopubic eminence

Pubic symphysis

Pubic tubercle,
Pubic crest

Sacral canal

Base of sacrum

Sacro-iliac joint

Linea terminalis

Ala of ilium

Coccyx

Linea terminalis

Ischial spine

Superior pubic ramus

Pectineal line of pubis
= Pecten pubis

174 Pelvic girdle (40 %)
Superior aspect
a Male pelvis
b Female pelvis

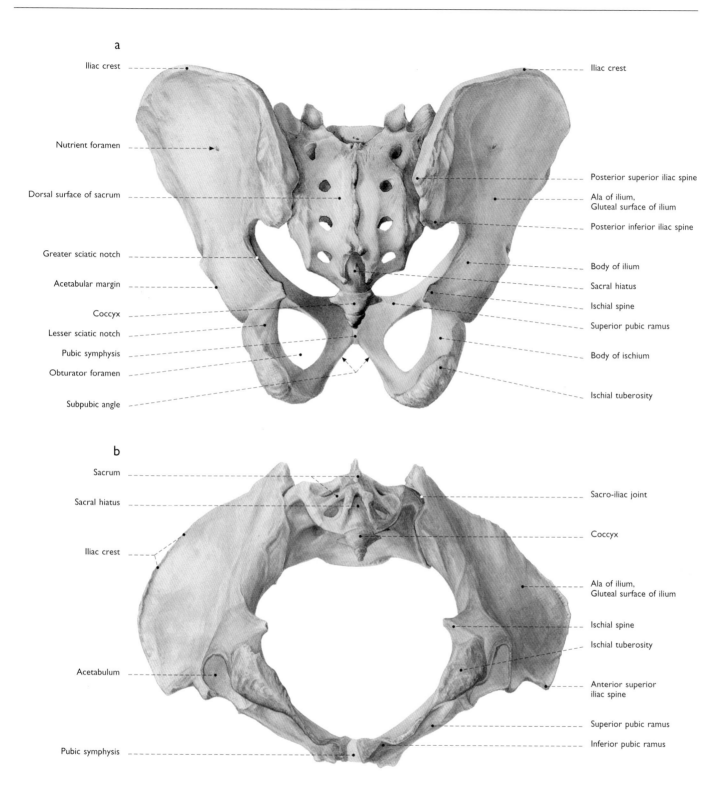

a

Iliac crest

Nutrient foramen

Dorsal surface of sacrum

Greater sciatic notch

Acetabular margin

Coccyx

Lesser sciatic notch

Pubic symphysis

Obturator foramen

Subpubic angle

Iliac crest

Posterior superior iliac spine

Ala of ilium,
Gluteal surface of ilium

Posterior inferior iliac spine

Body of ilium

Sacral hiatus

Ischial spine

Superior pubic ramus

Body of ischium

Ischial tuberosity

b

Sacrum

Sacral hiatus

Iliac crest

Acetabulum

Pubic symphysis

Sacro-iliac joint

Coccyx

Ala of ilium,
Gluteal surface of ilium

Ischial spine

Ischial tuberosity

Anterior superior
iliac spine

Superior pubic ramus

Inferior pubic ramus

175 Pelvic girdle of a female (40%)
a Dorsal aspect
b Inferior aspect

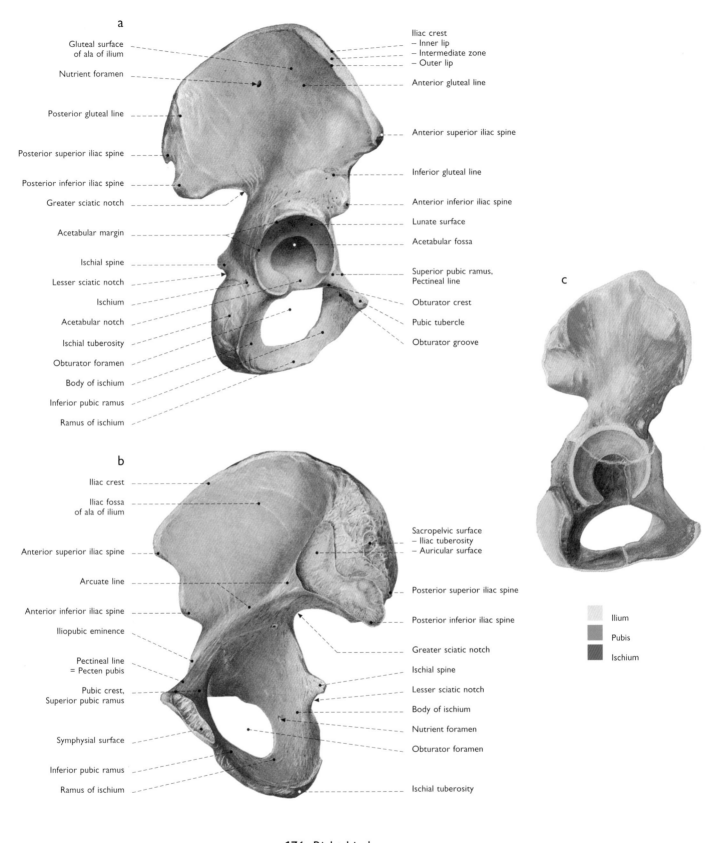

a

Gluteal surface of ala of ilium
Nutrient foramen
Posterior gluteal line
Posterior superior iliac spine
Posterior inferior iliac spine
Greater sciatic notch
Acetabular margin
Ischial spine
Lesser sciatic notch
Ischium
Acetabular notch
Ischial tuberosity
Obturator foramen
Body of ischium
Inferior pubic ramus
Ramus of ischium

Iliac crest
– Inner lip
– Intermediate zone
– Outer lip
Anterior gluteal line
Anterior superior iliac spine
Inferior gluteal line
Anterior inferior iliac spine
Lunate surface
Acetabular fossa
Superior pubic ramus, Pectineal line
Obturator crest
Pubic tubercle
Obturator groove

c

b

Iliac crest
Iliac fossa of ala of ilium
Anterior superior iliac spine
Arcuate line
Anterior inferior iliac spine
Iliopubic eminence
Pectineal line = Pecten pubis
Pubic crest, Superior pubic ramus
Symphysial surface
Inferior pubic ramus
Ramus of ischium

Sacropelvic surface
– Iliac tuberosity
– Auricular surface
Posterior superior iliac spine
Posterior inferior iliac spine
Greater sciatic notch
Ischial spine
Lesser sciatic notch
Body of ischium
Nutrient foramen
Obturator foramen
Ischial tuberosity

Ilium
Pubis
Ischium

176 Right hip bone

a, b Hip bone of an adult (40%)
a Lateral aspect
b Medial aspect
c Hip bone of a 10-year-old child with the typical Y-shaped epiphysial plate (50%), lateral aspect

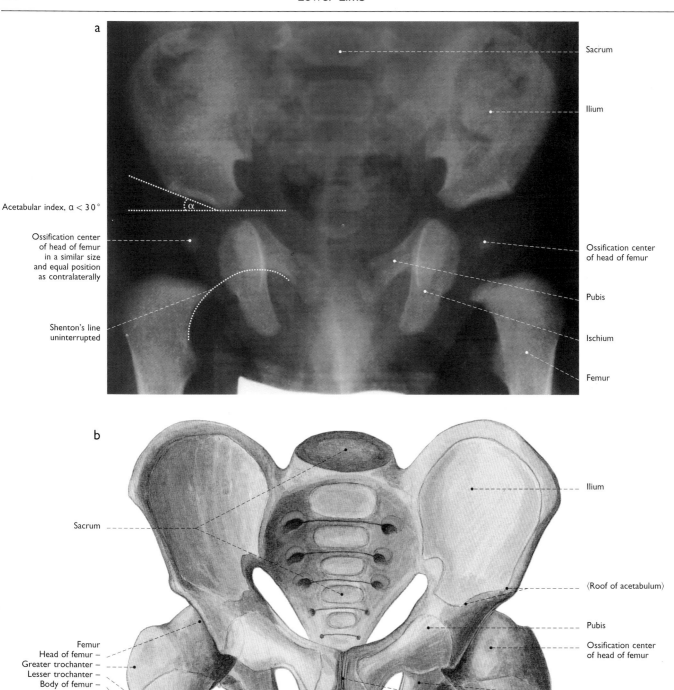

a

Sacrum

Ilium

Acetabular index, α < 30°

Ossification center
of head of femur
in a similar size
and equal position
as contralaterally

Ossification center
of head of femur

Pubis

Shenton's line
uninterrupted

Ischium

Femur

b

Sacrum

Ilium

⟨Roof of acetabulum⟩

Pubis

Femur
Head of femur –
Greater trochanter –
Lesser trochanter –
Body of femur –

Ossification center
of head of femur

Ischium

Pubic symphysis

**177 Pelvic girdle and proximal thigh bones (= femora)
of a 3-month-old child** (100%)

a   Anteroposterior radiograph. On the left side of the picture,
    the main radiological criteria for a normal development
    of the hip joint at this age are indicated.
b   Ventral aspect

a

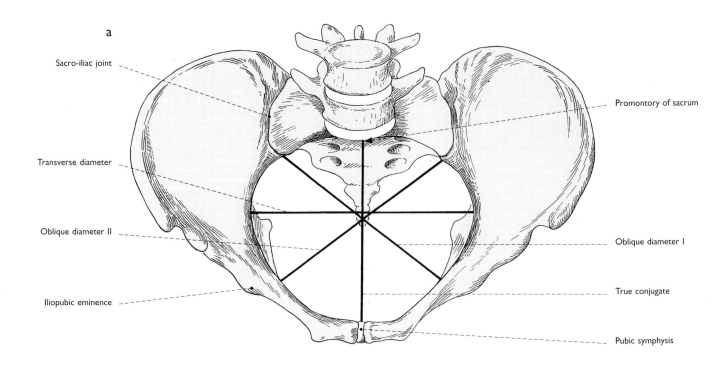

Sacro-iliac joint

Transverse diameter

Oblique diameter II

Iliopubic eminence

Promontory of sacrum

Oblique diameter I

True conjugate

Pubic symphysis

b

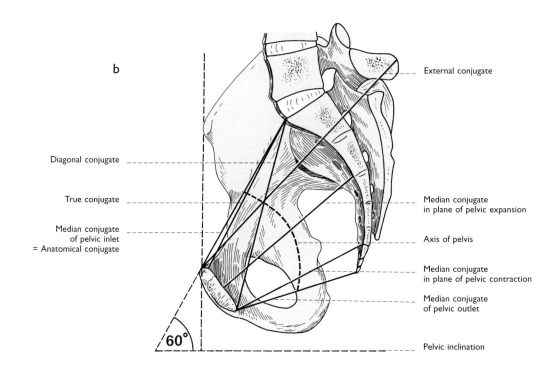

Diagonal conjugate

True conjugate

Median conjugate
of pelvic inlet
= Anatomical conjugate

External conjugate

Median conjugate
in plane of pelvic expansion

Axis of pelvis

Median conjugate
in plane of pelvic contraction

Median conjugate
of pelvic outlet

Pelvic inclination

60°

178 Pelvis of a female (40%)

Schematic representations
a Diameters of the pelvic inlet, cranial aspect
b Inclination of the pelvis and median conjugates,
medial aspect of a median section

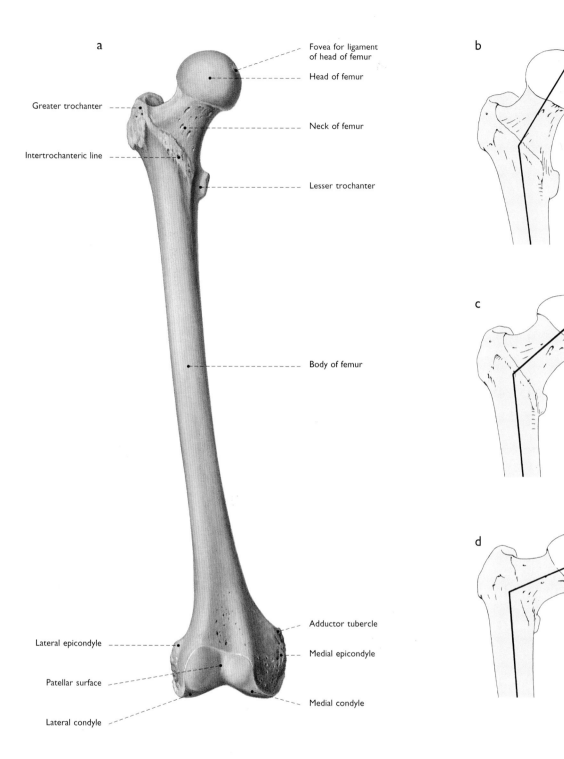

a

Fovea for ligament
of head of femur

Head of femur

Greater trochanter

Neck of femur

Intertrochanteric line

Lesser trochanter

Body of femur

Adductor tubercle

Lateral epicondyle

Medial epicondyle

Patellar surface

Medial condyle

Lateral condyle

b

c

d

179 Right thigh bone (= femur) (40%)

a Ventral aspect
b–d Neck-shaft angle
b 140°, coxa valga
c 124°, within the norm of an adult (120–130°)
d 108°, coxa vara

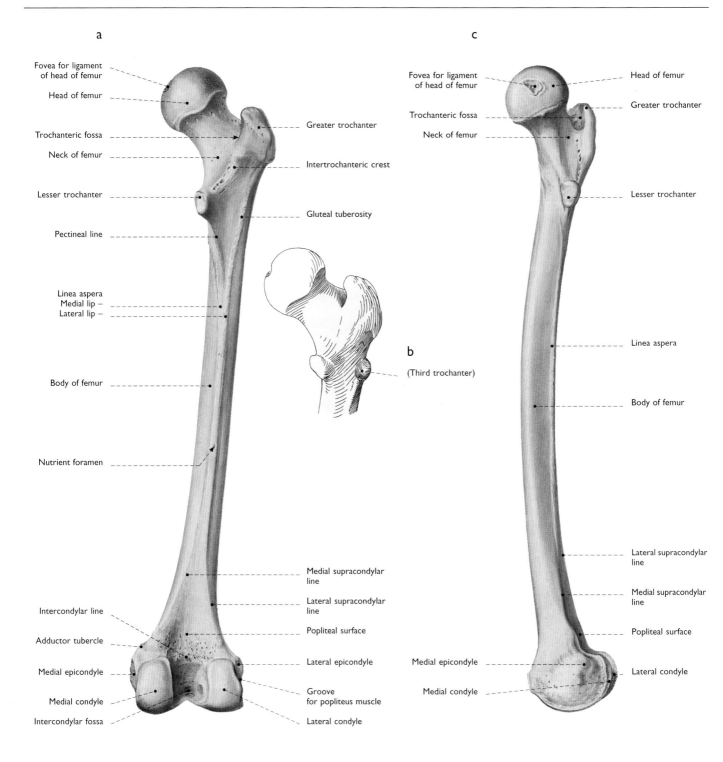

a

Fovea for ligament of head of femur

Head of femur

Trochanteric fossa

Neck of femur

Lesser trochanter

Pectineal line

Linea aspera
Medial lip —
Lateral lip —

Body of femur

Nutrient foramen

Greater trochanter

Intertrochanteric crest

Gluteal tuberosity

b

(Third trochanter)

Medial supracondylar line

Lateral supracondylar line

Popliteal surface

Lateral epicondyle

Groove for popliteus muscle

Lateral condyle

Intercondylar line

Adductor tubercle

Medial epicondyle

Medial condyle

Intercondylar fossa

c

Fovea for ligament of head of femur

Trochanteric fossa

Neck of femur

Head of femur

Greater trochanter

Lesser trochanter

Linea aspera

Body of femur

Lateral supracondylar line

Medial supracondylar line

Popliteal surface

Medial epicondyle

Medial condyle

Lateral condyle

180 Right thigh bone (= femur) (40%)

a Dorsal aspect
b Proximal end of the thigh bone
   with a third trochanter, dorsal aspect
c Medial aspect

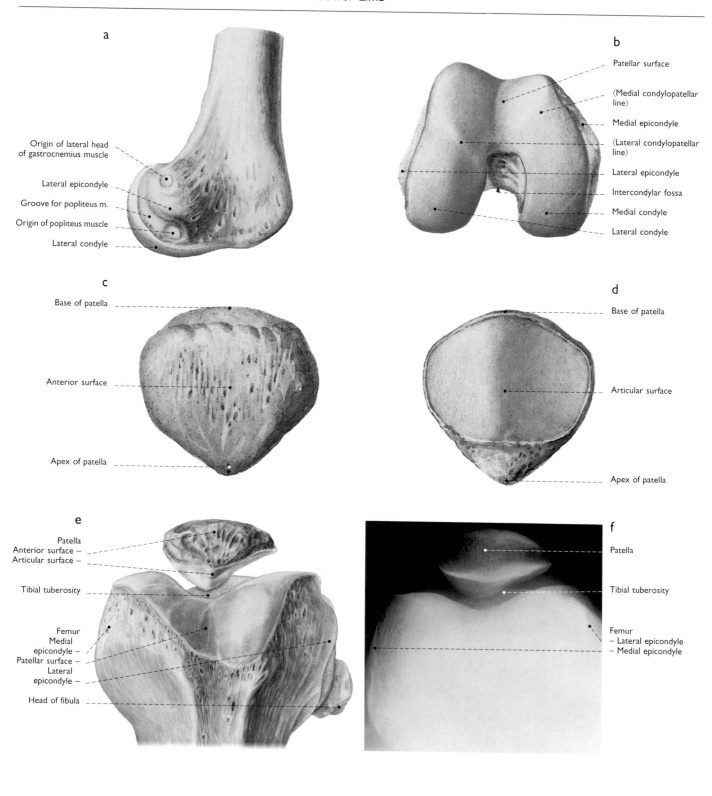

a

Origin of lateral head
of gastrocnemius muscle

Lateral epicondyle

Groove for popliteus m.

Origin of popliteus muscle

Lateral condyle

b

Patellar surface

⟨Medial condylopatellar
line⟩

Medial epicondyle

⟨Lateral condylopatellar
line⟩

Lateral epicondyle

Intercondylar fossa

Medial condyle

Lateral condyle

c

Base of patella

Anterior surface

Apex of patella

d

Base of patella

Articular surface

Apex of patella

e

Patella
Anterior surface –
Articular surface –

Tibial tuberosity

Femur
Medial
epicondyle –
Patellar surface –
Lateral
epicondyle –

Head of fibula

f

Patella

Tibial tuberosity

Femur
– Lateral epicondyle
– Medial epicondyle

181 Right thigh bone (= femur) and patella
a, b Distal end of the thigh bone (60%)
  a Lateral aspect
  b Distal aspect
  c, d Patella (100%)
  c Ventral aspect
  d Dorsal aspect
  e, f Patella and distal end of the thigh bone,
    knee joint in flexion (70%)
  e Ventral aspect
  f 'Tangential' radiograph (inferosuperior projection)

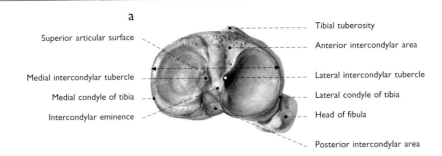

a

Superior articular surface

Medial intercondylar tubercle

Medial condyle of tibia

Intercondylar eminence

Tibial tuberosity

Anterior intercondylar area

Lateral intercondylar tubercle

Lateral condyle of tibia

Head of fibula

Posterior intercondylar area

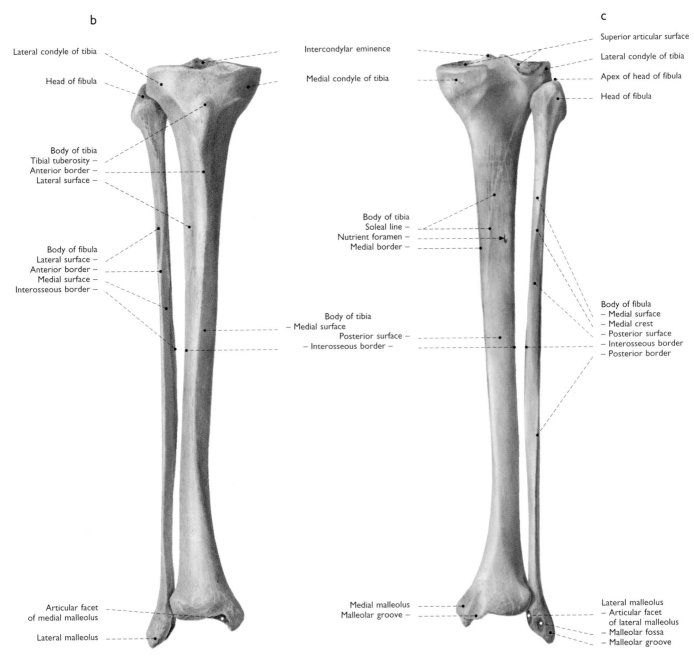

b

Lateral condyle of tibia

Head of fibula

Body of tibia
Tibial tuberosity –
Anterior border –
Lateral surface –

Body of fibula
Lateral surface –
Anterior border –
Medial surface –
Interosseous border –

Articular facet
of medial malleolus

Lateral malleolus

Intercondylar eminence

Medial condyle of tibia

Body of tibia
– Medial surface

Body of tibia
– Medial surface
Posterior surface –
– Interosseous border –

Medial malleolus
Malleolar groove –

c

Superior articular surface

Lateral condyle of tibia

Apex of head of fibula

Head of fibula

Body of tibia
Soleal line –
Nutrient foramen –
Medial border –

Body of fibula
– Medial surface
– Medial crest
– Posterior surface
– Interosseous border
– Posterior border

Lateral malleolus
– Articular facet
of lateral malleolus
– Malleolar fossa
– Malleolar groove

182 Bones of the right leg (40%)

a Proximal aspect
b Ventral aspect
c Dorsal aspect

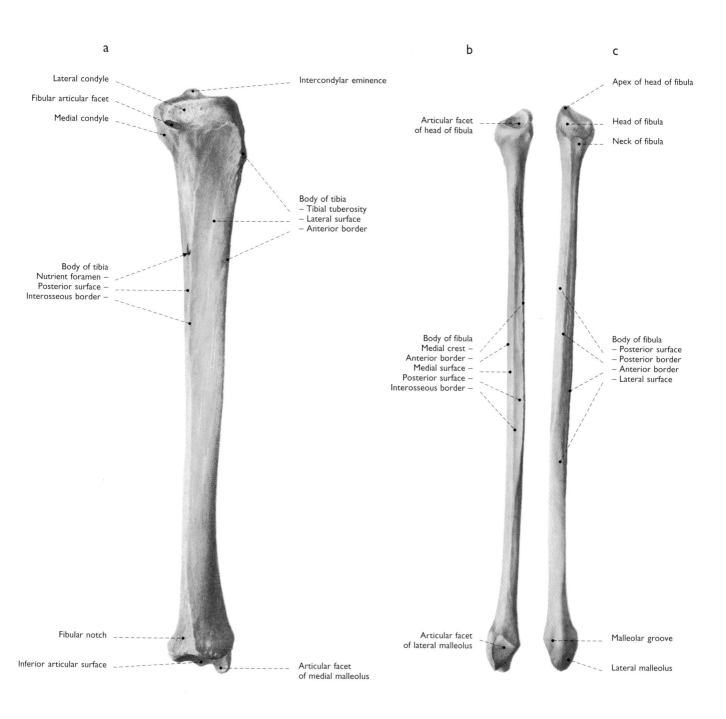

Lateral condyle

Fibular articular facet

Medial condyle

Intercondylar eminence

Apex of head of fibula

Articular facet
of head of fibula

Head of fibula

Neck of fibula

Body of tibia
– Tibial tuberosity
– Lateral surface
– Anterior border

Body of tibia
Nutrient foramen –
Posterior surface –
Interosseous border –

Body of fibula
Medial crest –
Anterior border –
Medial surface –
Posterior surface –
Interosseous border –

Body of fibula
– Posterior surface
– Posterior border
– Anterior border
– Lateral surface

Fibular notch

Inferior articular surface

Articular facet
of medial malleolus

Articular facet
of lateral malleolus

Malleolar groove

Lateral malleolus

183 Right tibia and fibula (40%)
a Tibia (= shin bone), lateral aspect
b Fibula (= calf bone), medial aspect
c Fibula (= calf bone), lateral aspect

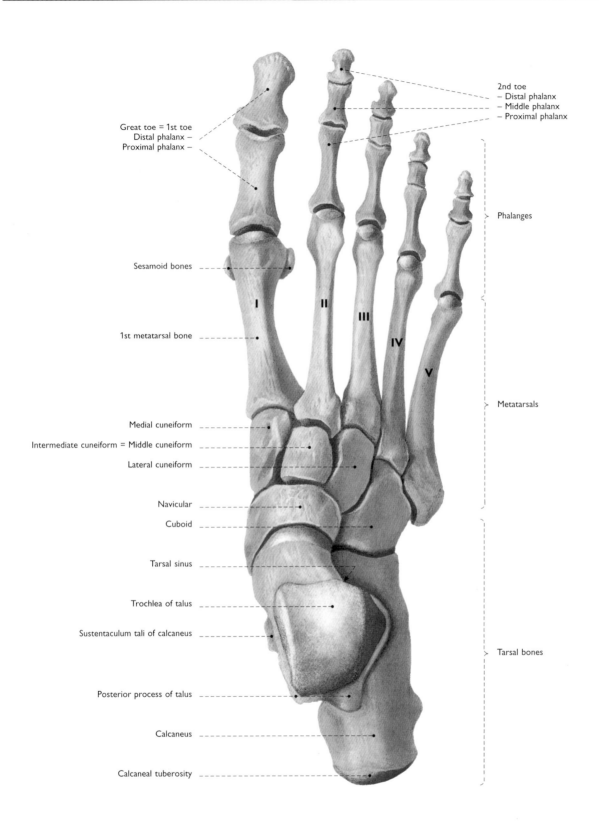

Great toe = 1st toe
Distal phalanx –
Proximal phalanx –

2nd toe
– Distal phalanx
– Middle phalanx
– Proximal phalanx

Sesamoid bones

Phalanges

I   II   III   IV   V

1st metatarsal bone

Metatarsals

Medial cuneiform

Intermediate cuneiform = Middle cuneiform

Lateral cuneiform

Navicular

Cuboid

Tarsal sinus

Trochlea of talus

Sustentaculum tali of calcaneus

Posterior process of talus

Calcaneus

Calcaneal tuberosity

Tarsal bones

184 Bones of the right foot (80%)
Dorsal aspect

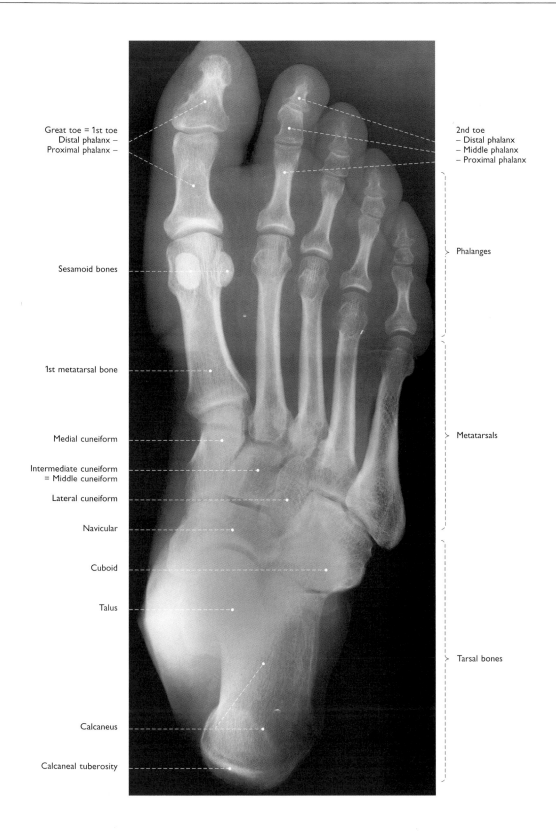

Great toe = 1st toe
Distal phalanx −
Proximal phalanx −

2nd toe
− Distal phalanx
− Middle phalanx
− Proximal phalanx

Sesamoid bones

Phalanges

1st metatarsal bone

Medial cuneiform

Metatarsals

Intermediate cuneiform
= Middle cuneiform

Lateral cuneiform

Navicular

Cuboid

Talus

Tarsal bones

Calcaneus

Calcaneal tuberosity

185 Bones of the right foot (80%)
Dorsoplantar radiograph

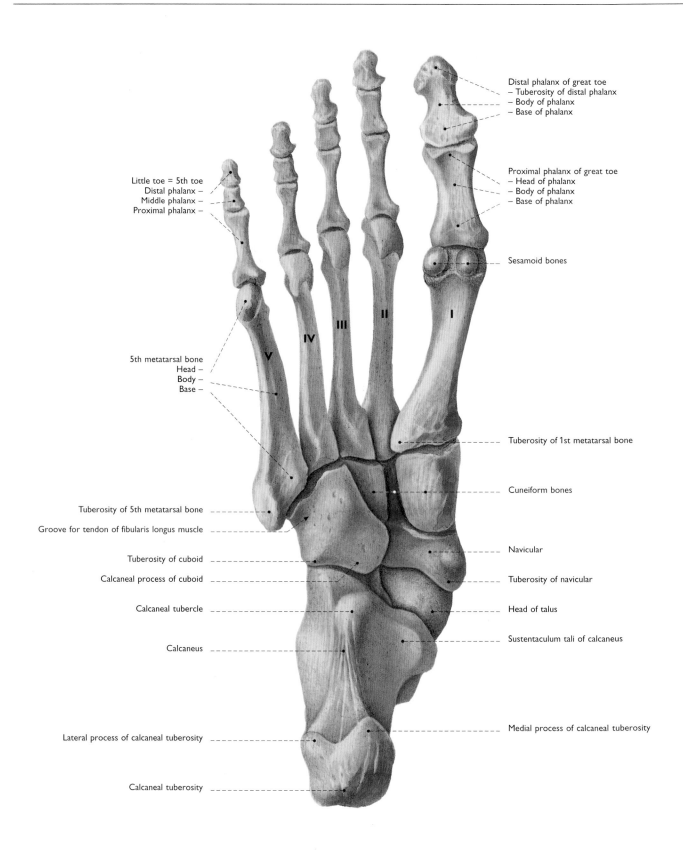

Distal phalanx of great toe
– Tuberosity of distal phalanx
– Body of phalanx
– Base of phalanx

Proximal phalanx of great toe
– Head of phalanx
– Body of phalanx
– Base of phalanx

Little toe = 5th toe
Distal phalanx –
Middle phalanx –
Proximal phalanx –

Sesamoid bones

V   IV   III   II   I

5th metatarsal bone
Head –
Body –
Base –

Tuberosity of 1st metatarsal bone

Cuneiform bones

Tuberosity of 5th metatarsal bone
Groove for tendon of fibularis longus muscle

Navicular

Tuberosity of cuboid

Tuberosity of navicular

Calcaneal process of cuboid

Head of talus

Calcaneal tubercle

Sustentaculum tali of calcaneus

Calcaneus

Lateral process of calcaneal tuberosity

Medial process of calcaneal tuberosity

Calcaneal tuberosity

186 Bones of the right foot (80%)
Plantar aspect

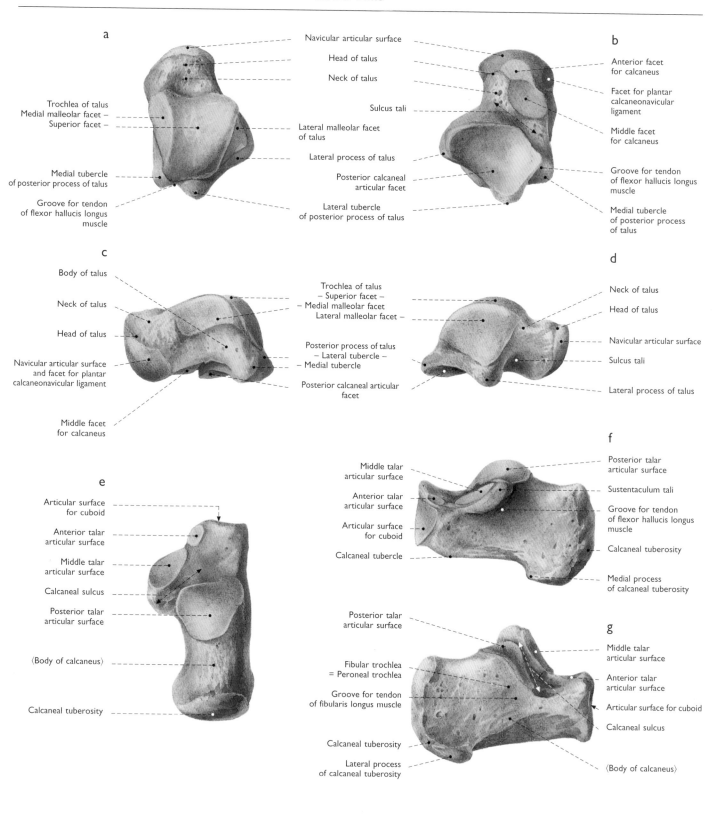

a

Navicular articular surface

Head of talus

Neck of talus

Trochlea of talus
Medial malleolar facet –
Superior facet –

Sulcus tali

Lateral malleolar facet
of talus

Lateral process of talus

Medial tubercle
of posterior process of talus

Posterior calcaneal
articular facet

Groove for tendon
of flexor hallucis longus
muscle

Lateral tubercle
of posterior process of talus

b

Anterior facet
for calcaneus

Facet for plantar
calcaneonavicular
ligament

Middle facet
for calcaneus

Groove for tendon
of flexor hallucis longus
muscle

Medial tubercle
of posterior process
of talus

c

Body of talus

Neck of talus

Head of talus

Navicular articular surface
and facet for plantar
calcaneonavicular ligament

Middle facet
for calcaneus

Trochlea of talus
– Superior facet –
– Medial malleolar facet
Lateral malleolar facet –

Posterior process of talus
– Lateral tubercle –
– Medial tubercle

Posterior calcaneal articular
facet

d

Neck of talus

Head of talus

Navicular articular surface

Sulcus tali

Lateral process of talus

e

Articular surface
for cuboid

Anterior talar
articular surface

Middle talar
articular surface

Calcaneal sulcus

Posterior talar
articular surface

⟨Body of calcaneus⟩

Calcaneal tuberosity

Middle talar
articular surface

Anterior talar
articular surface

Articular surface
for cuboid

Calcaneal tubercle

f

Posterior talar
articular surface

Sustentaculum tali

Groove for tendon
of flexor hallucis longus
muscle

Calcaneal tuberosity

Medial process
of calcaneal tuberosity

Posterior talar
articular surface

Fibular trochlea
= Peroneal trochlea

Groove for tendon
of fibularis longus muscle

Calcaneal tuberosity

Lateral process
of calcaneal tuberosity

g

Middle talar
articular surface

Anterior talar
articular surface

Articular surface for cuboid

Calcaneal sulcus

⟨Body of calcaneus⟩

187 Right talus and calcaneus (75%)

a–d Talus (= ankle bone)
e–g Calcaneus (= heel bone)
a, e Proximal aspect
b Plantar aspect
c, f Medial aspect
d, g Lateral aspect

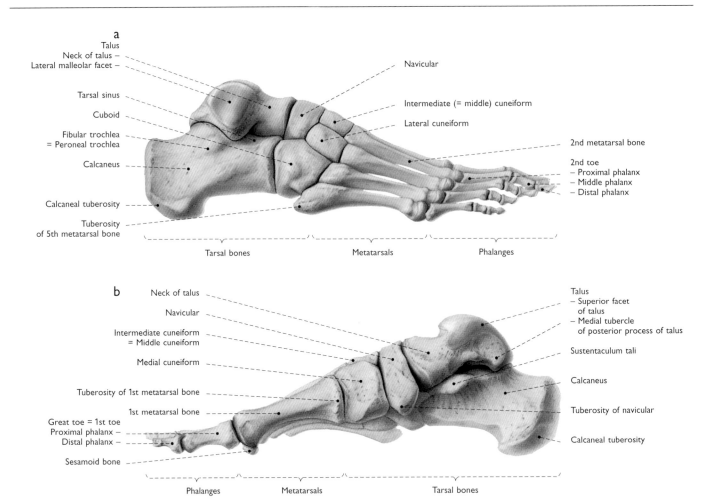

a

Talus
Neck of talus –
Lateral malleolar facet –

Tarsal sinus

Cuboid

Fibular trochlea
= Peroneal trochlea

Calcaneus –

Calcaneal tuberosity

Tuberosity
of 5th metatarsal bone

Navicular

Intermediate (= middle) cuneiform

Lateral cuneiform

2nd metatarsal bone

2nd toe
– Proximal phalanx
– Middle phalanx
– Distal phalanx

Tarsal bones · Metatarsals · Phalanges

b

Neck of talus

Navicular

Intermediate cuneiform
= Middle cuneiform

Medial cuneiform

Tuberosity of 1st metatarsal bone

1st metatarsal bone

Great toe = 1st toe
Proximal phalanx –
Distal phalanx –

Sesamoid bone

Talus
– Superior facet
of talus
– Medial tubercle
of posterior process of talus

Sustentaculum tali

Calcaneus

Tuberosity of navicular

Calcaneal tuberosity

Phalanges · Metatarsals · Tarsal bones

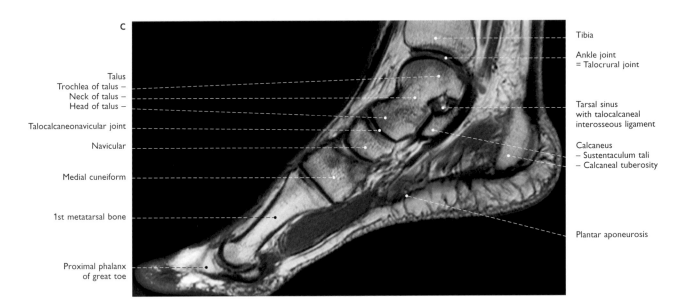

c

Talus
Trochlea of talus –
Neck of talus –
Head of talus –

Talocalcaneonavicular joint

Navicular

Medial cuneiform

1st metatarsal bone

Proximal phalanx
of great toe

Tibia

Ankle joint
= Talocrural joint

Tarsal sinus
with talocalcaneal
interosseous ligament

Calcaneus
– Sustentaculum tali
– Calcaneal tuberosity

Plantar aponeurosis

188 Bones of the right foot (45%)

a Lateral aspect
b Medial aspect
c Sagittal magnetic resonance image (MRI, T₁-weighted)
through the medial part of the right foot, medial aspect

a

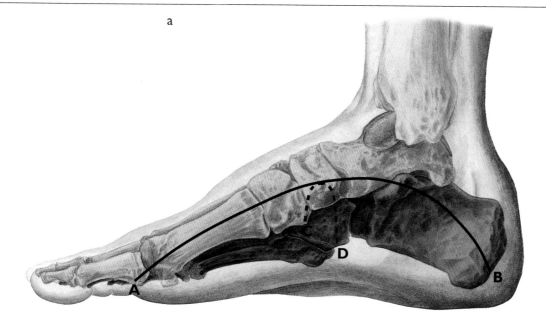

Bones of medial arch of foot

Bones of lateral arch of foot

c

Medial cuneiform

Intermediate cuneiform
= Middle cuneiform

Lateral cuneiform

Cuboid

b

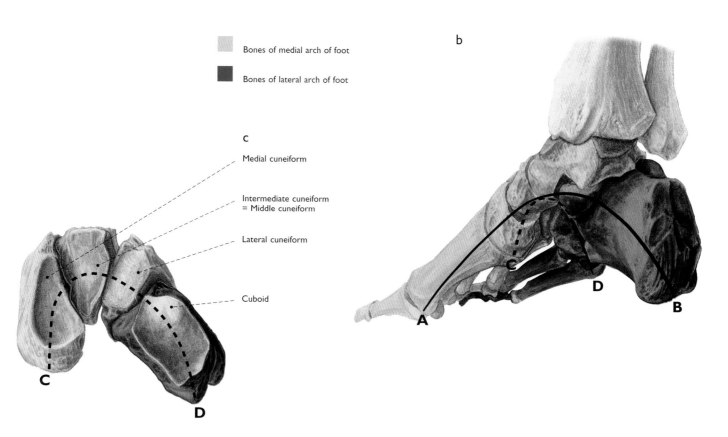

189 Longitudinal and transverse arches
of the skeleton of the right foot

The bones of the medial arch are illustrated in clear brown,
those of the lateral arch in dark brown color.
The longitudinal arch is shown by a continuous line (A–B),
the transverse arch by a broken line (C–D).
a Medial aspect (55%)
b Mediodorsal aspect (55%)
c Proximal aspect of the cuneiform bones and the cuboid bone (85%)

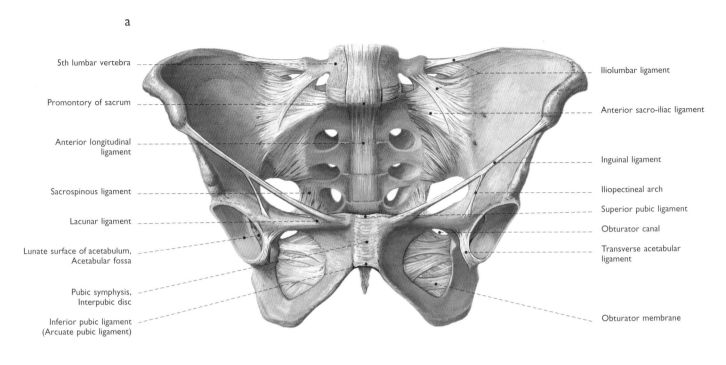

a

5th lumbar vertebra

Promontory of sacrum

Anterior longitudinal ligament

Sacrospinous ligament

Lacunar ligament

Lunate surface of acetabulum, Acetabular fossa

Pubic symphysis, Interpubic disc

Inferior pubic ligament (Arcuate pubic ligament)

Iliolumbar ligament

Anterior sacro-iliac ligament

Inguinal ligament

Iliopectineal arch

Superior pubic ligament

Obturator canal

Transverse acetabular ligament

Obturator membrane

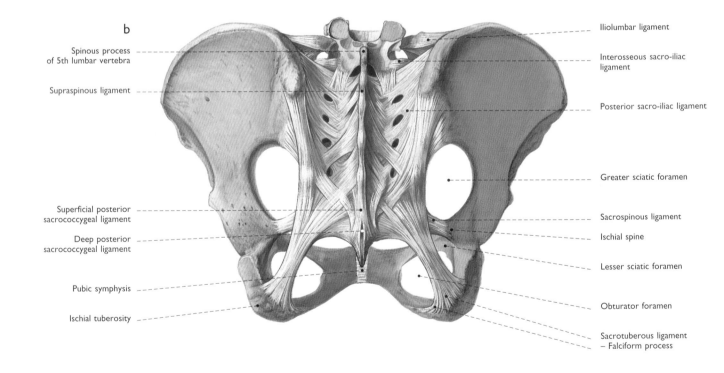

b

Spinous process of 5th lumbar vertebra

Supraspinous ligament

Superficial posterior sacrococcygeal ligament

Deep posterior sacrococcygeal ligament

Pubic symphysis

Ischial tuberosity

Iliolumbar ligament

Interosseous sacro-iliac ligament

Posterior sacro-iliac ligament

Greater sciatic foramen

Sacrospinous ligament

Ischial spine

Lesser sciatic foramen

Obturator foramen

Sacrotuberous ligament – Falciform process

190 Joints and ligaments of the pelvic girdle of a female (40%)

a   Ventral aspect
b   The obturator membrane was removed. Dorsal aspect

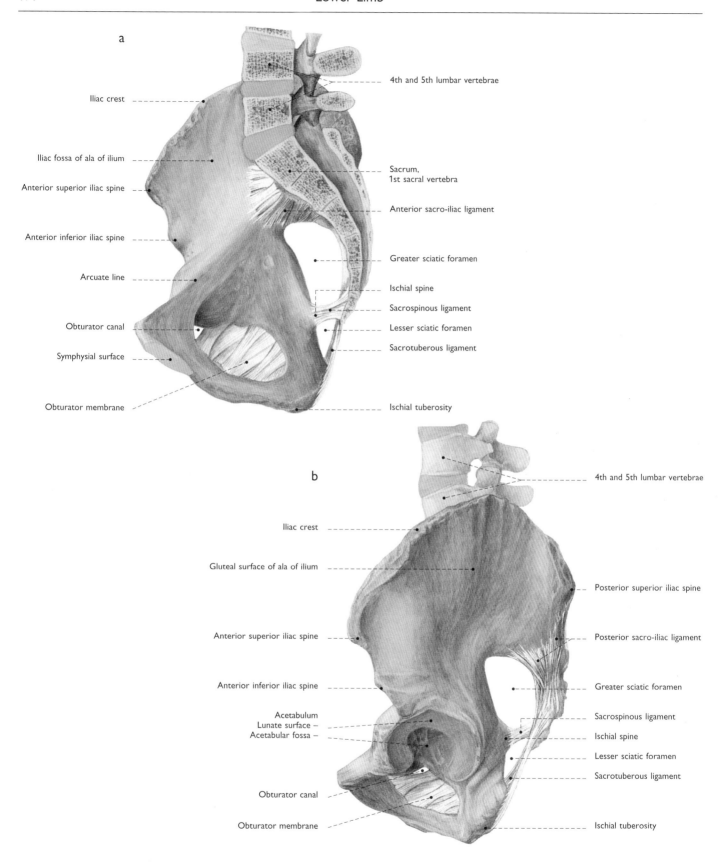

a

Iliac crest

Iliac fossa of ala of ilium

Anterior superior iliac spine

Anterior inferior iliac spine

Arcuate line

Obturator canal

Symphysial surface

Obturator membrane

4th and 5th lumbar vertebrae

Sacrum,
1st sacral vertebra

Anterior sacro-iliac ligament

Greater sciatic foramen

Ischial spine

Sacrospinous ligament

Lesser sciatic foramen

Sacrotuberous ligament

Ischial tuberosity

b

Iliac crest

Gluteal surface of ala of ilium

Anterior superior iliac spine

Anterior inferior iliac spine

Acetabulum
Lunate surface –
Acetabular fossa –

Obturator canal

Obturator membrane

4th and 5th lumbar vertebrae

Posterior superior iliac spine

Posterior sacro-iliac ligament

Greater sciatic foramen

Sacrospinous ligament

Ischial spine

Lesser sciatic foramen

Sacrotuberous ligament

Ischial tuberosity

191 Joints and ligaments of the pelvic girdle (45%)
a Medial aspect of the right half of the pelvis
b Left lateral aspect of the pelvis

a

Anterior superior iliac spine

Anterior inferior iliac spine

Greater trochanter

Iliofemoral ligament

Pubofemoral ligament

Intertrochanteric line

Lesser trochanter

Pectineal ligament

Obturator foramen

b

Sacrospinous ligament

Ischiofemoral ligament

Lesser sciatic foramen

Sacrotuberous ligament

Iliofemoral ligament

Greater trochanter

Intertrochanteric crest

Zona orbicularis

Lesser trochanter

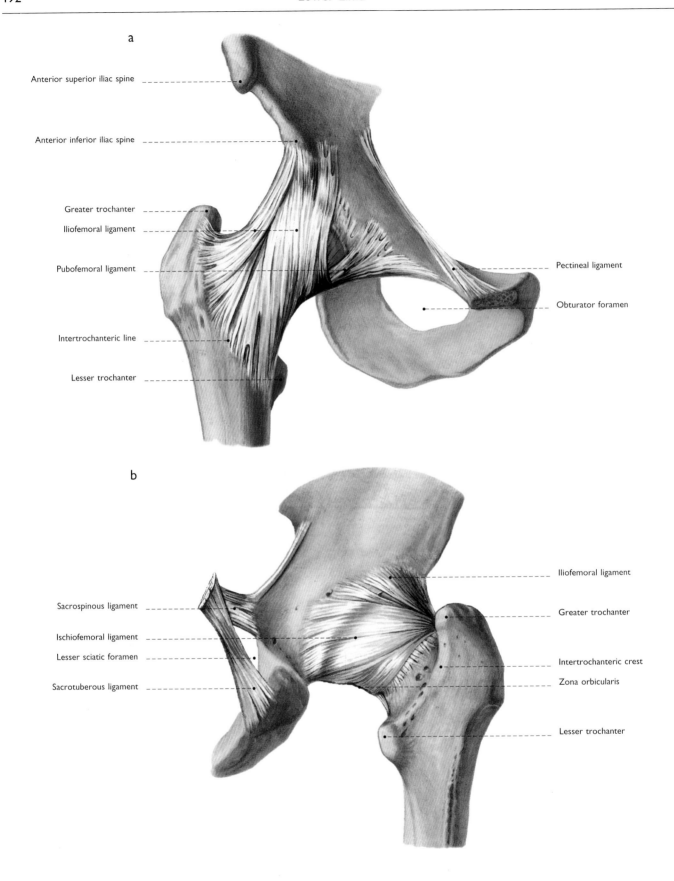

192 Right hip joint (70%)
a Ventral aspect
b Dorsal aspect

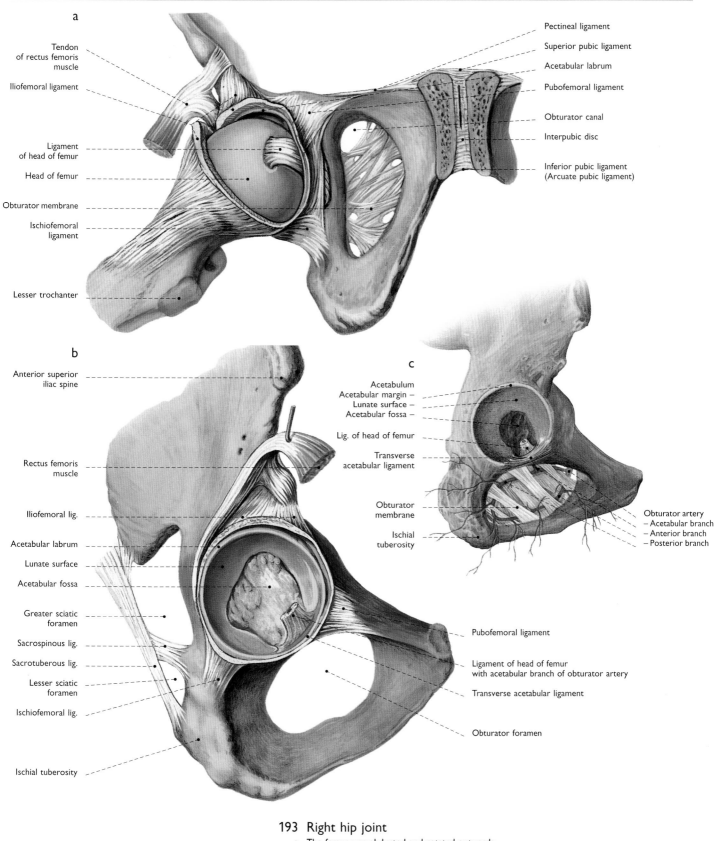

a

Tendon
of rectus femoris
muscle

Iliofemoral ligament

Ligament
of head of femur

Head of femur

Obturator membrane

Ischiofemoral
ligament

Lesser trochanter

Pectineal ligament

Superior pubic ligament

Acetabular labrum

Pubofemoral ligament

Obturator canal

Interpubic disc

Inferior pubic ligament
(Arcuate pubic ligament)

b

Anterior superior
iliac spine

Rectus femoris
muscle

Iliofemoral lig.

Acetabular labrum

Lunate surface

Acetabular fossa

Greater sciatic
foramen

Sacrospinous lig.

Sacrotuberous lig.

Lesser sciatic
foramen

Ischiofemoral lig.

Ischial tuberosity

c

Acetabulum
Acetabular margin —
Lunate surface —
Acetabular fossa —

Lig. of head of femur

Transverse
acetabular ligament

Obturator
membrane

Ischial
tuberosity

Obturator artery
– Acetabular branch
– Anterior branch
– Posterior branch

Pubofemoral ligament

Ligament of head of femur
with acetabular branch of obturator artery

Transverse acetabular ligament

Obturator foramen

193 Right hip joint

a   The femur was abducted and rotated outwards.
    The capsule of the hip joint was opened ventrally
    and the pubic symphysis cut frontally 60%).
    Ventral aspect
b   View of the socket of hip joint (60%), ventrolateral aspect
c   Ligament of the head of femur with acetabular artery (35%),
    ventrolateral aspect

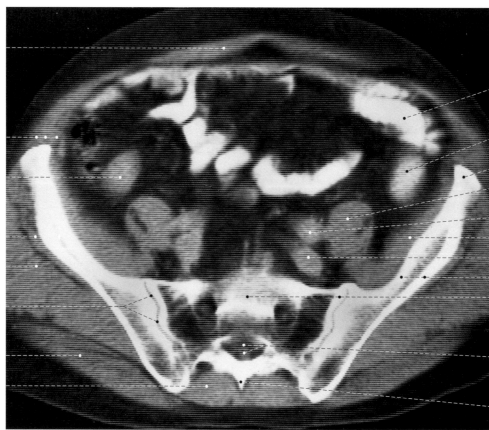

a

Rectus abdominis muscle

External and internal oblique muscles, Transversus abdominis m.

Cecum

Gluteus minimus muscle

Gluteus medius muscle

Sacro-iliac joint

Gluteus maximus muscle

Erector spinae muscle

Sigmoid colon

Descending colon

Iliac crest

Psoas major muscle

Common iliac artery

Iliacus muscle

Common iliac vein

Ilium

Sacrum
(1st sacral vertebra)

Sacral canal,
Cauda equina

Median sacral crest

b

Sartorius muscle

Rectus femoris muscle

Iliopsoas muscle

Tensor fasciae latae muscle

Gluteus medius muscle

Urinary bladder

Levator ani muscle

Rectum

Ischio-anal fossa

Gluteus maximus muscle

Rectus abdominis
muscle

Pubis

Femur
– Head of femur
– Neck of femur
– Greater trochanter
– Trochanteric fossa

Acetabular fossa

Ischium

Obturator internus
muscle

194 Sacro-iliac and hip joints (40%)

Inferior aspect

a Transverse computed tomogram (CT)
showing both sacro-iliac joints

b Transverse magnetic resonance image (MRI, T$_1$-weighted)
showing both hip joints

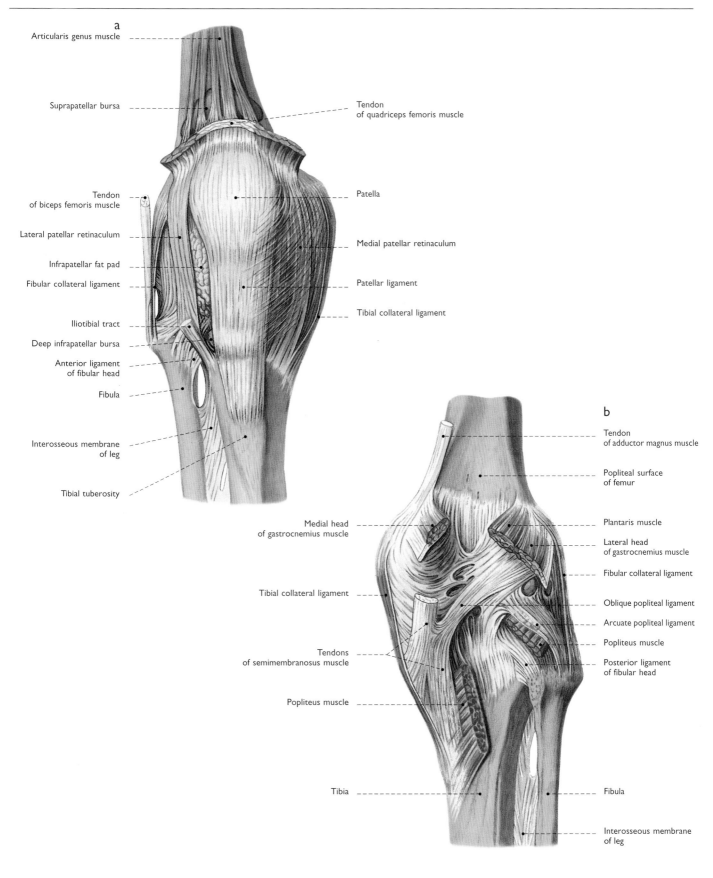

a

Articularis genus muscle

Suprapatellar bursa

Tendon
of biceps femoris muscle

Lateral patellar retinaculum

Infrapatellar fat pad

Fibular collateral ligament

Iliotibial tract

Deep infrapatellar bursa

Anterior ligament
of fibular head

Fibula

Interosseous membrane
of leg

Tibial tuberosity

Tendon
of quadriceps femoris muscle

Patella

Medial patellar retinaculum

Patellar ligament

Tibial collateral ligament

b

Medial head
of gastrocnemius muscle

Tibial collateral ligament

Tendons
of semimembranosus muscle

Popliteus muscle

Tibia

Tendon
of adductor magnus muscle

Popliteal surface
of femur

Plantaris muscle

Lateral head
of gastrocnemius muscle

Fibular collateral ligament

Oblique popliteal ligament

Arcuate popliteal ligament

Popliteus muscle

Posterior ligament
of fibular head

Fibula

Interosseous membrane
of leg

195 Right knee joint (70%)
a Ventral aspect
b Dorsal aspect

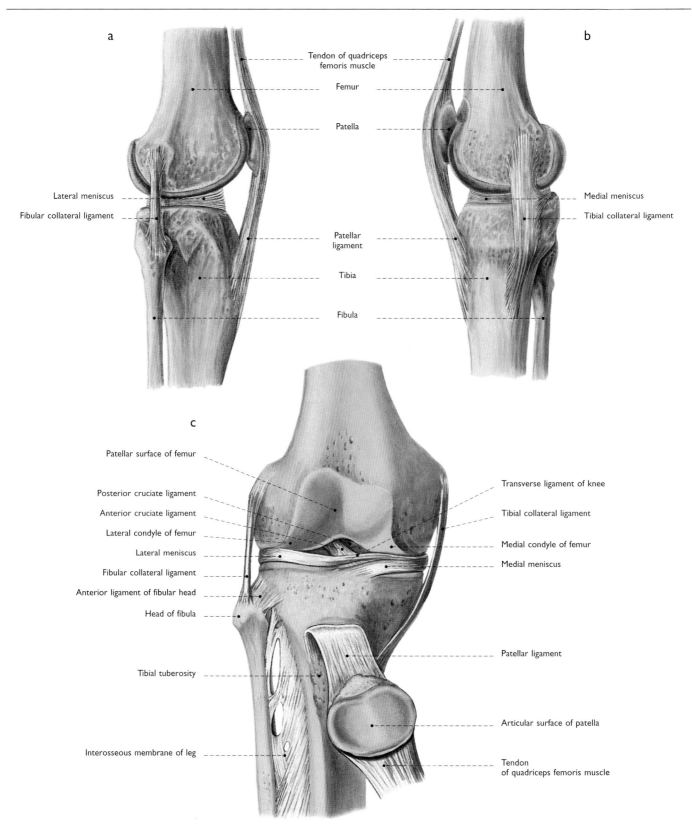

a

Tendon of quadriceps femoris muscle

Femur

Patella

Lateral meniscus

Fibular collateral ligament

Patellar ligament

Tibia

Fibula

b

Medial meniscus

Tibial collateral ligament

c

Patellar surface of femur

Posterior cruciate ligament

Anterior cruciate ligament

Lateral condyle of femur

Lateral meniscus

Fibular collateral ligament

Anterior ligament of fibular head

Head of fibula

Tibial tuberosity

Interosseous membrane of leg

Transverse ligament of knee

Tibial collateral ligament

Medial condyle of femur

Medial meniscus

Patellar ligament

Articular surface of patella

Tendon
of quadriceps femoris muscle

196 Right knee joint
The capsule was removed.
a Lateral aspect (50%)
b Medial aspect (50%)
c The patella was turned downwards (70%). Ventral aspect

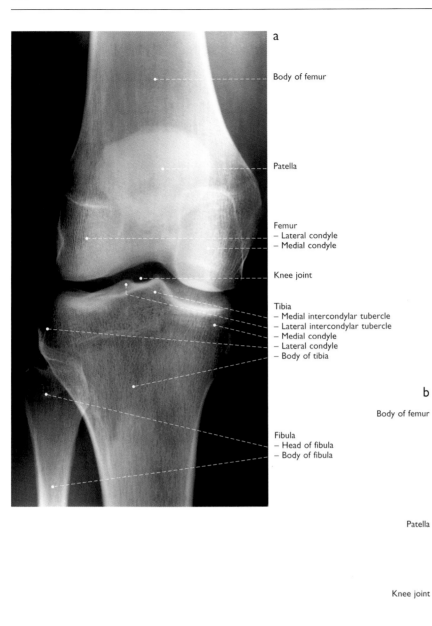

a

Body of femur

Patella

Femur
– Lateral condyle
– Medial condyle

Knee joint

Tibia
– Medial intercondylar tubercle
– Lateral intercondylar tubercle
– Medial condyle
– Lateral condyle
– Body of tibia

Fibula
– Head of fibula
– Body of fibula

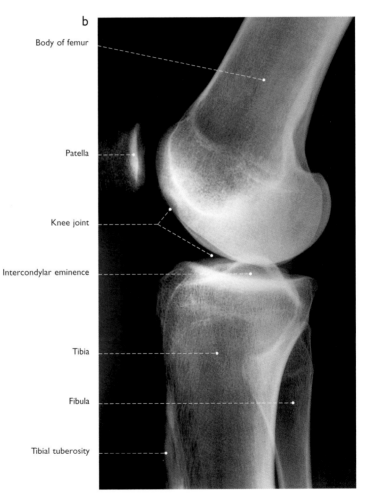

b

Body of femur

Patella

Knee joint

Intercondylar eminence

Tibia

Fibula

Tibial tuberosity

197 Right knee joint (80%)
a   Anteroposterior radiograph
b   Lateral radiograph

a

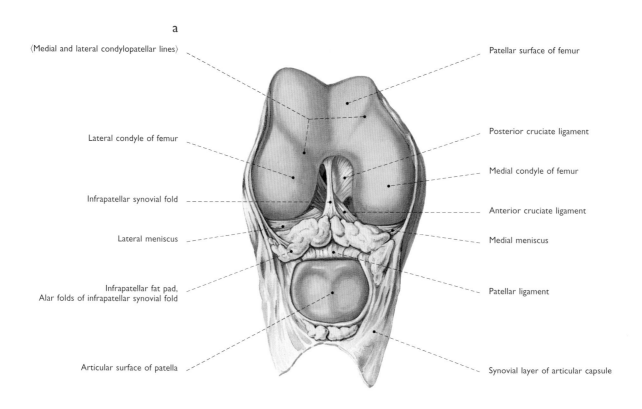

⟨Medial and lateral condylopatellar lines⟩

Lateral condyle of femur

Infrapatellar synovial fold

Lateral meniscus

Infrapatellar fat pad,
Alar folds of infrapatellar synovial fold

Articular surface of patella

Patellar surface of femur

Posterior cruciate ligament

Medial condyle of femur

Anterior cruciate ligament

Medial meniscus

Patellar ligament

Synovial layer of articular capsule

b

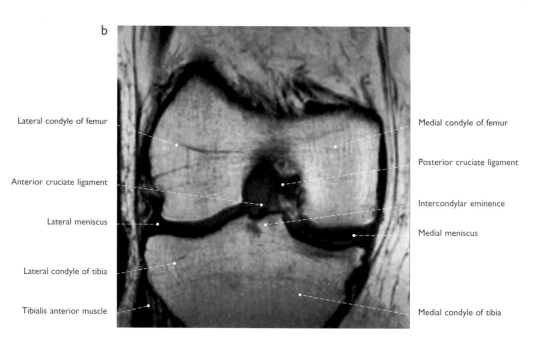

Lateral condyle of femur

Anterior cruciate ligament

Lateral meniscus

Lateral condyle of tibia

Tibialis anterior muscle

Medial condyle of femur

Posterior cruciate ligament

Intercondylar eminence

Medial meniscus

Medial condyle of tibia

198 Right knee joint

Ventral aspect
a The joint is flexed, the capsule was opened
   and the patella turned downwards (70%).
b Coronal magnetic resonance image (MRI, T$_1$-weighted)
   through ventral parts of the knee joint (90%)

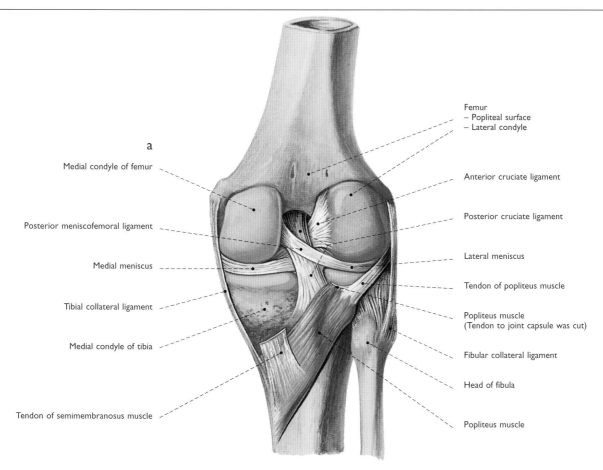

a

Medial condyle of femur

Posterior meniscofemoral ligament

Medial meniscus

Tibial collateral ligament

Medial condyle of tibia

Tendon of semimembranosus muscle

Femur
– Popliteal surface
– Lateral condyle

Anterior cruciate ligament

Posterior cruciate ligament

Lateral meniscus

Tendon of popliteus muscle

Popliteus muscle
(Tendon to joint capsule was cut)

Fibular collateral ligament

Head of fibula

Popliteus muscle

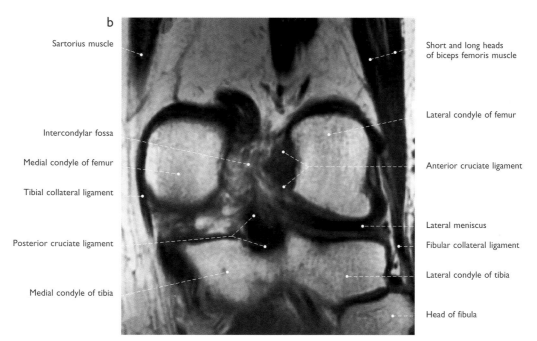

b

Sartorius muscle

Intercondylar fossa

Medial condyle of femur

Tibial collateral ligament

Posterior cruciate ligament

Medial condyle of tibia

Short and long heads
of biceps femoris muscle

Lateral condyle of femur

Anterior cruciate ligament

Lateral meniscus

Fibular collateral ligament

Lateral condyle of tibia

Head of fibula

199   Right knee joint

Dorsal aspect
a   The joint is extended, and the capsule was partially removed (70%).
b   Coronal magnetic resonance image (MRI, T_1-weighted)
    through dorsal parts of the knee joint (90%)

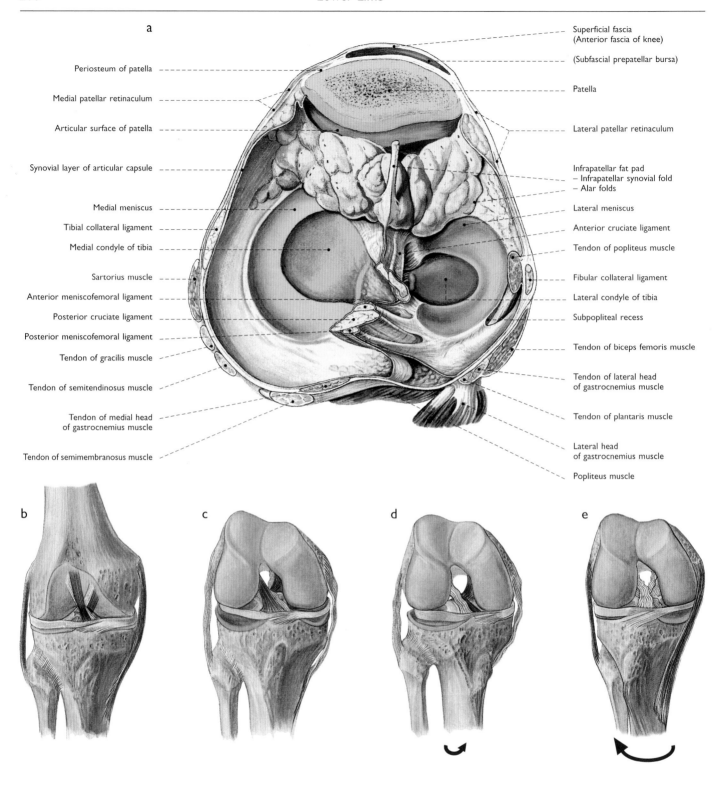

a

Periosteum of patella

Medial patellar retinaculum

Articular surface of patella

Synovial layer of articular capsule

Medial meniscus

Tibial collateral ligament

Medial condyle of tibia

Sartorius muscle

Anterior meniscofemoral ligament

Posterior cruciate ligament

Posterior meniscofemoral ligament

Tendon of gracilis muscle

Tendon of semitendinosus muscle

Tendon of medial head of gastrocnemius muscle

Tendon of semimembranosus muscle

Superficial fascia (Anterior fascia of knee)

(Subfascial prepatellar bursa)

Patella

Lateral patellar retinaculum

Infrapatellar fat pad – Infrapatellar synovial fold – Alar folds

Lateral meniscus

Anterior cruciate ligament

Tendon of popliteus muscle

Fibular collateral ligament

Lateral condyle of tibia

Subpopliteal recess

Tendon of biceps femoris muscle

Tendon of lateral head of gastrocnemius muscle

Tendon of plantaris muscle

Lateral head of gastrocnemius muscle

Popliteus muscle

b   c   d   e

200 Right knee joint
a The joint was cut transversally through the middle of the patella (100%). Cranial aspect of the distal part
b–e State of tautening of the cruciate and collateral ligaments (50%) (according to von Lanz and Wachsmuth, 1972)
b knee in extension
c knee in flexion
d knee in flexion and medial rotation
e knee in flexion and lateral rotation
The taut parts of ligaments are dark-colored. Ventral aspect

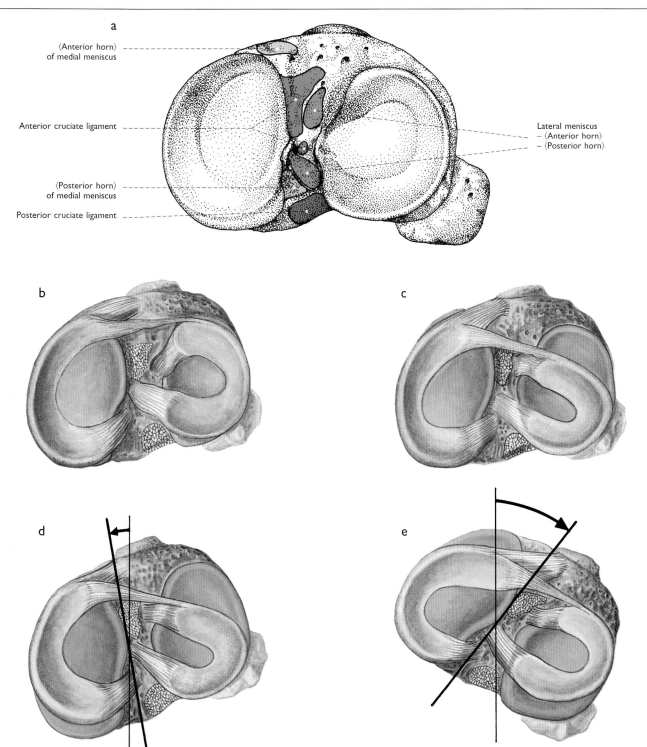

a

⟨Anterior horn⟩
of medial meniscus

Anterior cruciate ligament

⟨Posterior horn⟩
of medial meniscus

Posterior cruciate ligament

Lateral meniscus
– ⟨Anterior horn⟩
– ⟨Posterior horn⟩

b

c

d

e

201 Right knee joint
Cranial aspect
a Insertions of the cruciate ligaments and menisci (100%),
schematic representation
b–e Position of the menisci (80%)
(according to von Lanz and Wachsmuth, 1972)
b knee in extension
c knee in flexion
d knee in flexion and medial rotation
e knee in flexion and lateral rotation

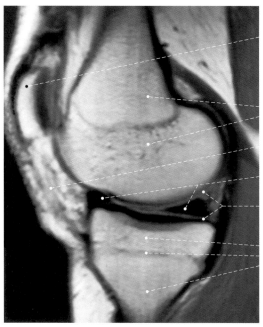

a

Patella

Femur
– Body of femur
– Medial condyle

Infrapatellar fat pad

Medial meniscus

Articular cartilage

Tibia
– Medial condyle
– Epiphysial line
– Body of tibia

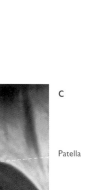

b

Quadriceps femoris muscle

Patella

Femur

Epiphysial line

Anterior cruciate ligament

Infrapatellar fat pad

Articular cartilage

Patellar ligament

Posterior cruciate ligament

Body of tibia

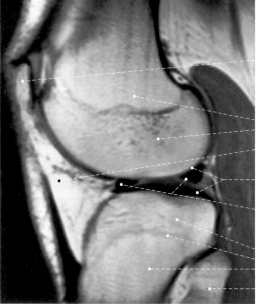

c

Patella

Femur
– Body of femur
– Lateral condyle

Infrapatellar fat pad

Articular cartilage

Lateral meniscus

Tibia
– Lateral condyle
– Epiphysial line
– Body of tibia

Head of fibula

202 Right knee joint (80%)

Sagittal magnetic resonance images (MRI, [1]H-weighted)
through the
a medial part of the knee joint
b middle part of the knee joint
c lateral part of the knee joint.
Bones and fat can be well recognized.

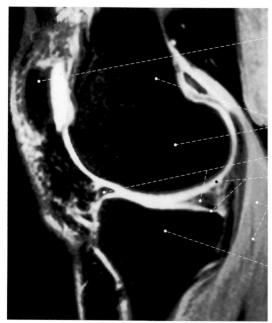

a

Patella

Femur
– Body of femur
– Medial condyle

Medial meniscus

Articular cartilage

Triceps surae muscle,
Medial head
of gastrocnemius muscle

Medial condyle of tibia

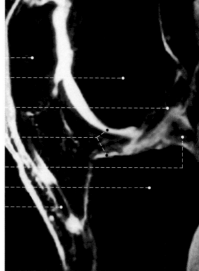

b

Patella

Femur

Anterior cruciate ligament

Articular cartilage

Posterior cruciate ligament

Tibia

Patellar ligament

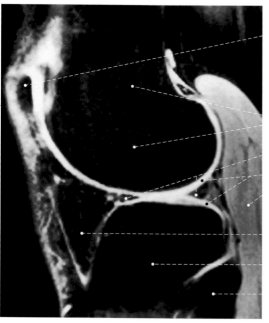

c

Patella

Femur
– Body of femur
– Lateral condyle

Lateral meniscus

Articular cartilage

Triceps surae muscle,
Lateral head
of gastrocnemius muscle

Infrapatellar fat pad

Lateral condyle of tibia

Head of fibula

203 Right knee joint (80%)

Sagittal magnetic resonance images (MRI, T$_1$-weighted,
fat-suppressed) through the
a medial part of the knee joint
b middle part of the knee joint
c lateral part of the knee joint.
Cartilaginous and muscular structures can be well recognized.

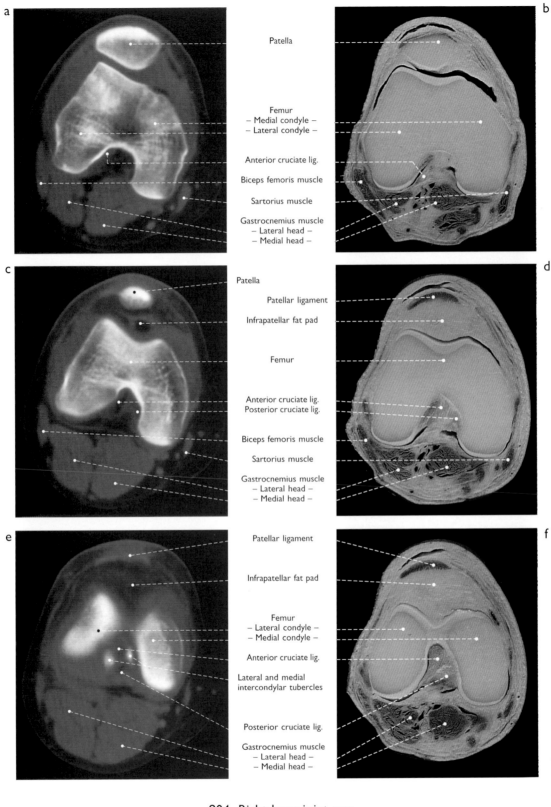

Patella

Femur
– Medial condyle –
– Lateral condyle –

Anterior cruciate lig.
Biceps femoris muscle
Sartorius muscle
Gastrocnemius muscle
– Lateral head –
– Medial head –

Patella
Patellar ligament
Infrapatellar fat pad

Femur

Anterior cruciate lig.
Posterior cruciate lig.

Biceps femoris muscle
Sartorius muscle
Gastrocnemius muscle
– Lateral head –
– Medial head –

Patellar ligament

Infrapatellar fat pad

Femur
– Lateral condyle –
– Medial condyle –

Anterior cruciate lig.

Lateral and medial
intercondylar tubercles

Posterior cruciate lig.

Gastrocnemius muscle
– Lateral head –
– Medial head –

204 Right knee joint (65%)
Inferior aspect
a, c, e Transverse magnetic resonance images (MRI, T$_1$-weighted)
b, d, f Transverse anatomical sections
through
a, b cranial parts
c, d middle parts
e, f caudal parts
of the knee joint

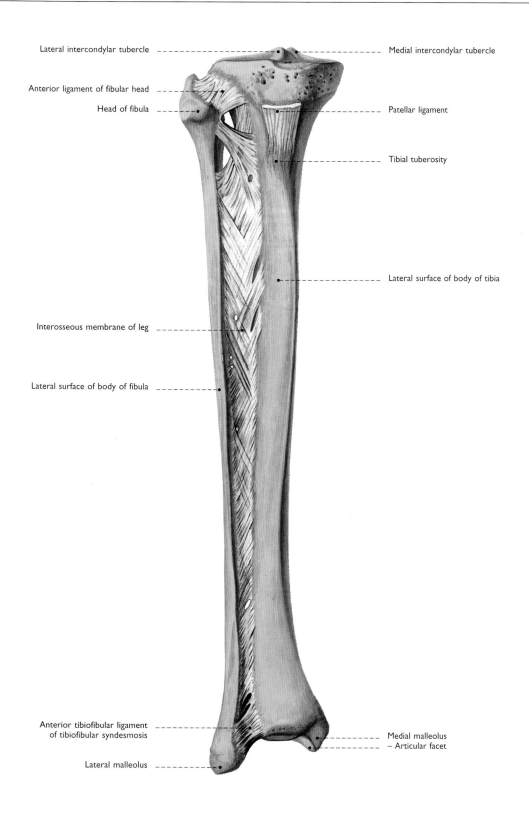

Lateral intercondylar tubercle

Anterior ligament of fibular head

Head of fibula

Interosseous membrane of leg

Lateral surface of body of fibula

Anterior tibiofibular ligament
of tibiofibular syndesmosis

Lateral malleolus

Medial intercondylar tubercle

Patellar ligament

Tibial tuberosity

Lateral surface of body of tibia

Medial malleolus
– Articular facet

**205 Tibiofibular joints and syndesmoses
of the right leg** (50%)
Ventral aspect

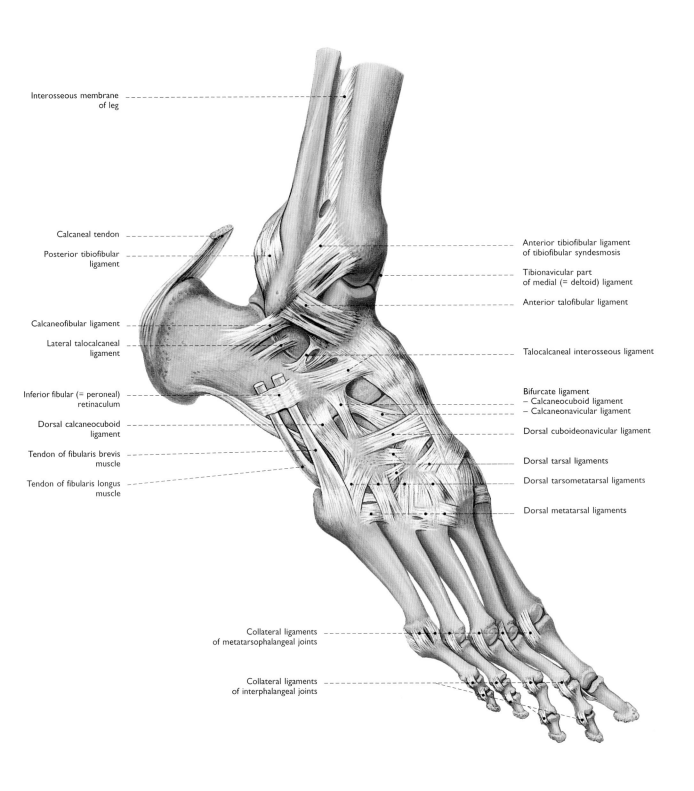

Interosseous membrane of leg

Calcaneal tendon

Posterior tibiofibular ligament

Calcaneofibular ligament

Lateral talocalcaneal ligament

Inferior fibular (= peroneal) retinaculum

Dorsal calcaneocuboid ligament

Tendon of fibularis brevis muscle

Tendon of fibularis longus muscle

Collateral ligaments of metatarsophalangeal joints

Collateral ligaments of interphalangeal joints

Anterior tibiofibular ligament of tibiofibular syndesmosis

Tibionavicular part of medial (= deltoid) ligament

Anterior talofibular ligament

Talocalcaneal interosseous ligament

Bifurcate ligament
– Calcaneocuboid ligament
– Calcaneonavicular ligament

Dorsal cuboideonavicular ligament

Dorsal tarsal ligaments

Dorsal tarsometatarsal ligaments

Dorsal metatarsal ligaments

206 Joints and ligaments of the right foot (70%)
Lateral aspect

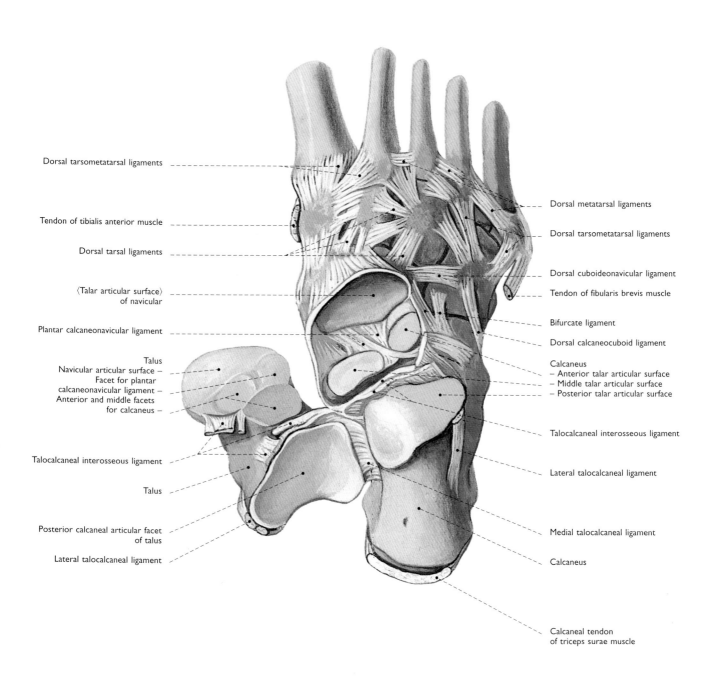

Dorsal tarsometatarsal ligaments

Tendon of tibialis anterior muscle

Dorsal tarsal ligaments

⟨Talar articular surface⟩
of navicular

Plantar calcaneonavicular ligament

Talus
Navicular articular surface –
Facet for plantar
calcaneonavicular ligament –
Anterior and middle facets
for calcaneus –

Talocalcaneal interosseous ligament

Talus

Posterior calcaneal articular facet
of talus

Lateral talocalcaneal ligament

Dorsal metatarsal ligaments

Dorsal tarsometatarsal ligaments

Dorsal cuboideonavicular ligament

Tendon of fibularis brevis muscle

Bifurcate ligament

Dorsal calcaneocuboid ligament

Calcaneus
– Anterior talar articular surface
– Middle talar articular surface
– Posterior talar articular surface

Talocalcaneal interosseous ligament

Lateral talocalcaneal ligament

Medial talocalcaneal ligament

Calcaneus

Calcaneal tendon
of triceps surae muscle

207 Subtalar (= talocalcaneal), talocalcaneonavicular,
and tarsometatarsal joint of the right foot (90%)
The talus was turned medially. Dorsal aspect

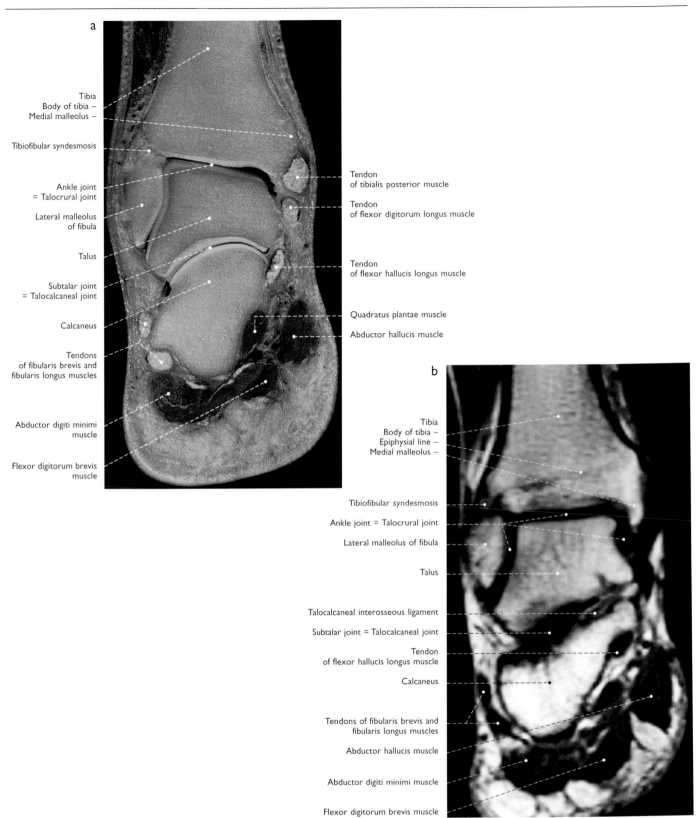

a

Tibia
Body of tibia –
Medial malleolus –

Tibiofibular syndesmosis

Ankle joint
= Talocrural joint

Lateral malleolus
of fibula

Talus

Subtalar joint
= Talocalcaneal joint

Calcaneus

Tendons
of fibularis brevis and
fibularis longus muscles

Abductor digiti minimi
muscle

Flexor digitorum brevis
muscle

Tendon
of tibialis posterior muscle

Tendon
of flexor digitorum longus muscle

Tendon
of flexor hallucis longus muscle

Quadratus plantae muscle

Abductor hallucis muscle

b

Tibia
Body of tibia –
Epiphysial line –
Medial malleolus –

Tibiofibular syndesmosis

Ankle joint = Talocrural joint

Lateral malleolus of fibula

Talus

Talocalcaneal interosseous ligament

Subtalar joint = Talocalcaneal joint

Tendon
of flexor hallucis longus muscle

Calcaneus

Tendons of fibularis brevis and
fibularis longus muscles

Abductor hallucis muscle

Abductor digiti minimi muscle

Flexor digitorum brevis muscle

208 Bones, joints, and ligaments of the right foot (80%)

Coronal sections, distal aspect
a Anatomical section
b Magnetic resonance image (MRI, T$_1$-weighted)

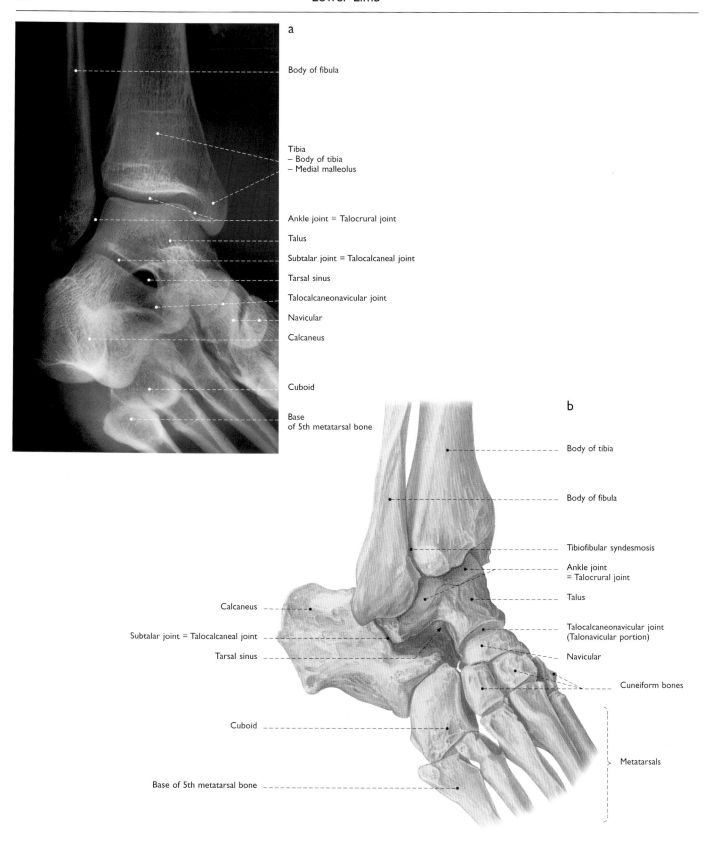

a

Body of fibula

Tibia
– Body of tibia
– Medial malleolus

Ankle joint = Talocrural joint

Talus

Subtalar joint = Talocalcaneal joint

Tarsal sinus

Talocalcaneonavicular joint

Navicular

Calcaneus

Cuboid

Base
of 5th metatarsal bone

b

Body of tibia

Body of fibula

Tibiofibular syndesmosis

Ankle joint
= Talocrural joint

Talus

Talocalcaneonavicular joint
(Talonavicular portion)

Navicular

Cuneiform bones

Metatarsals

Calcaneus

Subtalar joint = Talocalcaneal joint

Tarsal sinus

Cuboid

Base of 5th metatarsal bone

209 Bones and joints of the right foot (75%)
Oblique laterodistal view
a Radiograph showing the ankle (= talocrural),
   subtalar (= talocalcaneal), and talocalcaneonavicular joints
   as well as the tarsal sinus
b Corresponding anatomical representation

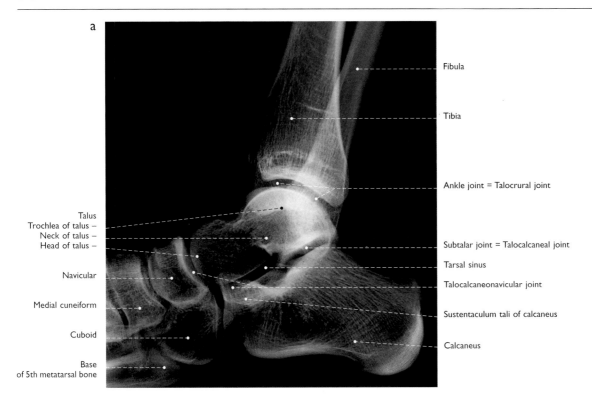

a

Fibula

Tibia

Ankle joint = Talocrural joint

Talus
Trochlea of talus –
Neck of talus –
Head of talus –

Subtalar joint = Talocalcaneal joint

Tarsal sinus

Navicular

Talocalcaneonavicular joint

Medial cuneiform

Sustentaculum tali of calcaneus

Cuboid

Calcaneus

Base
of 5th metatarsal bone

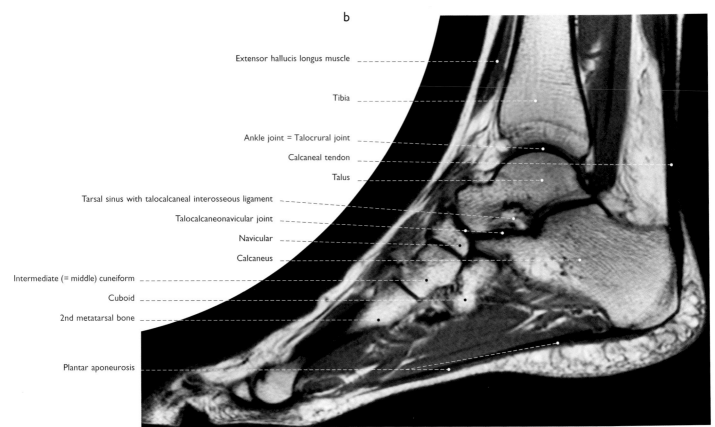

b

Extensor hallucis longus muscle

Tibia

Ankle joint = Talocrural joint

Calcaneal tendon

Talus

Tarsal sinus with talocalcaneal interosseous ligament

Talocalcaneonavicular joint

Navicular

Calcaneus

Intermediate (= middle) cuneiform

Cuboid

2nd metatarsal bone

Plantar aponeurosis

210 Bones and joints of the right foot (70%)

a Mediolateral radiograph
b Sagittal magnetic resonance image (MRI, T$_1$-weighted)
through the medial part of the bones of the right foot, medial aspect

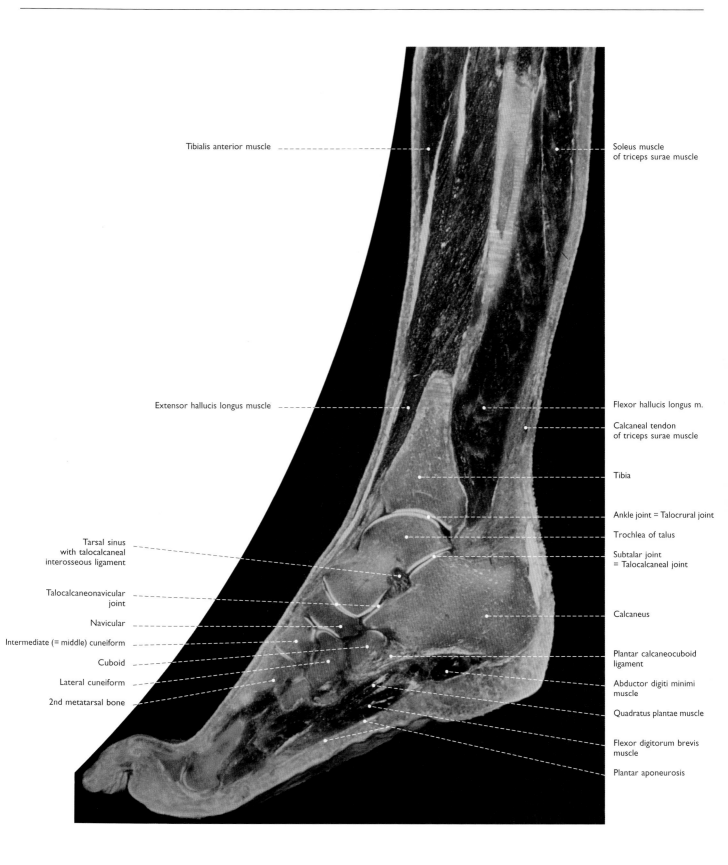

Tibialis anterior muscle

Soleus muscle
of triceps surae muscle

Extensor hallucis longus muscle

Flexor hallucis longus m.

Calcaneal tendon
of triceps surae muscle

Tibia

Ankle joint = Talocrural joint

Trochlea of talus

Subtalar joint
= Talocalcaneal joint

Tarsal sinus
with talocalcaneal
interosseous ligament

Talocalcaneonavicular
joint

Navicular

Intermediate (= middle) cuneiform

Cuboid

Lateral cuneiform

2nd metatarsal bone

Calcaneus

Plantar calcaneocuboid
ligament

Abductor digiti minimi
muscle

Quadratus plantae muscle

Flexor digitorum brevis
muscle

Plantar aponeurosis

211 Bones and joints of the right foot (60%)
Sagittal anatomical section through the medial part
of the bones of the right foot, medial aspect

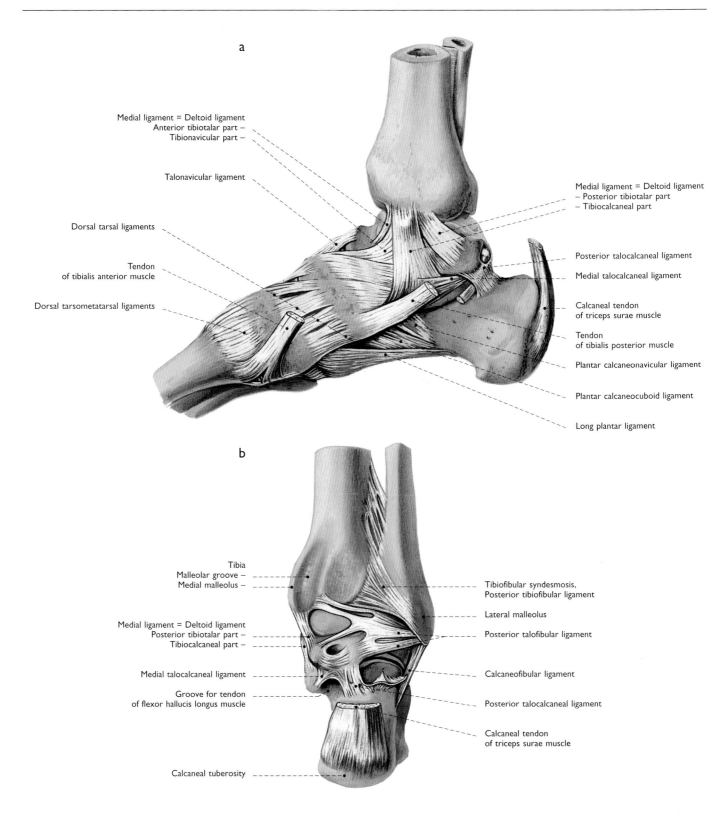

a

Medial ligament = Deltoid ligament
Anterior tibiotalar part –
Tibionavicular part –

Talonavicular ligament

Dorsal tarsal ligaments

Tendon
of tibialis anterior muscle

Dorsal tarsometatarsal ligaments

Medial ligament = Deltoid ligament
– Posterior tibiotalar part
– Tibiocalcaneal part

Posterior talocalcaneal ligament

Medial talocalcaneal ligament

Calcaneal tendon
of triceps surae muscle

Tendon
of tibialis posterior muscle

Plantar calcaneonavicular ligament

Plantar calcaneocuboid ligament

Long plantar ligament

b

Tibia
Malleolar groove –
Medial malleolus –

Medial ligament = Deltoid ligament
Posterior tibiotalar part –
Tibiocalcaneal part –

Medial talocalcaneal ligament

Groove for tendon
of flexor hallucis longus muscle

Calcaneal tuberosity

Tibiofibular syndesmosis,
Posterior tibiofibular ligament

Lateral malleolus

Posterior talofibular ligament

Calcaneofibular ligament

Posterior talocalcaneal ligament

Calcaneal tendon
of triceps surae muscle

212 Joints and ligaments of the right foot (60%)
    a Medial aspect
    b Dorsal aspect

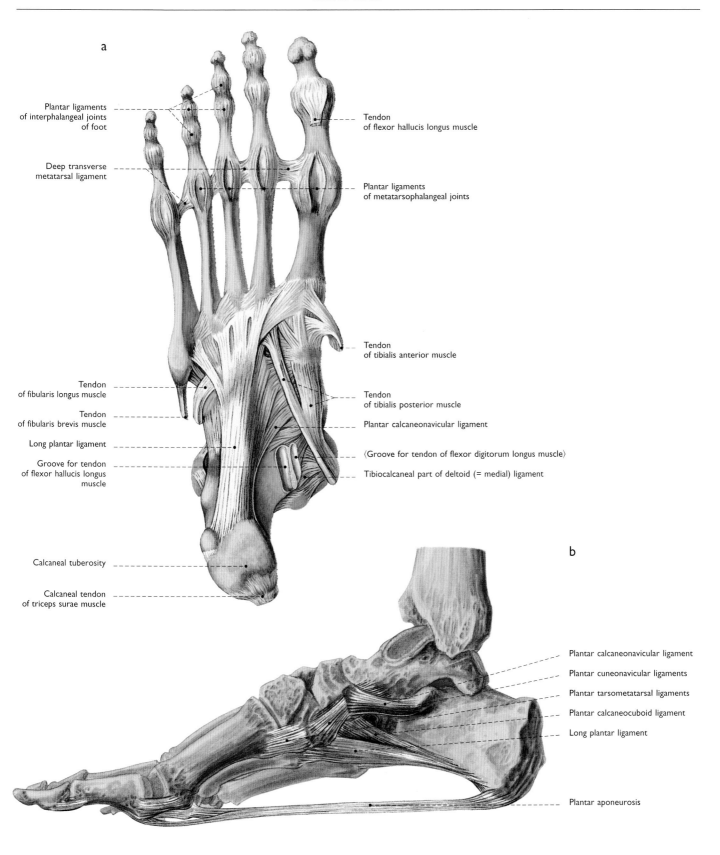

a

Plantar ligaments
of interphalangeal joints
of foot

Deep transverse
metatarsal ligament

Tendon
of flexor hallucis longus muscle

Plantar ligaments
of metatarsophalangeal joints

Tendon
of tibialis anterior muscle

Tendon
of fibularis longus muscle

Tendon
of fibularis brevis muscle

Tendon
of tibialis posterior muscle

Long plantar ligament

Plantar calcaneonavicular ligament

Groove for tendon
of flexor hallucis longus
muscle

⟨Groove for tendon of flexor digitorum longus muscle⟩

Tibiocalcaneal part of deltoid (= medial) ligament

Calcaneal tuberosity

Calcaneal tendon
of triceps surae muscle

b

Plantar calcaneonavicular ligament

Plantar cuneonavicular ligaments

Plantar tarsometatarsal ligaments

Plantar calcaneocuboid ligament

Long plantar ligament

Plantar aponeurosis

213 Joints and ligaments of the right foot (60%)
a Plantar aspect
b Ligaments stabilizing the subtalar (= talocalcaneal)
and talocalcaneonavicular joints, medial aspect

a

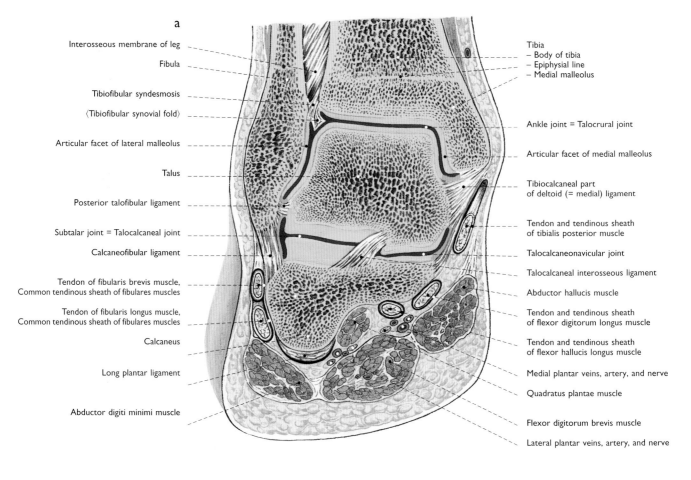

Interosseous membrane of leg

Fibula

Tibiofibular syndesmosis

⟨Tibiofibular synovial fold⟩

Articular facet of lateral malleolus

Talus

Posterior talofibular ligament

Subtalar joint = Talocalcaneal joint

Calcaneofibular ligament

Tendon of fibularis brevis muscle,
Common tendinous sheath of fibulares muscles

Tendon of fibularis longus muscle,
Common tendinous sheath of fibulares muscles

Calcaneus

Long plantar ligament

Abductor digiti minimi muscle

Tibia
− Body of tibia
− Epiphysial line
− Medial malleolus

Ankle joint = Talocrural joint

Articular facet of medial malleolus

Tibiocalcaneal part
of deltoid (= medial) ligament

Tendon and tendinous sheath
of tibialis posterior muscle

Talocalcaneonavicular joint

Talocalcaneal interosseous ligament

Abductor hallucis muscle

Tendon and tendinous sheath
of flexor digitorum longus muscle

Tendon and tendinous sheath
of flexor hallucis longus muscle

Medial plantar veins, artery, and nerve

Quadratus plantae muscle

Flexor digitorum brevis muscle

Lateral plantar veins, artery, and nerve

b

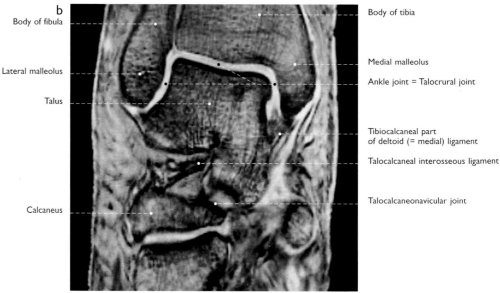

Body of fibula

Lateral malleolus

Talus

Calcaneus

Body of tibia

Medial malleolus

Ankle joint = Talocrural joint

Tibiocalcaneal part
of deltoid (= medial) ligament

Talocalcaneal interosseous ligament

Talocalcaneonavicular joint

**214 Ankle (= talocrural), subtalar,
and talocalcaneonavicular joints
of the right foot** (100%)
Coronal sections, distal aspect
a Anatomical section
b Magnetic resonance image (MRI, T$_2$-weighted)

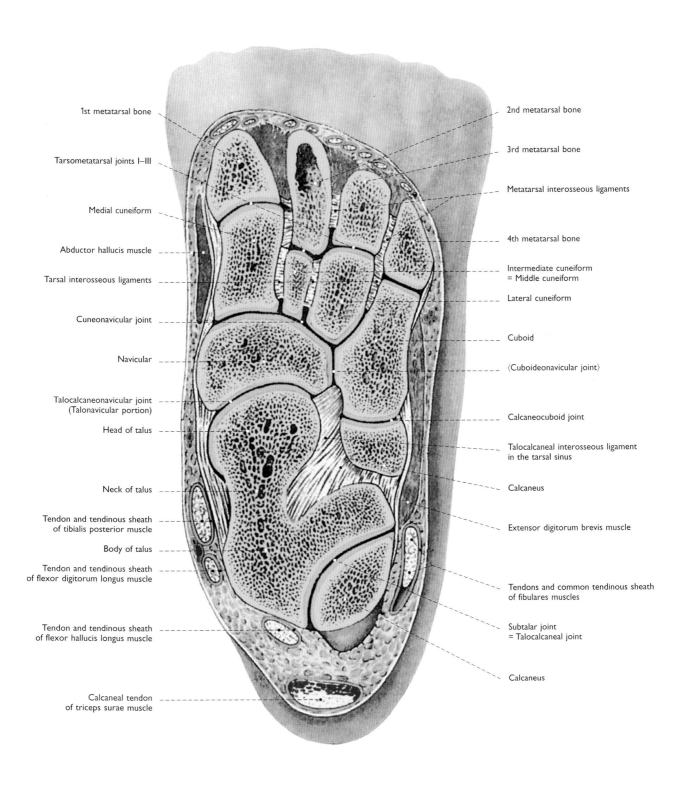

1st metatarsal bone

Tarsometatarsal joints I–III

Medial cuneiform

Abductor hallucis muscle

Tarsal interosseous ligaments

Cuneonavicular joint

Navicular

Talocalcaneonavicular joint
(Talonavicular portion)

Head of talus

Neck of talus

Tendon and tendinous sheath
of tibialis posterior muscle

Body of talus

Tendon and tendinous sheath
of flexor digitorum longus muscle

Tendon and tendinous sheath
of flexor hallucis longus muscle

Calcaneal tendon
of triceps surae muscle

2nd metatarsal bone

3rd metatarsal bone

Metatarsal interosseous ligaments

4th metatarsal bone

Intermediate cuneiform
= Middle cuneiform

Lateral cuneiform

Cuboid

(Cuboideonavicular joint)

Calcaneocuboid joint

Talocalcaneal interosseous ligament
in the tarsal sinus

Calcaneus

Extensor digitorum brevis muscle

Tendons and common tendinous sheath
of fibulares muscles

Subtalar joint
= Talocalcaneal joint

Calcaneus

215 Joints of the right foot (100%)
Horizontal section through the right foot,
proximal aspect of the plantar part

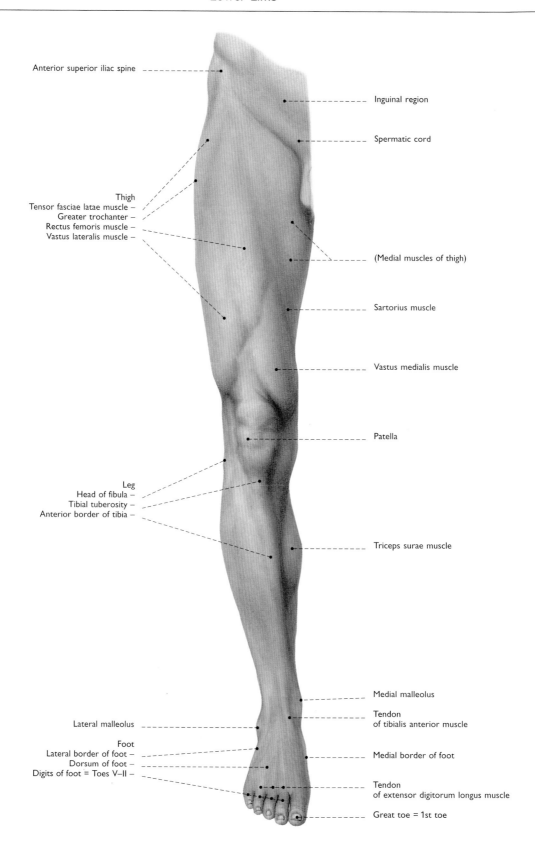

Anterior superior iliac spine

Inguinal region

Spermatic cord

Thigh
Tensor fasciae latae muscle –
Greater trochanter –
Rectus femoris muscle –
Vastus lateralis muscle –

(Medial muscles of thigh)

Sartorius muscle

Vastus medialis muscle

Patella

Leg
Head of fibula –
Tibial tuberosity –
Anterior border of tibia –

Triceps surae muscle

Medial malleolus

Tendon
of tibialis anterior muscle

Lateral malleolus

Foot
Lateral border of foot –
Dorsum of foot –
Digits of foot = Toes V–II –

Medial border of foot

Tendon
of extensor digitorum longus muscle

Great toe = 1st toe

216 Surface anatomy of the right lower limb (20%)
Ventral aspect

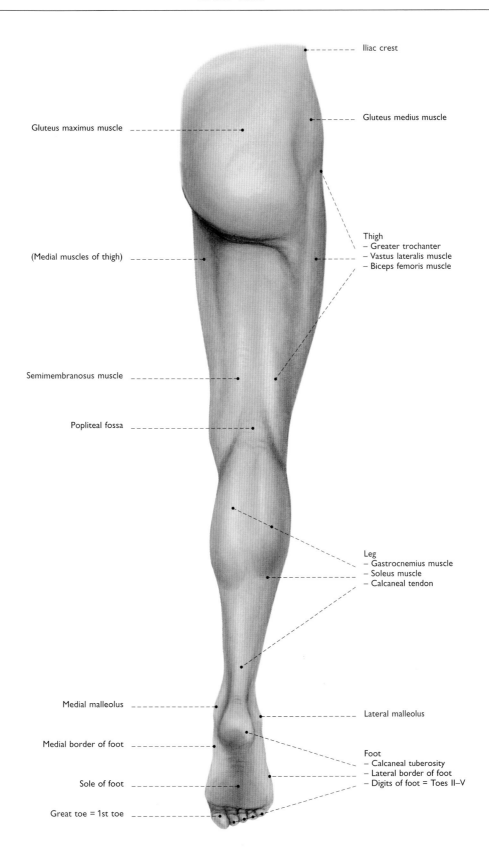

Iliac crest

Gluteus medius muscle

Gluteus maximus muscle

Thigh
– Greater trochanter
– Vastus lateralis muscle
– Biceps femoris muscle

(Medial muscles of thigh)

Semimembranosus muscle

Popliteal fossa

Leg
– Gastrocnemius muscle
– Soleus muscle
– Calcaneal tendon

Medial malleolus

Lateral malleolus

Medial border of foot

Foot
– Calcaneal tuberosity
– Lateral border of foot
– Digits of foot = Toes II–V

Sole of foot

Great toe = 1st toe

217 Surface anatomy of the right lower limb (20%)
Dorsal aspect

a

b

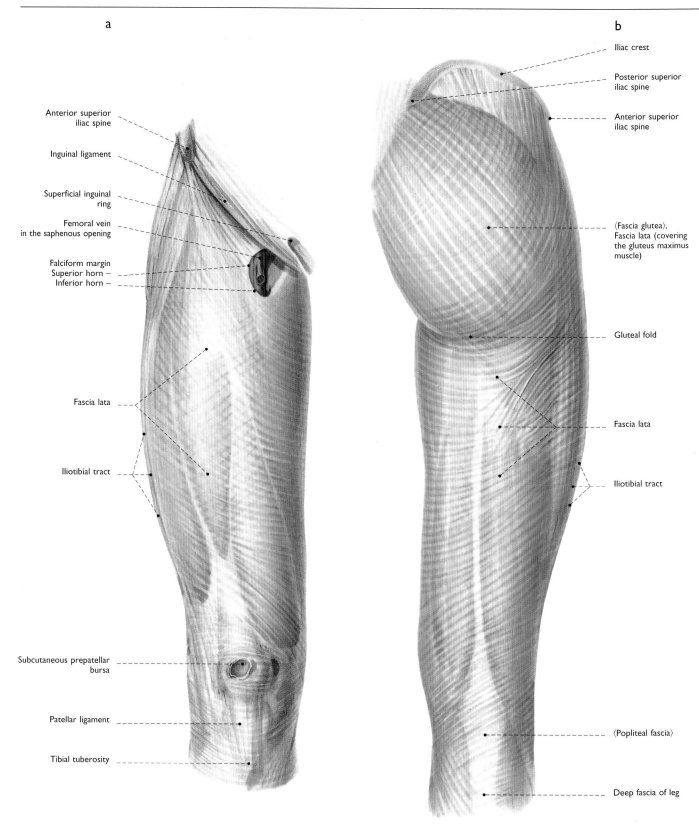

Anterior superior
iliac spine

Inguinal ligament

Superficial inguinal
ring

Femoral vein
in the saphenous opening

Falciform margin
Superior horn –
Inferior horn –

Fascia lata

Iliotibial tract

Subcutaneous prepatellar
bursa

Patellar ligament

Tibial tuberosity

Iliac crest

Posterior superior
iliac spine

Anterior superior
iliac spine

⟨Fascia glutea⟩,
Fascia lata (covering
the gluteus maximus
muscle)

Gluteal fold

Fascia lata

Iliotibial tract

⟨Popliteal fascia⟩

Deep fascia of leg

218 Fascia lata of the right thigh (30%)

a The cribriform fascia in the saphenous opening
   was removed. Ventral aspect
b Dorsal aspect

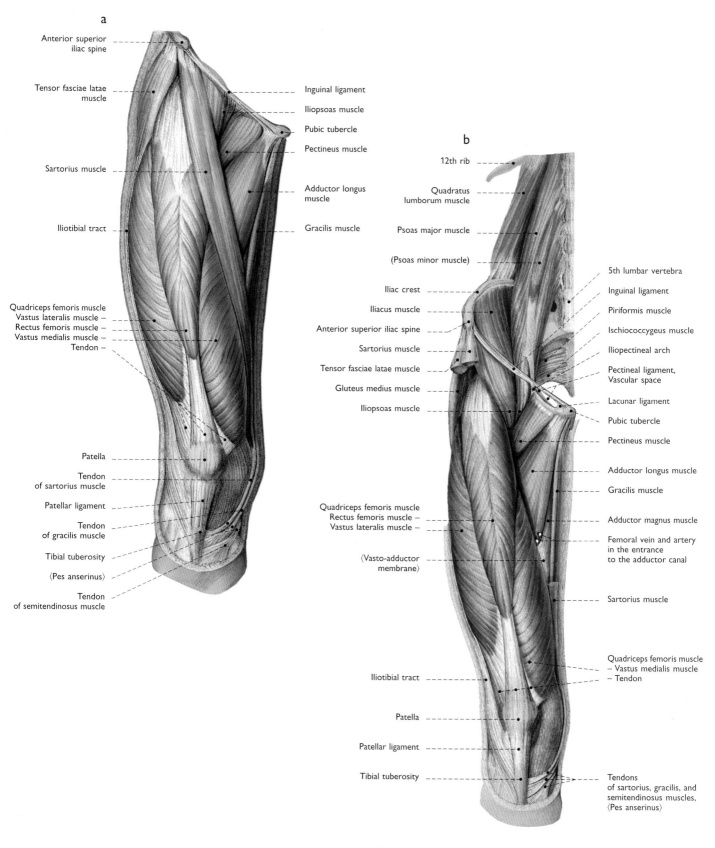

a

Anterior superior iliac spine

Tensor fasciae latae muscle

Sartorius muscle

Iliotibial tract

Quadriceps femoris muscle
Vastus lateralis muscle –
Rectus femoris muscle –
Vastus medialis muscle –
Tendon –

Patella

Tendon of sartorius muscle

Patellar ligament

Tendon of gracilis muscle

Tibial tuberosity

⟨Pes anserinus⟩

Tendon of semitendinosus muscle

Inguinal ligament

Iliopsoas muscle

Pubic tubercle

Pectineus muscle

Adductor longus muscle

Gracilis muscle

b

12th rib

Quadratus lumborum muscle

Psoas major muscle

(Psoas minor muscle)

Iliac crest

Iliacus muscle

Anterior superior iliac spine

Sartorius muscle

Tensor fasciae latae muscle

Gluteus medius muscle

Iliopsoas muscle

Quadriceps femoris muscle
Rectus femoris muscle –
Vastus lateralis muscle –

⟨Vasto-adductor membrane⟩

Iliotibial tract

Patella

Patellar ligament

Tibial tuberosity

5th lumbar vertebra

Inguinal ligament

Piriformis muscle

Ischiococcygeus muscle

Iliopectineal arch

Pectineal ligament, Vascular space

Lacunar ligament

Pubic tubercle

Pectineus muscle

Adductor longus muscle

Gracilis muscle

Adductor magnus muscle

Femoral vein and artery in the entrance to the adductor canal

Sartorius muscle

Quadriceps femoris muscle
– Vastus medialis muscle
– Tendon

Tendons of sartorius, gracilis, and semitendinosus muscles, ⟨Pes anserinus⟩

219 Muscles of the right thigh (25%)

Ventral aspect
a Anterior muscles of thigh
b The sartorius and tensor fasciae latae muscles were partially removed. Some muscles of the pelvis are additionally shown.

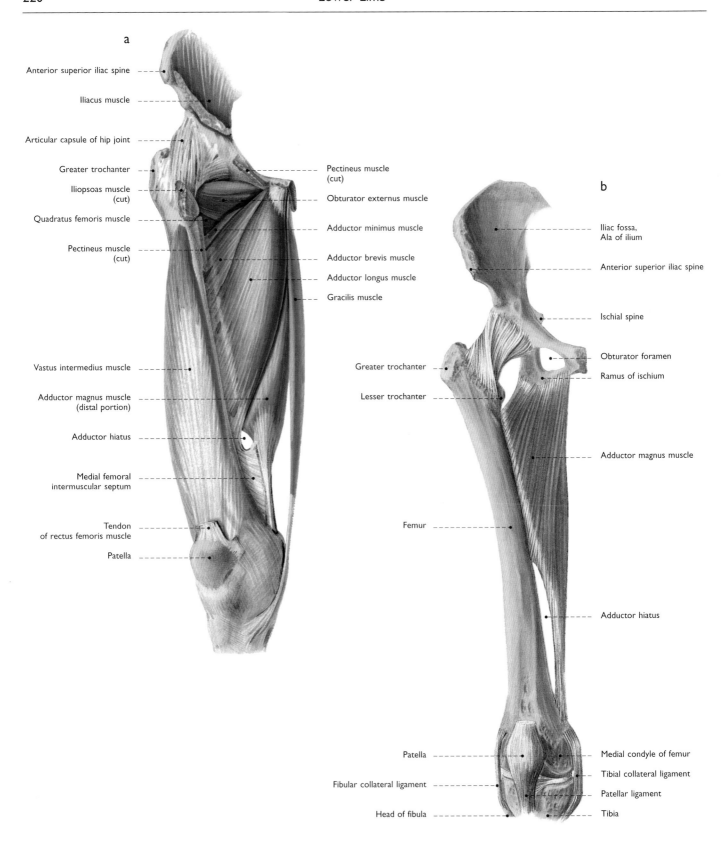

a

Anterior superior iliac spine

Iliacus muscle

Articular capsule of hip joint

Greater trochanter

Iliopsoas muscle
(cut)

Quadratus femoris muscle

Pectineus muscle
(cut)

Vastus intermedius muscle

Adductor magnus muscle
(distal portion)

Adductor hiatus

Medial femoral
intermuscular septum

Tendon
of rectus femoris muscle

Patella

Pectineus muscle
(cut)

Obturator externus muscle

Adductor minimus muscle

Adductor brevis muscle

Adductor longus muscle

Gracilis muscle

b

Iliac fossa,
Ala of ilium

Anterior superior iliac spine

Ischial spine

Obturator foramen

Ramus of ischium

Greater trochanter

Lesser trochanter

Adductor magnus muscle

Femur

Adductor hiatus

Patella

Fibular collateral ligament

Head of fibula

Medial condyle of femur

Tibial collateral ligament

Patellar ligament

Tibia

220 Muscles of the right thigh (25%)

Ventral aspect
a Medial muscles (adductors) of thigh
   and deep part of the quadriceps femoris muscle
b Adductor magnus muscle

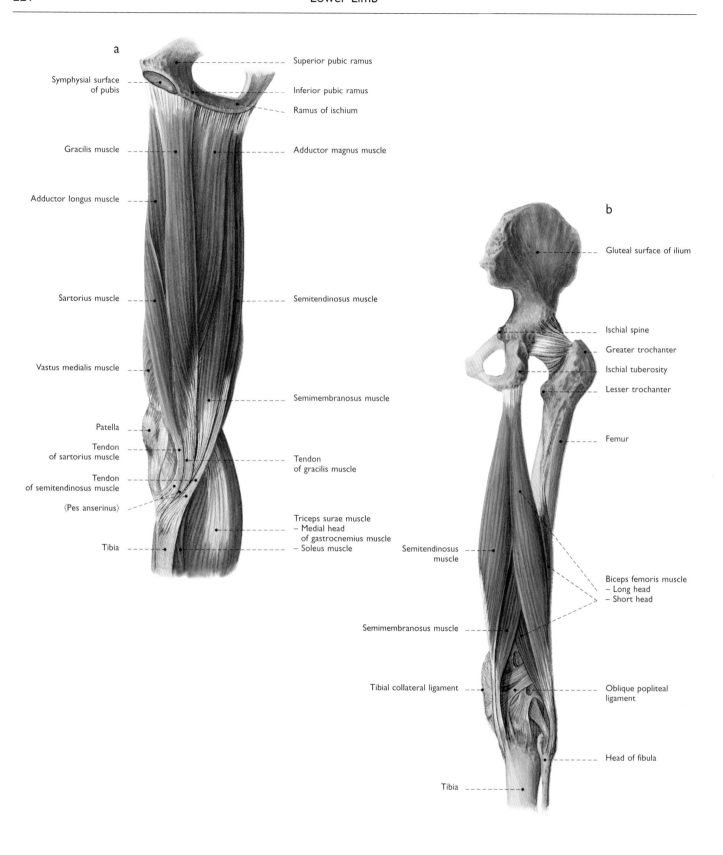

a

Symphysial surface of pubis

Gracilis muscle

Adductor longus muscle

Sartorius muscle

Vastus medialis muscle

Patella

Tendon of sartorius muscle

Tendon of semitendinosus muscle

⟨Pes anserinus⟩

Tibia

Superior pubic ramus

Inferior pubic ramus

Ramus of ischium

Adductor magnus muscle

Semitendinosus muscle

Semimembranosus muscle

Tendon of gracilis muscle

Triceps surae muscle
– Medial head of gastrocnemius muscle
– Soleus muscle

b

Gluteal surface of ilium

Ischial spine

Greater trochanter

Ischial tuberosity

Lesser trochanter

Femur

Semitendinosus muscle

Biceps femoris muscle
– Long head
– Short head

Semimembranosus muscle

Tibial collateral ligament

Oblique popliteal ligament

Head of fibula

Tibia

221 Muscles of the right thigh (25%)
a Medial muscles (adductors) of thigh, medial aspect
b Posterior muscles of thigh ('hamstrings'), dorsal aspect

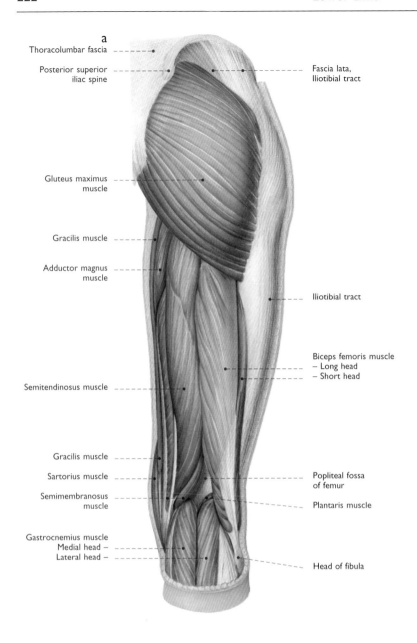

a

Thoracolumbar fascia

Posterior superior
iliac spine

Gluteus maximus
muscle

Gracilis muscle

Adductor magnus
muscle

Semitendinosus muscle

Gracilis muscle

Sartorius muscle

Semimembranosus
muscle

Gastrocnemius muscle
Medial head –
Lateral head –

Fascia lata,
Iliotibial tract

Iliotibial tract

Biceps femoris muscle
– Long head
– Short head

Popliteal fossa
of femur

Plantaris muscle

Head of fibula

b

Gluteus maximus muscle

Long head
of biceps femoris muscle

Semitendinosus muscle

Adductor magnus muscle

Gracilis muscle

Semimembranosus muscle

222   Muscles of the right thigh and
superficial layer of the muscles of the hip
a   Dorsal aspect (20%)
b   Coronal magnetic resonance image (MRI, T$_1$-weighted)

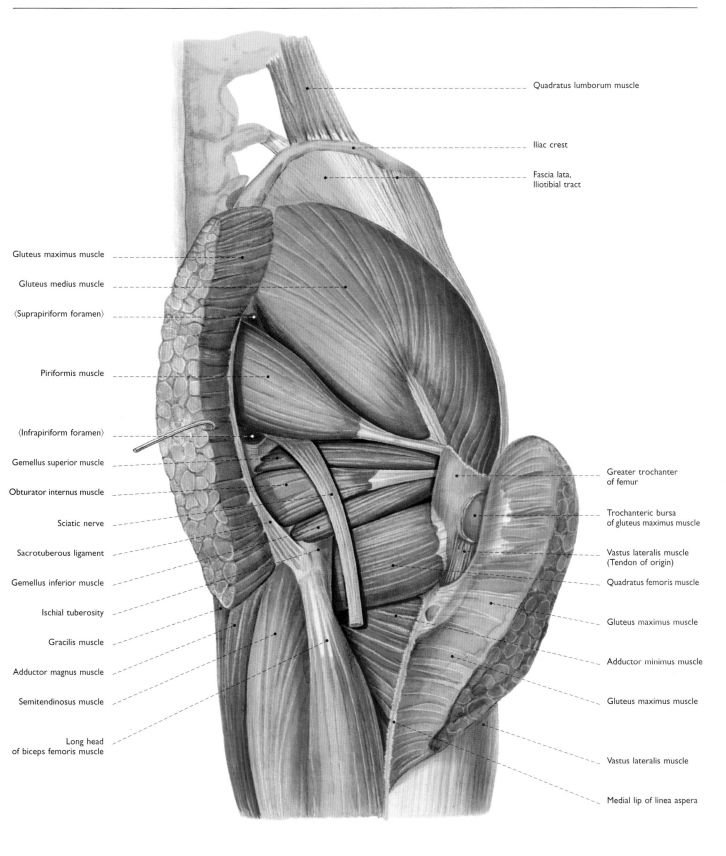

Quadratus lumborum muscle

Iliac crest

Fascia lata,
Iliotibial tract

Gluteus maximus muscle

Gluteus medius muscle

⟨Suprapiriform foramen⟩

Piriformis muscle

⟨Infrapiriform foramen⟩

Gemellus superior muscle

Obturator internus muscle

Sciatic nerve

Sacrotuberous ligament

Gemellus inferior muscle

Ischial tuberosity

Gracilis muscle

Adductor magnus muscle

Semitendinosus muscle

Long head
of biceps femoris muscle

Greater trochanter
of femur

Trochanteric bursa
of gluteus maximus muscle

Vastus lateralis muscle
(Tendon of origin)

Quadratus femoris muscle

Gluteus maximus muscle

Adductor minimus muscle

Gluteus maximus muscle

Vastus lateralis muscle

Medial lip of linea aspera

223 Muscles of the right hip (50%)
Deep layer. The gluteus maximus muscle was divided.
Dorsal aspect

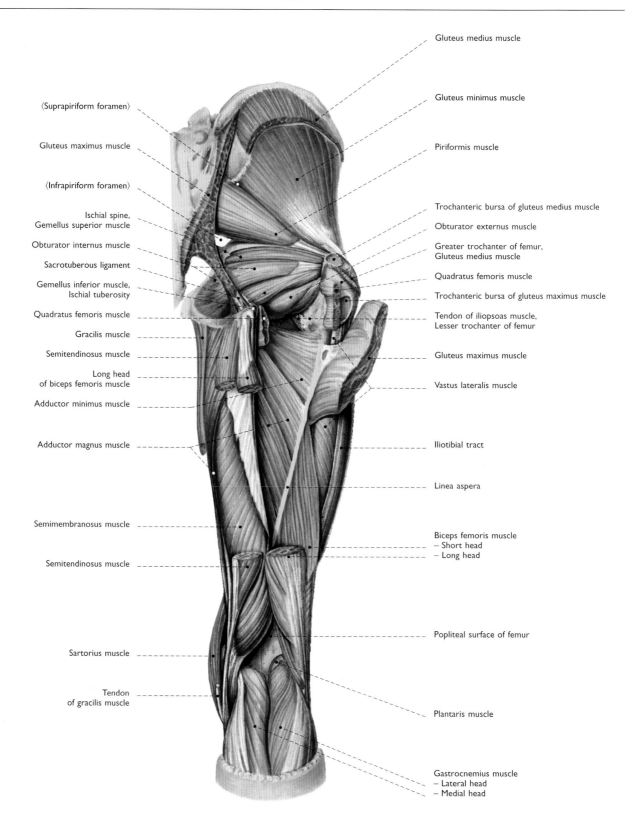

⟨Suprapiriform foramen⟩

Gluteus maximus muscle

⟨Infrapiriform foramen⟩

Ischial spine,
Gemellus superior muscle

Obturator internus muscle

Sacrotuberous ligament

Gemellus inferior muscle,
Ischial tuberosity

Quadratus femoris muscle

Gracilis muscle

Semitendinosus muscle

Long head
of biceps femoris muscle

Adductor minimus muscle

Adductor magnus muscle

Semimembranosus muscle

Semitendinosus muscle

Sartorius muscle

Tendon
of gracilis muscle

Gluteus medius muscle

Gluteus minimus muscle

Piriformis muscle

Trochanteric bursa of gluteus medius muscle

Obturator externus muscle

Greater trochanter of femur,
Gluteus medius muscle

Quadratus femoris muscle

Trochanteric bursa of gluteus maximus muscle

Tendon of iliopsoas muscle,
Lesser trochanter of femur

Gluteus maximus muscle

Vastus lateralis muscle

Iliotibial tract

Linea aspera

Biceps femoris muscle
– Short head
– Long head

Popliteal surface of femur

Plantaris muscle

Gastrocnemius muscle
– Lateral head
– Medial head

224 Muscles of the right thigh and hip (30%)
Deep muscular layer. The superficial muscles were partially removed.
Dorsal aspect

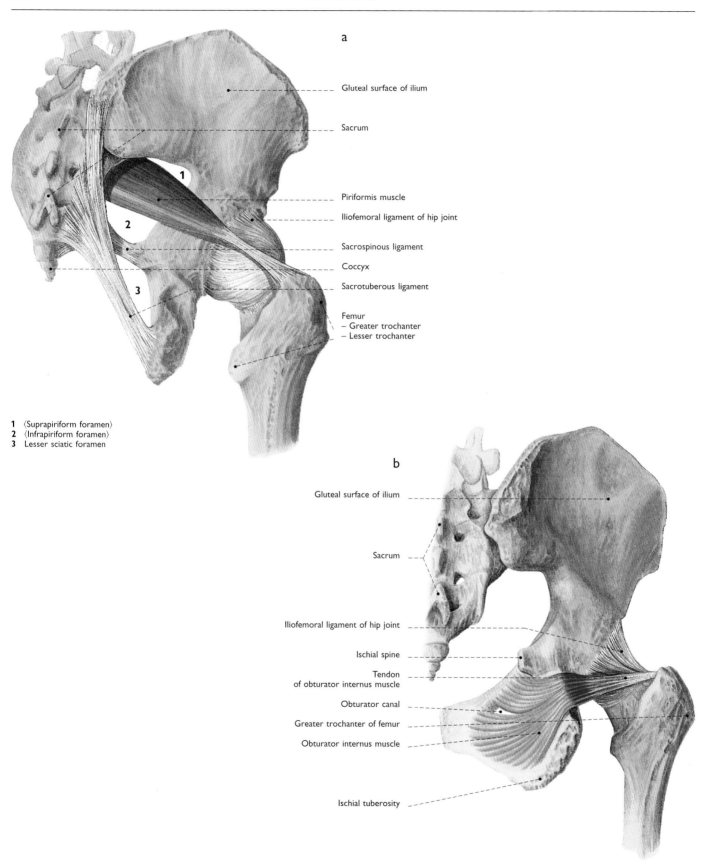

a

Gluteal surface of ilium

Sacrum

Piriformis muscle

Iliofemoral ligament of hip joint

Sacrospinous ligament

Coccyx

Sacrotuberous ligament

Femur
– Greater trochanter
– Lesser trochanter

1 ⟨Suprapiriform foramen⟩
2 ⟨Infrapiriform foramen⟩
3 Lesser sciatic foramen

b

Gluteal surface of ilium

Sacrum

Iliofemoral ligament of hip joint

Ischial spine

Tendon
of obturator internus muscle

Obturator canal

Greater trochanter of femur

Obturator internus muscle

Ischial tuberosity

225 Muscles of the right hip (40%)
Dorsal aspect
a Piriformis muscle
b Obturator internus muscle

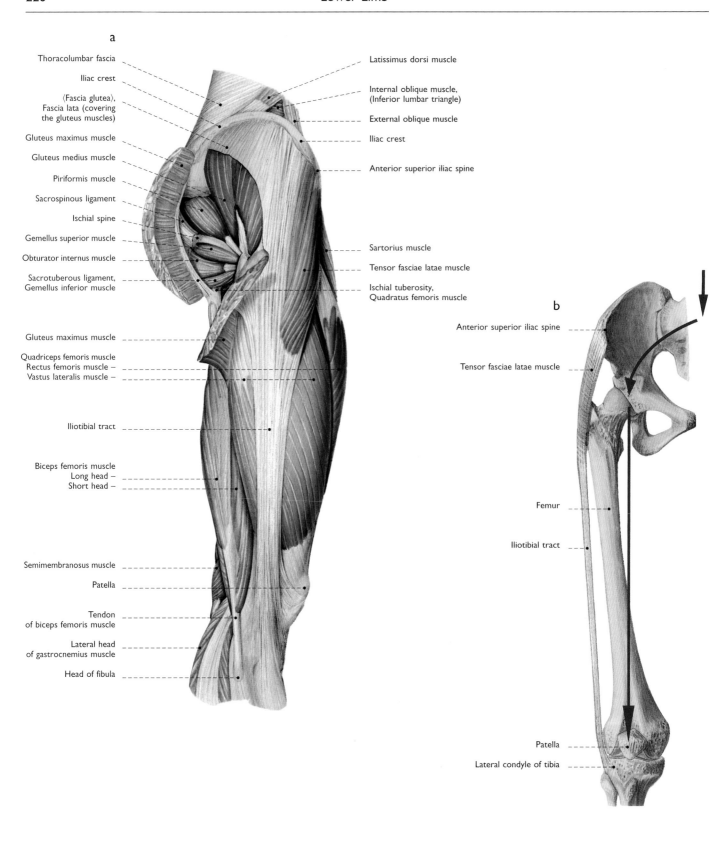

a

Thoracolumbar fascia

Iliac crest

⟨Fascia glutea⟩,
Fascia lata (covering
the gluteus muscles)

Gluteus maximus muscle

Gluteus medius muscle

Piriformis muscle

Sacrospinous ligament

Ischial spine

Gemellus superior muscle

Obturator internus muscle

Sacrotuberous ligament,
Gemellus inferior muscle

Gluteus maximus muscle

Quadriceps femoris muscle
Rectus femoris muscle –
Vastus lateralis muscle –

Iliotibial tract

Biceps femoris muscle
Long head –
Short head –

Semimembranosus muscle

Patella

Tendon
of biceps femoris muscle

Lateral head
of gastrocnemius muscle

Head of fibula

Latissimus dorsi muscle

Internal oblique muscle,
(Inferior lumbar triangle)

External oblique muscle

Iliac crest

Anterior superior iliac spine

Sartorius muscle

Tensor fasciae latae muscle

Ischial tuberosity,
Quadratus femoris muscle

b

Anterior superior iliac spine

Tensor fasciae latae muscle

Femur

Iliotibial tract

Patella

Lateral condyle of tibia

226 Muscles of the right thigh and hip (20%)

a The gluteus maximus muscle was divided and turned up. Lateral aspect
b Tensor fasciae latae muscle and iliotibial tract, ventral aspect.
The arrow indicates the weight line in erect posture.

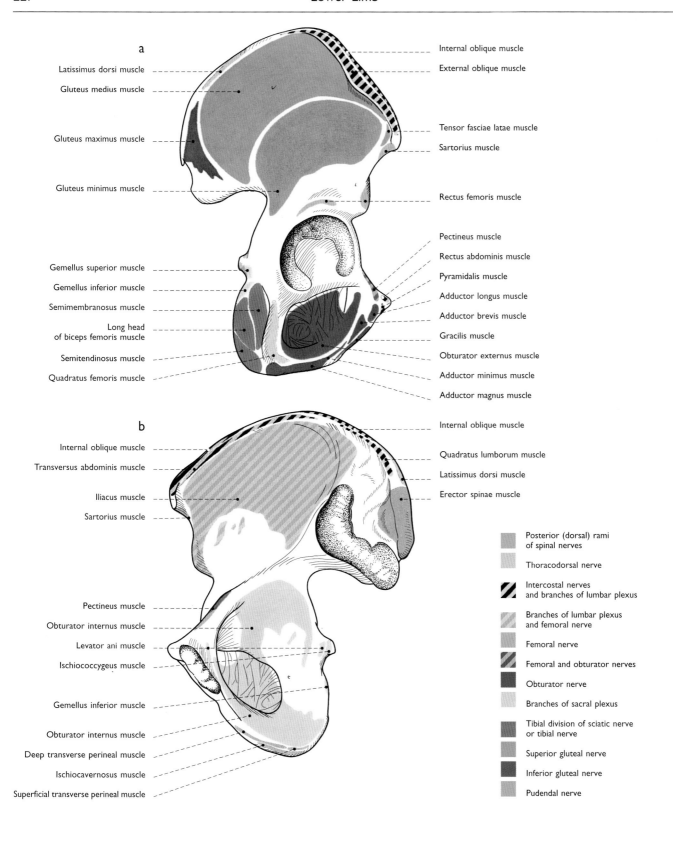

a

Latissimus dorsi muscle
Gluteus medius muscle

Gluteus maximus muscle

Gluteus minimus muscle

Gemellus superior muscle
Gemellus inferior muscle
Semimembranosus muscle
Long head
of biceps femoris muscle
Semitendinosus muscle
Quadratus femoris muscle

Internal oblique muscle
External oblique muscle

Tensor fasciae latae muscle
Sartorius muscle

Rectus femoris muscle

Pectineus muscle
Rectus abdominis muscle
Pyramidalis muscle
Adductor longus muscle
Adductor brevis muscle
Gracilis muscle
Obturator externus muscle
Adductor minimus muscle
Adductor magnus muscle

b

Internal oblique muscle
Transversus abdominis muscle

Iliacus muscle
Sartorius muscle

Pectineus muscle
Obturator internus muscle
Levator ani muscle
Ischiococcygeus muscle

Gemellus inferior muscle

Obturator internus muscle
Deep transverse perineal muscle
Ischiocavernosus muscle
Superficial transverse perineal muscle

Internal oblique muscle

Quadratus lumborum muscle
Latissimus dorsi muscle
Erector spinae muscle

Posterior (dorsal) rami
of spinal nerves

Thoracodorsal nerve

Intercostal nerves
and branches of lumbar plexus

Branches of lumbar plexus
and femoral nerve

Femoral nerve

Femoral and obturator nerves

Obturator nerve

Branches of sacral plexus

Tibial division of sciatic nerve
or tibial nerve

Superior gluteal nerve

Inferior gluteal nerve

Pudendal nerve

227 Muscle attachments to the right hip bone
The colors indicate the innervation of the muscles
attaching to the
a outer surface
b inner surface.

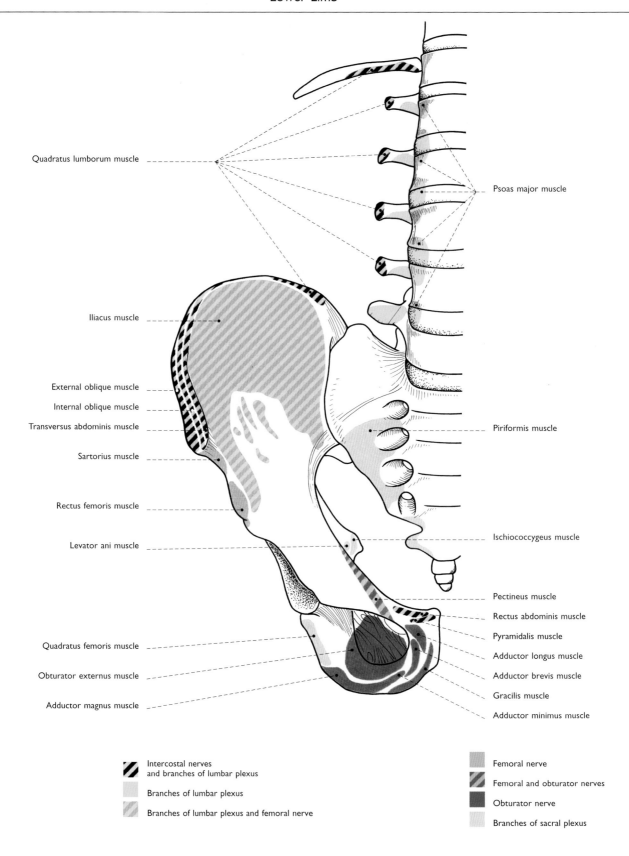

Quadratus lumborum muscle

Psoas major muscle

Iliacus muscle

External oblique muscle
Internal oblique muscle
Transversus abdominis muscle

Piriformis muscle

Sartorius muscle

Rectus femoris muscle

Levator ani muscle

Ischiococcygeus muscle

Pectineus muscle
Rectus abdominis muscle
Pyramidalis muscle
Adductor longus muscle
Adductor brevis muscle
Gracilis muscle
Adductor minimus muscle

Quadratus femoris muscle

Obturator externus muscle

Adductor magnus muscle

Intercostal nerves
and branches of lumbar plexus

Branches of lumbar plexus

Branches of lumbar plexus and femoral nerve

Femoral nerve

Femoral and obturator nerves

Obturator nerve

Branches of sacral plexus

228 Muscle attachments to the lumbar spine
and the pelvic girdle on the right side
The colors indicate the innervation.
Ventral aspect

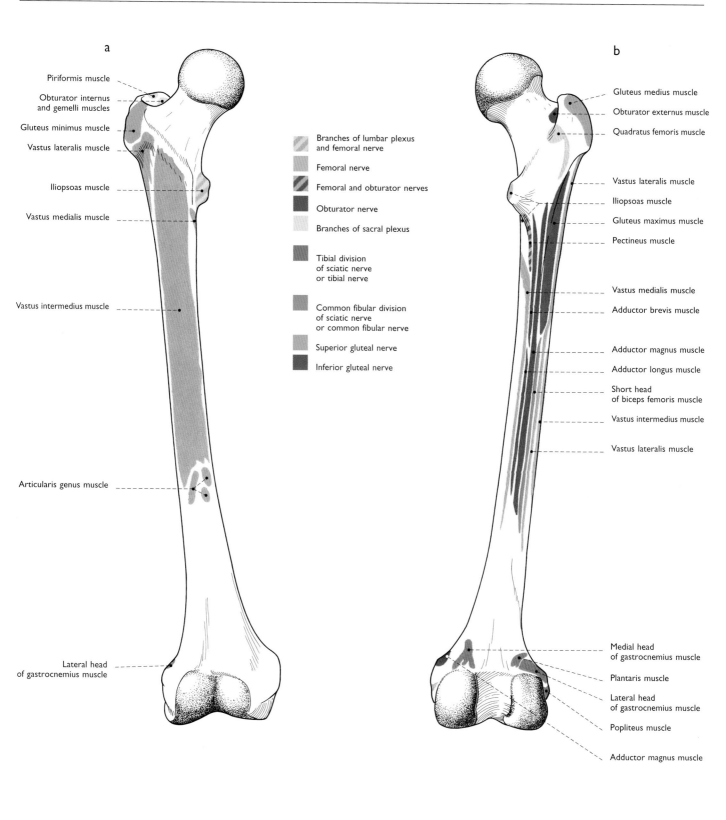

a

Piriformis muscle

Obturator internus and gemelli muscles

Gluteus minimus muscle

Vastus lateralis muscle

Iliopsoas muscle

Vastus medialis muscle

Vastus intermedius muscle

Articularis genus muscle

Lateral head of gastrocnemius muscle

b

Gluteus medius muscle

Obturator externus muscle

Quadratus femoris muscle

Vastus lateralis muscle

Iliopsoas muscle

Gluteus maximus muscle

Pectineus muscle

Vastus medialis muscle

Adductor brevis muscle

Adductor magnus muscle

Adductor longus muscle

Short head of biceps femoris muscle

Vastus intermedius muscle

Vastus lateralis muscle

Medial head of gastrocnemius muscle

Plantaris muscle

Lateral head of gastrocnemius muscle

Popliteus muscle

Adductor magnus muscle

Branches of lumbar plexus and femoral nerve

Femoral nerve

Femoral and obturator nerves

Obturator nerve

Branches of sacral plexus

Tibial division of sciatic nerve or tibial nerve

Common fibular division of sciatic nerve or common fibular nerve

Superior gluteal nerve

Inferior gluteal nerve

229 Muscle attachments to the right thigh bone (= femur)
The colors indicate the innervation of the muscles attaching to the
a ventral surface
b dorsal surface.

a

Fascia lata

Iliotibial tract

Subcutaneous prepatellar
bursa

Patella

Patellar ligament

Tibia
– Tibial tuberosity
– Anterior border
– Medial surface
– Medial malleolus

Deep fascia of leg

Superior extensor
retinaculum

Inferior extensor
retinaculum

Dorsal fascia of foot

b

Fascia lata

⟨Popliteal fascia⟩

Deep fascia of leg

Calcaneal tendon
of triceps surae muscle

Lateral malleolus
of fibula

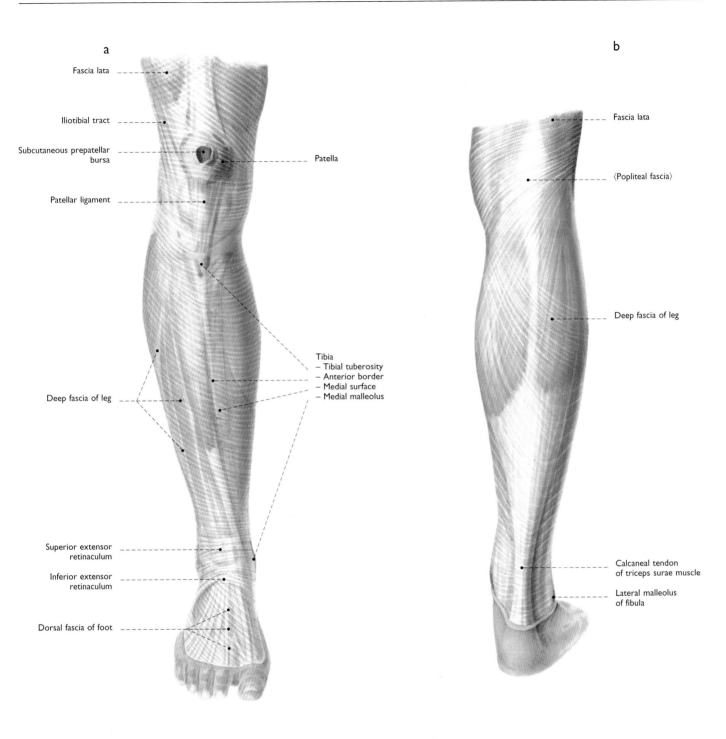

**230 Fasciae of the right leg
and the dorsum of foot** (25%)

a   Ventral aspect
b   Dorsal aspect

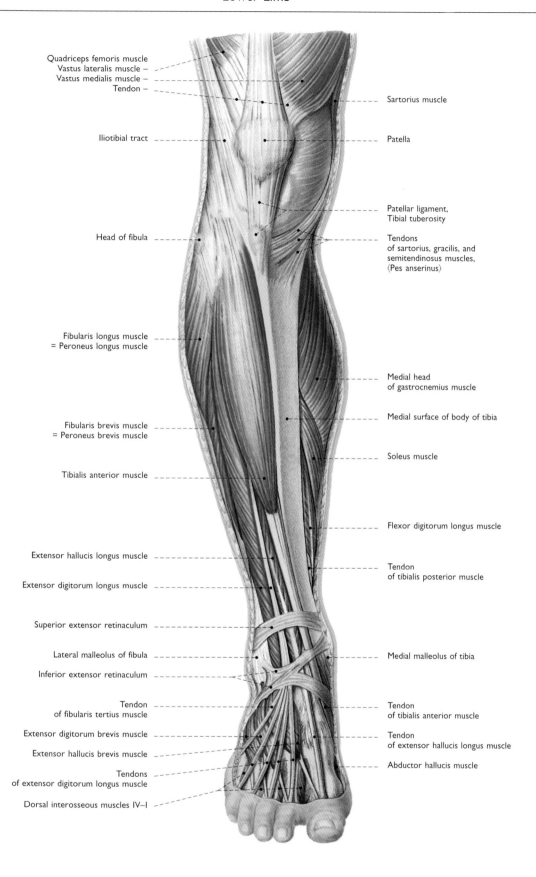

Quadriceps femoris muscle
Vastus lateralis muscle –
Vastus medialis muscle –
Tendon –

Iliotibial tract

Head of fibula

Fibularis longus muscle
= Peroneus longus muscle

Fibularis brevis muscle
= Peroneus brevis muscle

Tibialis anterior muscle

Extensor hallucis longus muscle

Extensor digitorum longus muscle

Superior extensor retinaculum

Lateral malleolus of fibula

Inferior extensor retinaculum

Tendon
of fibularis tertius muscle

Extensor digitorum brevis muscle

Extensor hallucis brevis muscle

Tendons
of extensor digitorum longus muscle

Dorsal interosseous muscles IV–I

Sartorius muscle

Patella

Patellar ligament,
Tibial tuberosity

Tendons
of sartorius, gracilis, and
semitendinosus muscles,
(Pes anserinus)

Medial head
of gastrocnemius muscle

Medial surface of body of tibia

Soleus muscle

Flexor digitorum longus muscle

Tendon
of tibialis posterior muscle

Medial malleolus of tibia

Tendon
of tibialis anterior muscle

Tendon
of extensor hallucis longus muscle

Abductor hallucis muscle

**231 Muscles of the right leg
and the dorsum of foot** (30%)
Ventral aspect

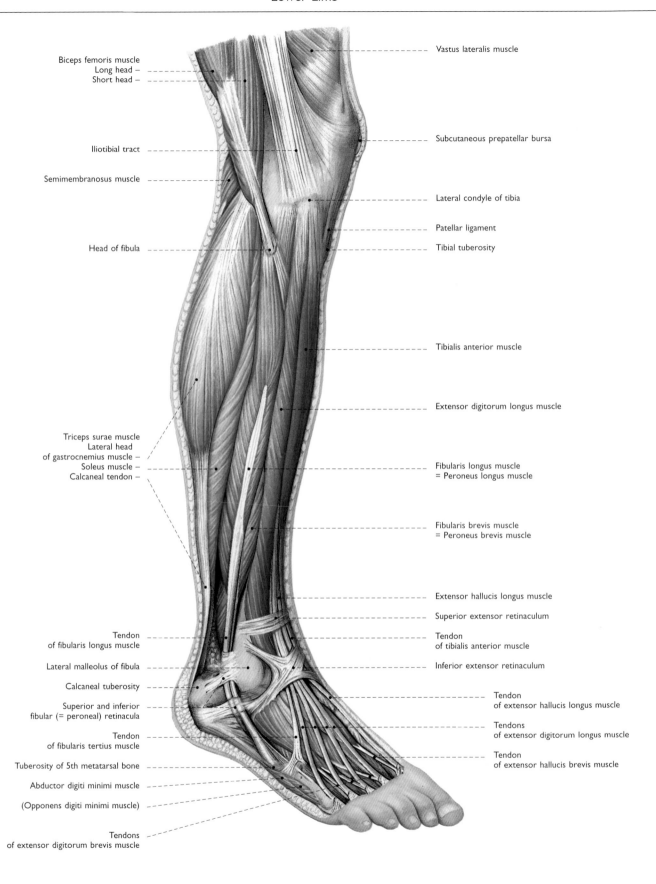

Biceps femoris muscle
Long head –
Short head –

Iliotibial tract

Semimembranosus muscle

Head of fibula

Triceps surae muscle
Lateral head
of gastrocnemius muscle –
Soleus muscle –
Calcaneal tendon –

Tendon
of fibularis longus muscle

Lateral malleolus of fibula

Calcaneal tuberosity

Superior and inferior
fibular (= peroneal) retinacula

Tendon
of fibularis tertius muscle

Tuberosity of 5th metatarsal bone

Abductor digiti minimi muscle

(Opponens digiti minimi muscle)

Tendons
of extensor digitorum brevis muscle

Vastus lateralis muscle

Subcutaneous prepatellar bursa

Lateral condyle of tibia

Patellar ligament

Tibial tuberosity

Tibialis anterior muscle

Extensor digitorum longus muscle

Fibularis longus muscle
= Peroneus longus muscle

Fibularis brevis muscle
= Peroneus brevis muscle

Extensor hallucis longus muscle

Superior extensor retinaculum

Tendon
of tibialis anterior muscle

Inferior extensor retinaculum

Tendon
of extensor hallucis longus muscle

Tendons
of extensor digitorum longus muscle

Tendon
of extensor hallucis brevis muscle

**232 Muscles of the right leg and
the dorsum of foot** (30%)
Lateral aspect

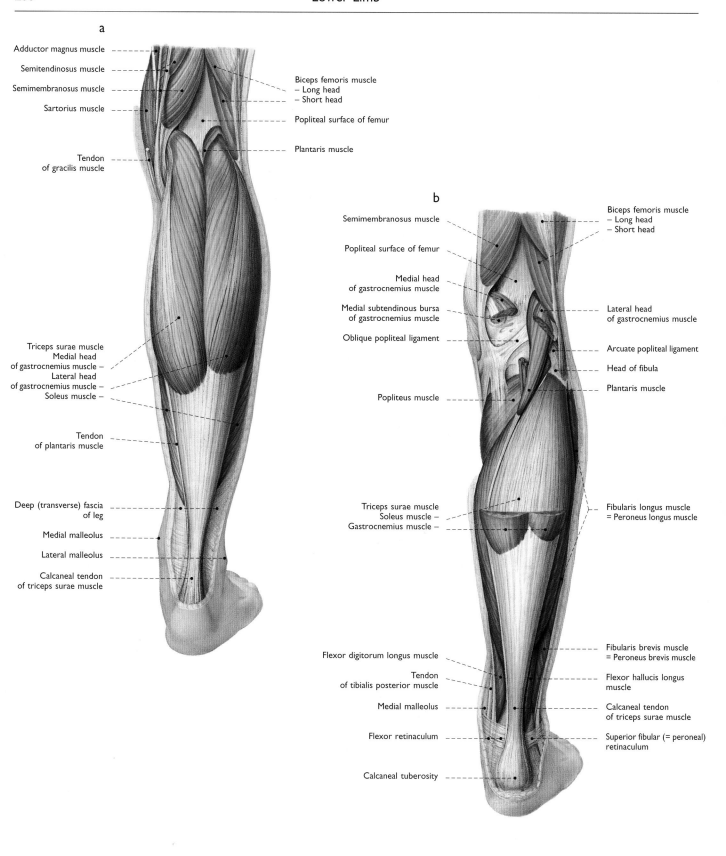

a

Adductor magnus muscle

Semitendinosus muscle

Semimembranosus muscle

Sartorius muscle

Tendon
of gracilis muscle

Biceps femoris muscle
– Long head
– Short head

Popliteal surface of femur

Plantaris muscle

Triceps surae muscle
Medial head
of gastrocnemius muscle –
Lateral head
of gastrocnemius muscle –
Soleus muscle –

Tendon
of plantaris muscle

Deep (transverse) fascia
of leg

Medial malleolus

Lateral malleolus

Calcaneal tendon
of triceps surae muscle

b

Semimembranosus muscle

Popliteal surface of femur

Medial head
of gastrocnemius muscle

Medial subtendinous bursa
of gastrocnemius muscle

Oblique popliteal ligament

Popliteus muscle

Triceps surae muscle
Soleus muscle –
Gastrocnemius muscle –

Biceps femoris muscle
– Long head
– Short head

Lateral head
of gastrocnemius muscle

Arcuate popliteal ligament

Head of fibula

Plantaris muscle

Fibularis longus muscle
= Peroneus longus muscle

Flexor digitorum longus muscle

Tendon
of tibialis posterior muscle

Medial malleolus

Flexor retinaculum

Calcaneal tuberosity

Fibularis brevis muscle
= Peroneus brevis muscle

Flexor hallucis longus
muscle

Calcaneal tendon
of triceps surae muscle

Superior fibular (= peroneal)
retinaculum

233 Muscles of the right leg (25%)
     Dorsal aspect
a   Most superficial layer
b   Superficial layer after partial removal
    of the gastrocnemius muscle

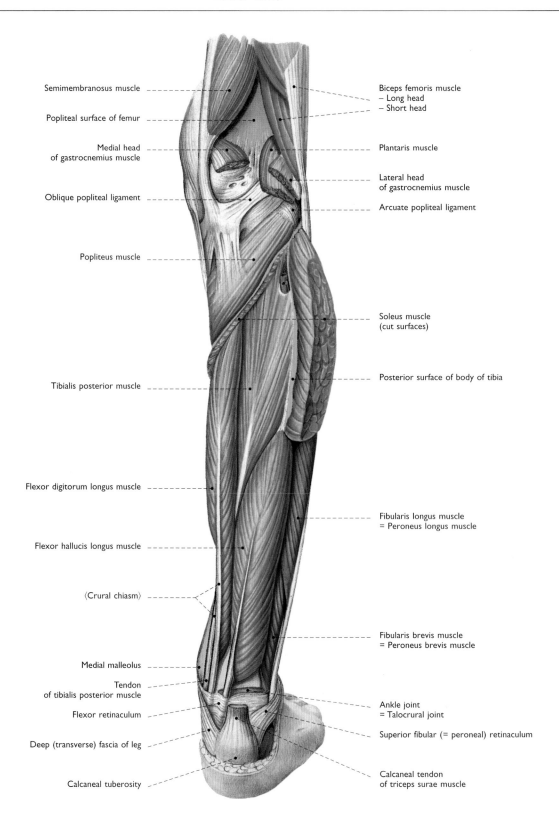

Semimembranosus muscle

Popliteal surface of femur

Medial head
of gastrocnemius muscle

Oblique popliteal ligament

Popliteus muscle

Tibialis posterior muscle

Flexor digitorum longus muscle

Flexor hallucis longus muscle

⟨Crural chiasm⟩

Medial malleolus

Tendon
of tibialis posterior muscle

Flexor retinaculum

Deep (transverse) fascia of leg

Calcaneal tuberosity

Biceps femoris muscle
– Long head
– Short head

Plantaris muscle

Lateral head
of gastrocnemius muscle

Arcuate popliteal ligament

Soleus muscle
(cut surfaces)

Posterior surface of body of tibia

Fibularis longus muscle
= Peroneus longus muscle

Fibularis brevis muscle
= Peroneus brevis muscle

Ankle joint
= Talocrural joint

Superior fibular (= peroneal) retinaculum

Calcaneal tendon
of triceps surae muscle

234 Muscles of the right leg (30%)
Deep layer, dorsal aspect

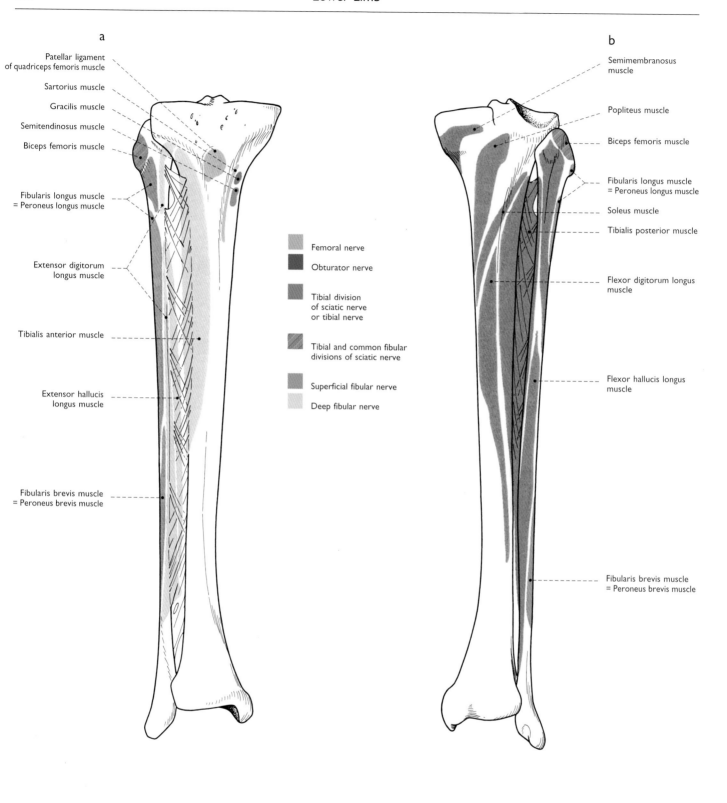

a

Patellar ligament
of quadriceps femoris muscle

Sartorius muscle

Gracilis muscle

Semitendinosus muscle

Biceps femoris muscle

Fibularis longus muscle
= Peroneus longus muscle

Extensor digitorum
longus muscle

Tibialis anterior muscle

Extensor hallucis
longus muscle

Fibularis brevis muscle
= Peroneus brevis muscle

b

Semimembranosus
muscle

Popliteus muscle

Biceps femoris muscle

Fibularis longus muscle
= Peroneus longus muscle

Soleus muscle

Tibialis posterior muscle

Flexor digitorum longus
muscle

Flexor hallucis longus
muscle

Fibularis brevis muscle
= Peroneus brevis muscle

Femoral nerve

Obturator nerve

Tibial division
of sciatic nerve
or tibial nerve

Tibial and common fibular
divisions of sciatic nerve

Superficial fibular nerve

Deep fibular nerve

235 Muscle attachments to the right tibia, fibula,
and the interosseous membrane of leg
The colors indicate the innervation of the muscles
attaching to the
a ventral surface
b dorsal surface.

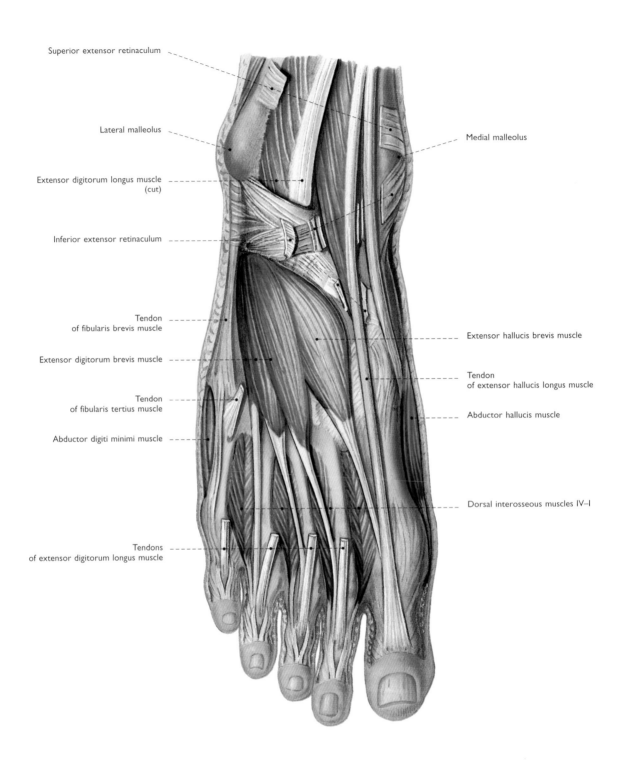

Superior extensor retinaculum

Lateral malleolus

Medial malleolus

Extensor digitorum longus muscle (cut)

Inferior extensor retinaculum

Tendon of fibularis brevis muscle

Extensor hallucis brevis muscle

Extensor digitorum brevis muscle

Tendon of extensor hallucis longus muscle

Tendon of fibularis tertius muscle

Abductor hallucis muscle

Abductor digiti minimi muscle

Dorsal interosseous muscles IV–I

Tendons of extensor digitorum longus muscle

236 Muscles of the dorsum of the right foot (75%)
The extensor digitorum longus muscle and the retinacula
were partially removed. Ventral aspect

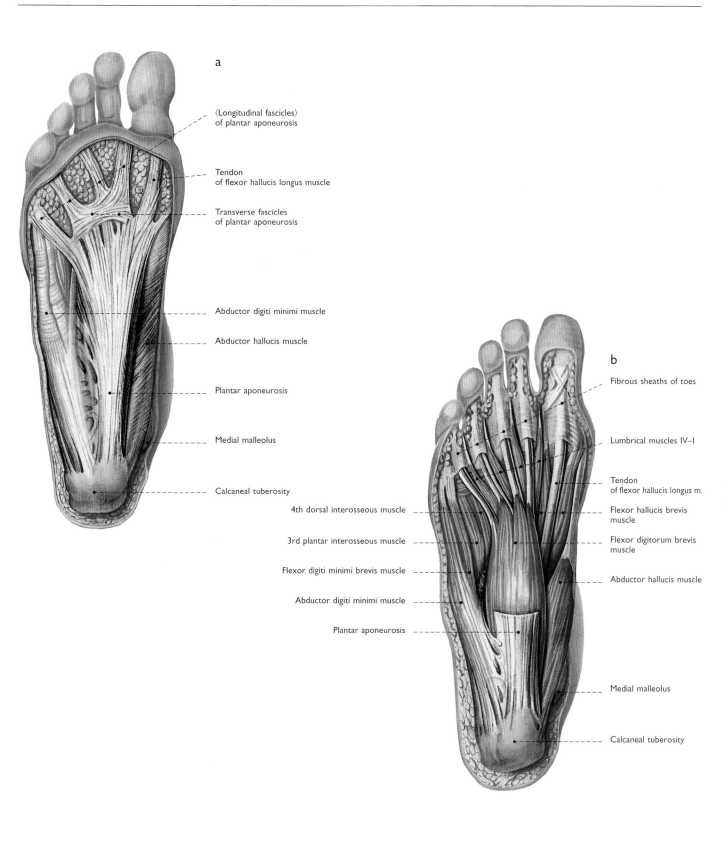

a

⟨Longitudinal fascicles⟩
of plantar aponeurosis

Tendon
of flexor hallucis longus muscle

Transverse fascicles
of plantar aponeurosis

Abductor digiti minimi muscle

Abductor hallucis muscle

Plantar aponeurosis

Medial malleolus

Calcaneal tuberosity

b

Fibrous sheaths of toes

Lumbrical muscles IV–I

Tendon
of flexor hallucis longus m.

Flexor hallucis brevis
muscle

Flexor digitorum brevis
muscle

Abductor hallucis muscle

Medial malleolus

Calcaneal tuberosity

4th dorsal interosseous muscle

3rd plantar interosseous muscle

Flexor digiti minimi brevis muscle

Abductor digiti minimi muscle

Plantar aponeurosis

237 Muscles of the sole of the right foot (50%)
Plantar aspect
a   Plantar aponeurosis and superficial muscles
b   Superficial layer after partial removal of the plantar aponeurosis

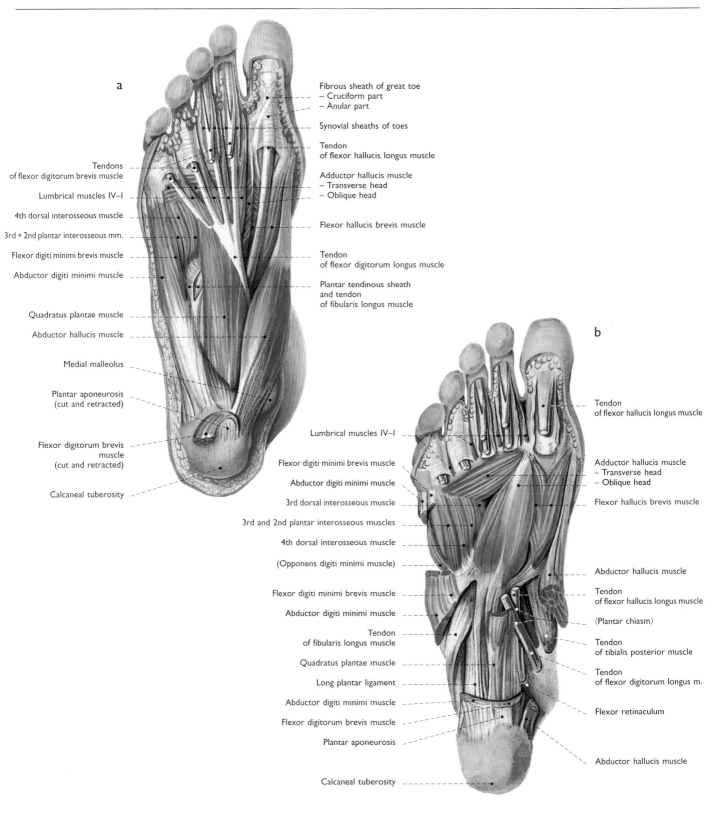

a

Tendons
of flexor digitorum brevis muscle

Lumbrical muscles IV–I

4th dorsal interosseous muscle

3rd + 2nd plantar interosseous mm.

Flexor digiti minimi brevis muscle

Abductor digiti minimi muscle

Quadratus plantae muscle

Abductor hallucis muscle

Medial malleolus

Plantar aponeurosis
(cut and retracted)

Flexor digitorum brevis
muscle
(cut and retracted)

Calcaneal tuberosity

Fibrous sheath of great toe
– Cruciform part
– Anular part

Synovial sheaths of toes

Tendon
of flexor hallucis longus muscle

Adductor hallucis muscle
– Transverse head
– Oblique head

Flexor hallucis brevis muscle

Tendon
of flexor digitorum longus muscle

Plantar tendinous sheath
and tendon
of fibularis longus muscle

b

Lumbrical muscles IV–I

Flexor digiti minimi brevis muscle

Abductor digiti minimi muscle

3rd dorsal interosseous muscle

3rd and 2nd plantar interosseous muscles

4th dorsal interosseous muscle

(Opponens digiti minimi muscle)

Flexor digiti minimi brevis muscle

Abductor digiti minimi muscle

Tendon
of fibularis longus muscle

Quadratus plantae muscle

Long plantar ligament

Abductor digiti minimi muscle

Flexor digitorum brevis muscle

Plantar aponeurosis

Calcaneal tuberosity

Tendon
of flexor hallucis longus muscle

Adductor hallucis muscle
– Transverse head
– Oblique head

Flexor hallucis brevis muscle

Abductor hallucis muscle

Tendon
of flexor hallucis longus muscle

⟨Plantar chiasm⟩

Tendon
of tibialis posterior muscle

Tendon
of flexor digitorum longus m.

Flexor retinaculum

Abductor hallucis muscle

238 Muscles of the sole of the right foot (50%)
Plantar aspect
a Deep layer after partial removal of the plantar aponeurosis
and the flexor digitorum brevis muscle
b Deepest layer after extensive removal of the muscles
of the superficial and deep layers

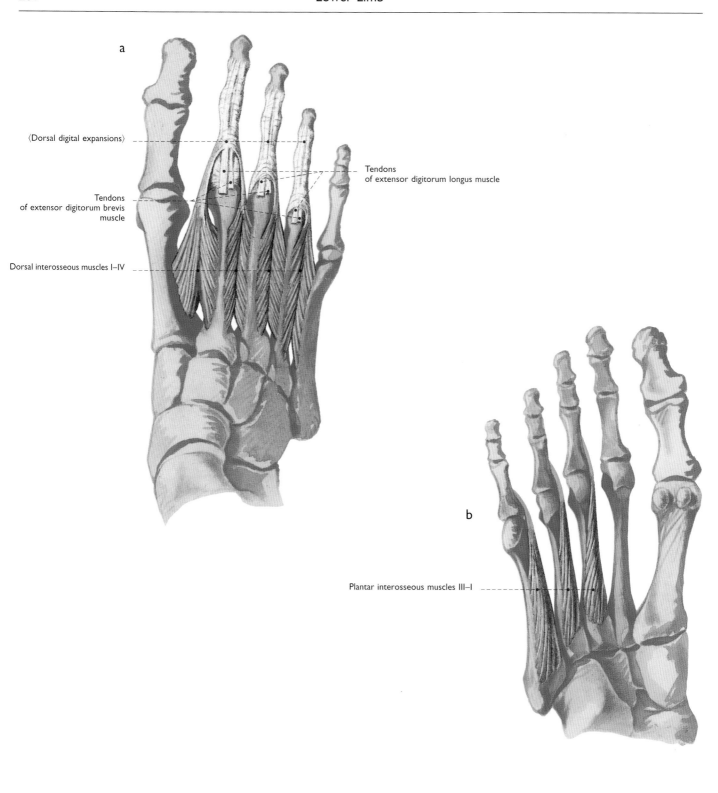

a

⟨Dorsal digital expansions⟩

Tendons
of extensor digitorum longus muscle

Tendons
of extensor digitorum brevis
muscle

Dorsal interosseous muscles I–IV

b

Plantar interosseous muscles III–I

239 Interosseous muscles of the right foot (75%)
  a Dorsal interosseous muscles, dorsal aspect
  b Plantar interosseous muscles, plantar aspect

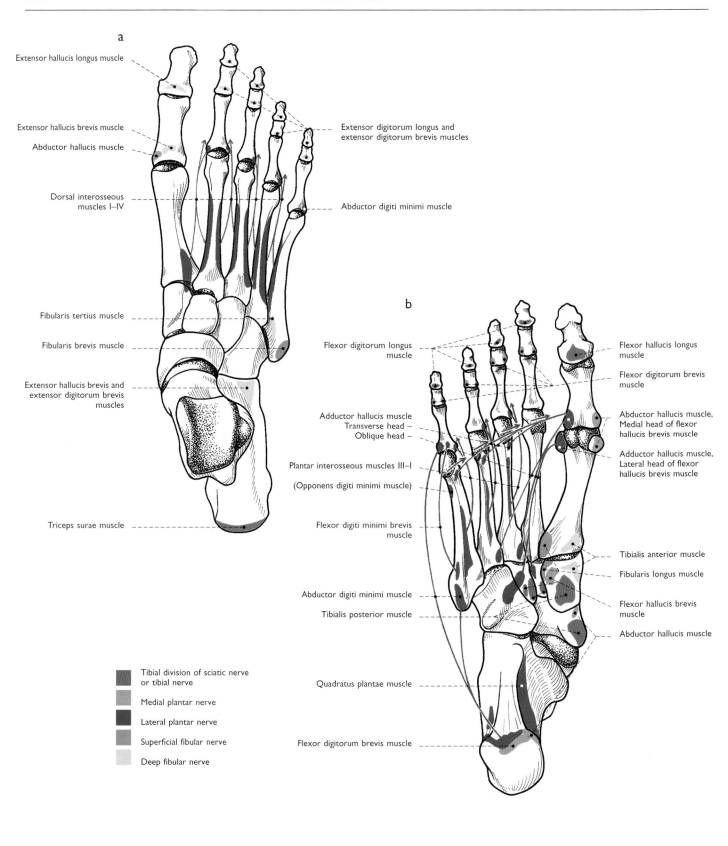

a

Extensor hallucis longus muscle

Extensor hallucis brevis muscle

Abductor hallucis muscle

Extensor digitorum longus and extensor digitorum brevis muscles

Dorsal interosseous muscles I–IV

Abductor digiti minimi muscle

Fibularis tertius muscle

Fibularis brevis muscle

Extensor hallucis brevis and extensor digitorum brevis muscles

Triceps surae muscle

b

Flexor digitorum longus muscle

Flexor hallucis longus muscle

Flexor digitorum brevis muscle

Adductor hallucis muscle
Transverse head –
Oblique head –

Abductor hallucis muscle, Medial head of flexor hallucis brevis muscle

Plantar interosseous muscles III–I

Adductor hallucis muscle, Lateral head of flexor hallucis brevis muscle

(Opponens digiti minimi muscle)

Flexor digiti minimi brevis muscle

Tibialis anterior muscle

Fibularis longus muscle

Abductor digiti minimi muscle

Flexor hallucis brevis muscle

Tibialis posterior muscle

Abductor hallucis muscle

Quadratus plantae muscle

Flexor digitorum brevis muscle

Tibial division of sciatic nerve or tibial nerve

Medial plantar nerve

Lateral plantar nerve

Superficial fibular nerve

Deep fibular nerve

240 Muscle attachments to the bones of the right foot
The colors indicate the innervation of the muscles attaching to the
a dorsal surface
b plantar surface.

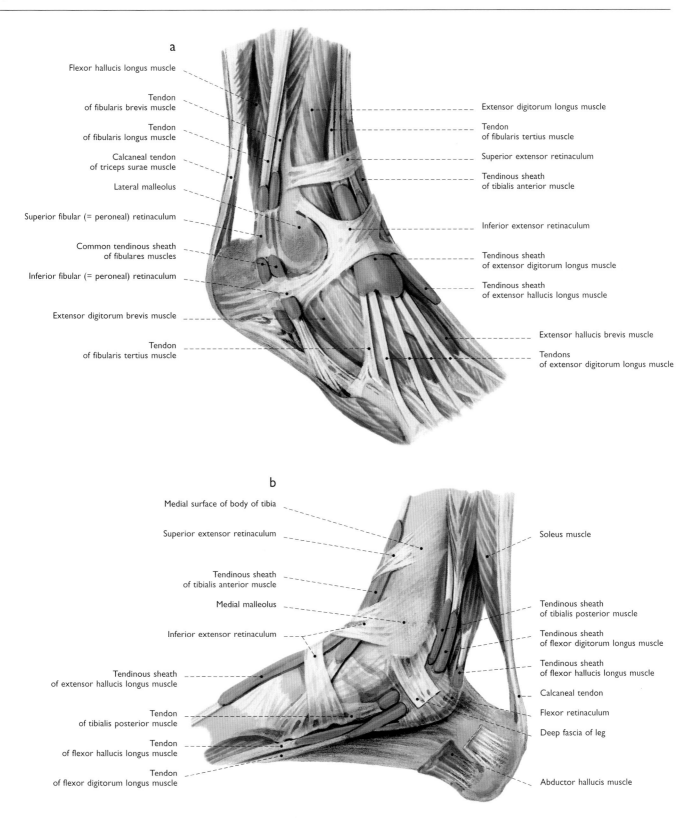

a

Flexor hallucis longus muscle

Tendon
of fibularis brevis muscle

Tendon
of fibularis longus muscle

Calcaneal tendon
of triceps surae muscle

Lateral malleolus

Superior fibular (= peroneal) retinaculum

Common tendinous sheath
of fibulares muscles

Inferior fibular (= peroneal) retinaculum

Extensor digitorum brevis muscle

Tendon
of fibularis tertius muscle

Extensor digitorum longus muscle

Tendon
of fibularis tertius muscle

Superior extensor retinaculum

Tendinous sheath
of tibialis anterior muscle

Inferior extensor retinaculum

Tendinous sheath
of extensor digitorum longus muscle

Tendinous sheath
of extensor hallucis longus muscle

Extensor hallucis brevis muscle

Tendons
of extensor digitorum longus muscle

b

Medial surface of body of tibia

Superior extensor retinaculum

Tendinous sheath
of tibialis anterior muscle

Medial malleolus

Inferior extensor retinaculum

Tendinous sheath
of extensor hallucis longus muscle

Tendon
of tibialis posterior muscle

Tendon
of flexor hallucis longus muscle

Tendon
of flexor digitorum longus muscle

Soleus muscle

Tendinous sheath
of tibialis posterior muscle

Tendinous sheath
of flexor digitorum longus muscle

Tendinous sheath
of flexor hallucis longus muscle

Calcaneal tendon

Flexor retinaculum

Deep fascia of leg

Abductor hallucis muscle

241 Tarsal tendinous sheaths of the right foot (50%)
a Lateral aspect
b Medial aspect

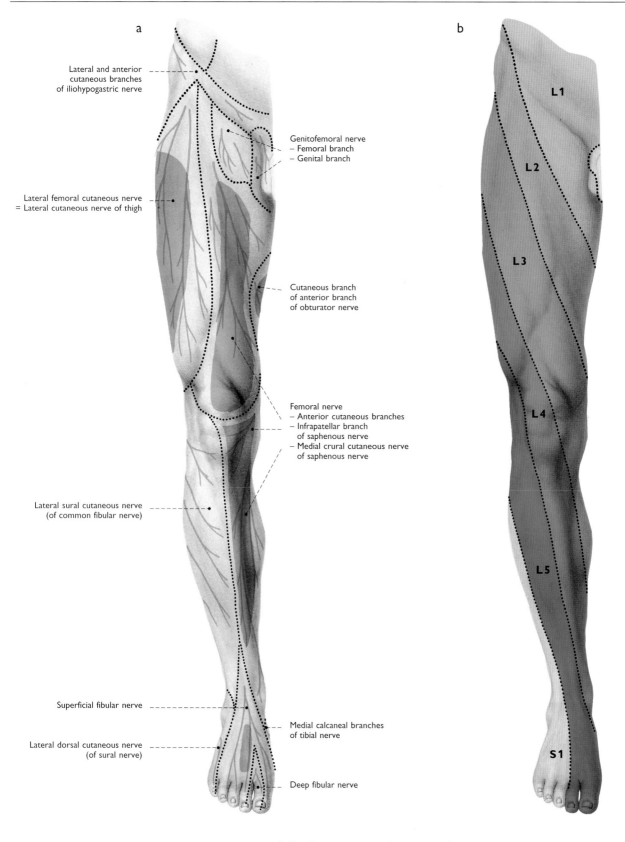

a

Lateral and anterior
cutaneous branches
of iliohypogastric nerve

Genitofemoral nerve
– Femoral branch
– Genital branch

Lateral femoral cutaneous nerve
= Lateral cutaneous nerve of thigh

Cutaneous branch
of anterior branch
of obturator nerve

Femoral nerve
– Anterior cutaneous branches
– Infrapatellar branch
of saphenous nerve
– Medial crural cutaneous nerve
of saphenous nerve

Lateral sural cutaneous nerve
(of common fibular nerve)

Superficial fibular nerve

Medial calcaneal branches
of tibial nerve

Lateral dorsal cutaneous nerve
(of sural nerve)

Deep fibular nerve

b

L1
L2
L3
L4
L5
S1

242 Cutaneous and segmental innervation
of the right lower limb (20%)
Schematic representations, ventral aspect
a Cutaneous nerves and areas of distribution, the autonomic
areas of the different nerves are given in a darker gray.
b Segmental innervation (dermatomes)

a

Superior clunial nerves

Medial clunial nerves

Pudendal nerve

Posterior femoral cutaneous nerve
= Posterior cutaneous nerve of thigh

Cutaneous branch
of anterior branch
of obturator nerve

Medial crural cutaneous nerve
(of saphenous nerve)

Sural nerve

Medial plantar nerve
(of tibial nerve)

b

Lateral cutaneous branch
of iliohypogastric nerve

Inferior clunial nerves
(of posterior femoral
cutaneous nerve)

Lateral femoral
cutaneous nerve
= Lateral cutaneous
nerve of thigh

Lateral sural cutaneous nerve
(of common fibular nerve)

Lateral plantar nerve
(of tibial nerve)

L1
L2
L3
L4
L5
S4
S5
S3
S1
L1
S2
L2
L3
L4
S1
L5

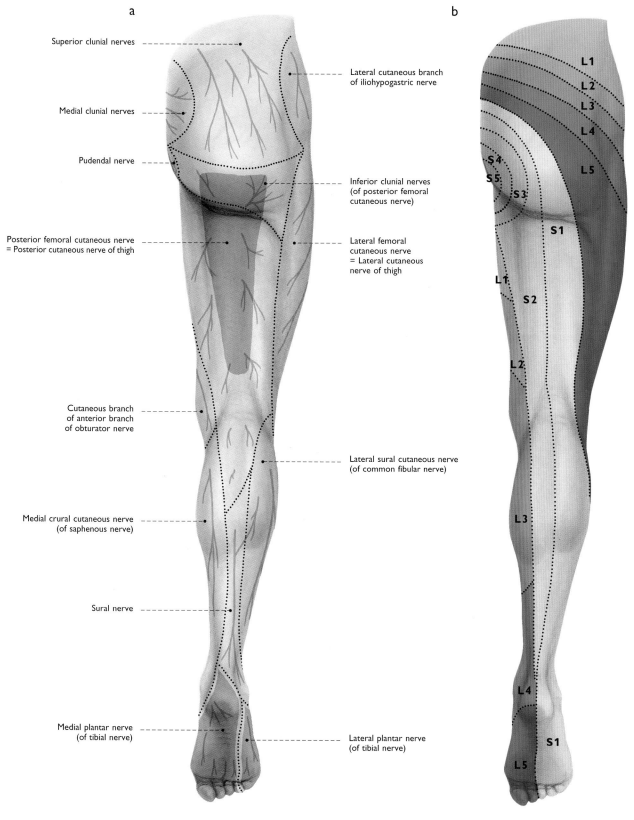

**243   Cutaneous and segmental innervation
of the right lower limb** (20%)

Schematic representations, dorsal aspect

a   Cutaneous nerves and areas of distribution, the autonomic
    areas of the different nerves are given in a darker gray.

b   Segmental innervation (dermatomes)

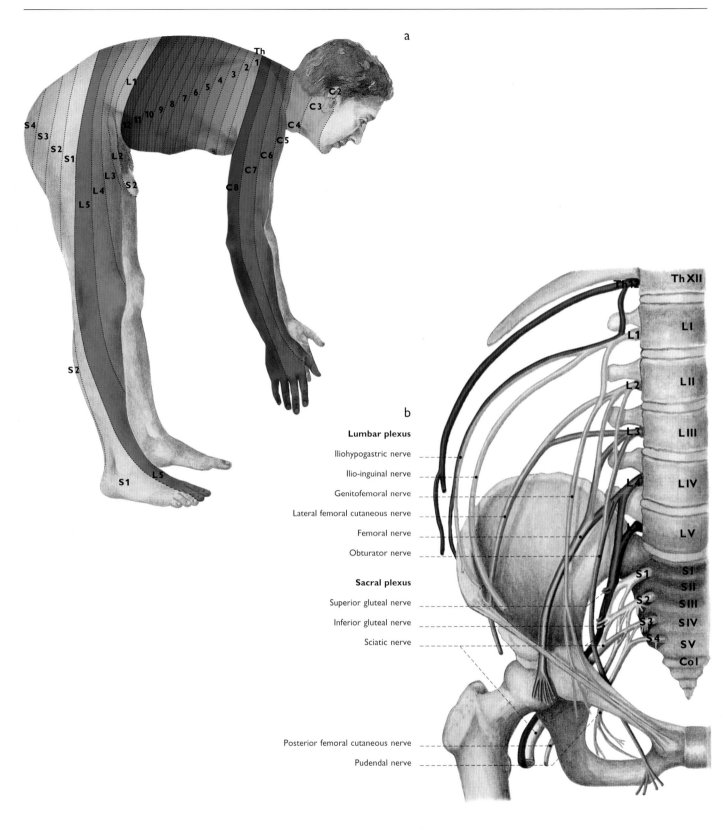

a

b

Lumbar plexus

Iliohypogastric nerve

Ilio-inguinal nerve

Genitofemoral nerve

Lateral femoral cutaneous nerve

Femoral nerve

Obturator nerve

Sacral plexus

Superior gluteal nerve

Inferior gluteal nerve

Sciatic nerve

Posterior femoral cutaneous nerve

Pudendal nerve

244 Segmental innervation and lumbosacral plexus

a Segmental innervation (dermatomes) of the upper limb, trunk,
    and lower limb (according to von Lanz and Wachsmuth, 1972)
b Plan of the lumbosacral plexus

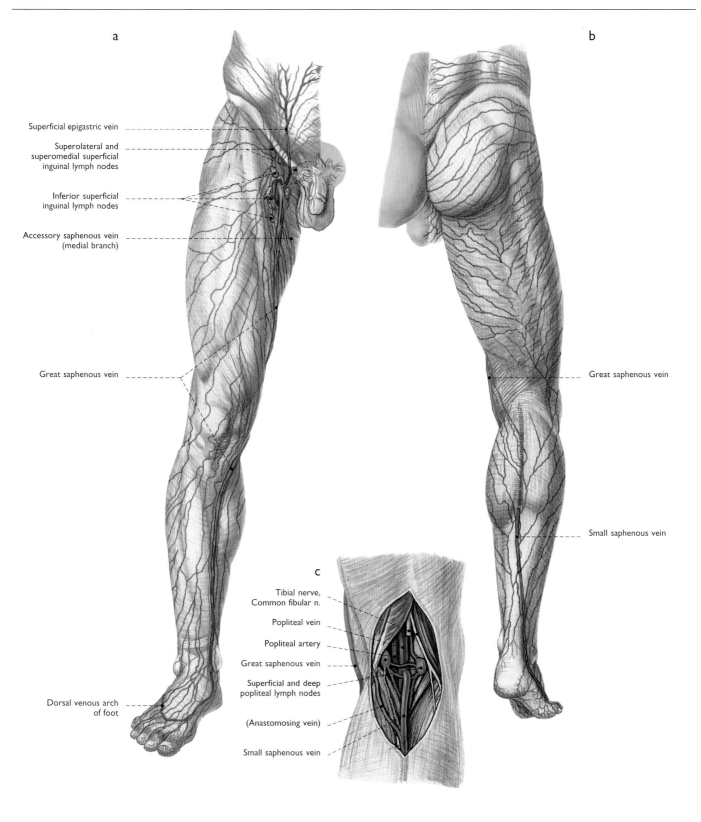

Superficial epigastric vein

Superolateral and superomedial superficial inguinal lymph nodes

Inferior superficial inguinal lymph nodes

Accessory saphenous vein (medial branch)

Great saphenous vein

Dorsal venous arch of foot

Great saphenous vein

Small saphenous vein

c

Tibial nerve, Common fibular n.

Popliteal vein

Popliteal artery

Great saphenous vein

Superficial and deep popliteal lymph nodes

(Anastomosing vein)

Small saphenous vein

245 Lymphatic vessels and lymph nodes of the right lower limb

a Ventral aspect (20%)
b Dorsal aspect (20%)
c Lymphatic vessels of the popliteal fossa (30%), dorsal aspect

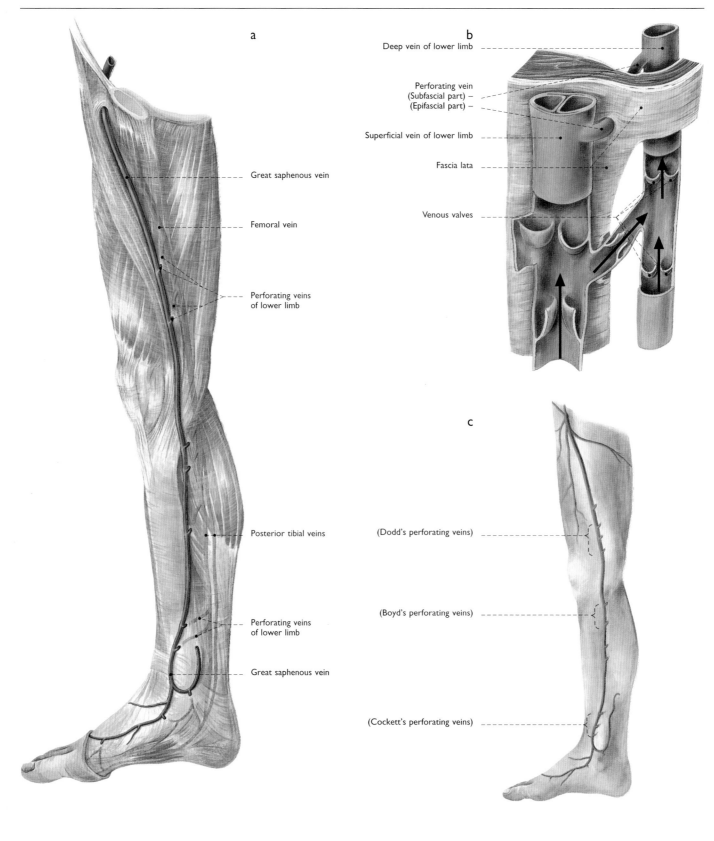

a

Great saphenous vein

Femoral vein

Perforating veins
of lower limb

Posterior tibial veins

Perforating veins
of lower limb

Great saphenous vein

b

Deep vein of lower limb

Perforating vein
(Subfascial part) –
(Epifascial part) –

Superficial vein of lower limb

Fascia lata

Venous valves

c

(Dodd's perforating veins)

(Boyd's perforating veins)

(Cockett's perforating veins)

246 Veins of the right lower limb
  a Superficial and deep veins of the lower limb (20%), medial aspect
  b Connection between superficial and deep veins of the lower limb
     by perforating veins (200%), schematic representation
  c Main localization of perforating veins over the lower limb (10%),
     medial aspect

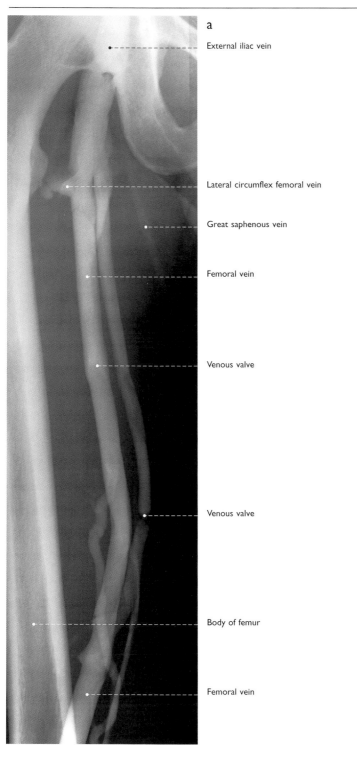

a

External iliac vein

Lateral circumflex femoral vein

Great saphenous vein

Femoral vein

Venous valve

Venous valve

Body of femur

Femoral vein

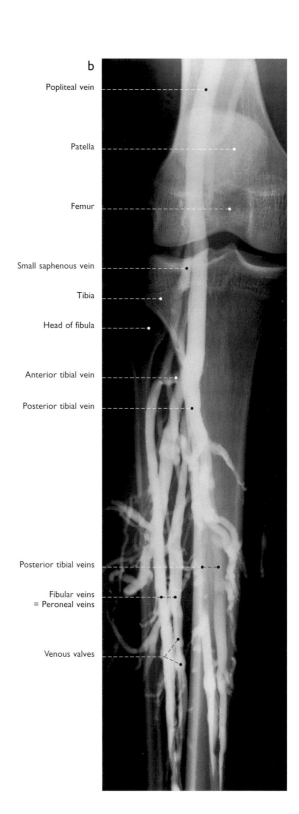

b

Popliteal vein

Patella

Femur

Small saphenous vein

Tibia

Head of fibula

Anterior tibial vein

Posterior tibial vein

Posterior tibial veins

Fibular veins
= Peroneal veins

Venous valves

247 Veins of the right lower limb (45%)
a Anteroposterior venogram of the thigh
b Anteroposterior venogram of the leg

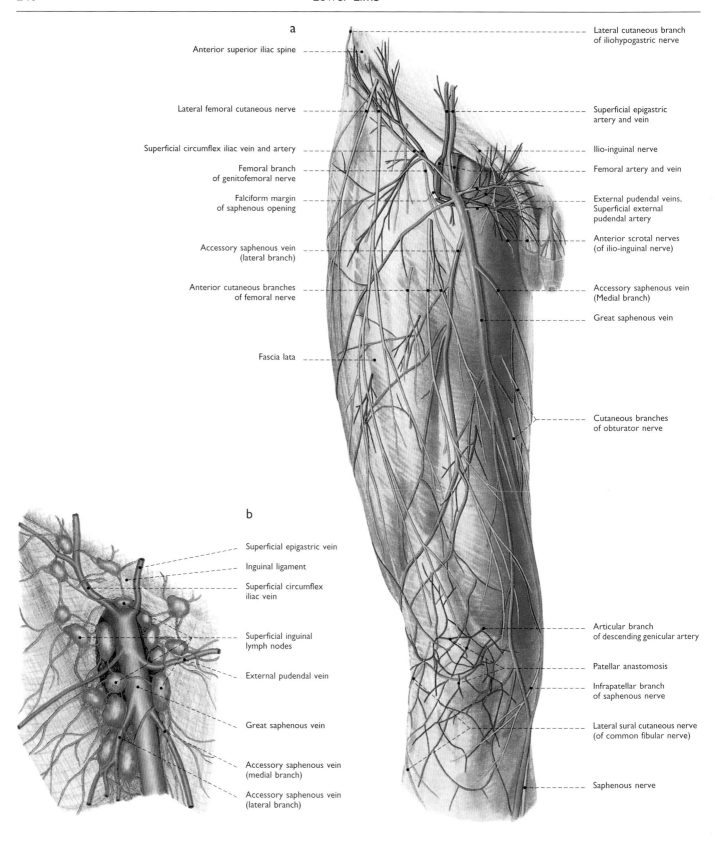

a

Anterior superior iliac spine

Lateral femoral cutaneous nerve

Superficial circumflex iliac vein and artery

Femoral branch
of genitofemoral nerve

Falciform margin
of saphenous opening

Accessory saphenous vein
(lateral branch)

Anterior cutaneous branches
of femoral nerve

Fascia lata

Lateral cutaneous branch
of iliohypogastric nerve

Superficial epigastric
artery and vein

Ilio-inguinal nerve

Femoral artery and vein

External pudendal veins,
Superficial external
pudendal artery

Anterior scrotal nerves
(of ilio-inguinal nerve)

Accessory saphenous vein
(Medial branch)

Great saphenous vein

Cutaneous branches
of obturator nerve

b

Superficial epigastric vein

Inguinal ligament

Superficial circumflex
iliac vein

Superficial inguinal
lymph nodes

External pudendal vein

Great saphenous vein

Accessory saphenous vein
(medial branch)

Accessory saphenous vein
(lateral branch)

Articular branch
of descending genicular artery

Patellar anastomosis

Infrapatellar branch
of saphenous nerve

Lateral sural cutaneous nerve
(of common fibular nerve)

Saphenous nerve

248 Subcutaneous blood vessels, nerves,
and lymph nodes of the right thigh
a Ventral aspect (30%)
b Superficial veins and lymph nodes in and around
the saphenous opening (70%)

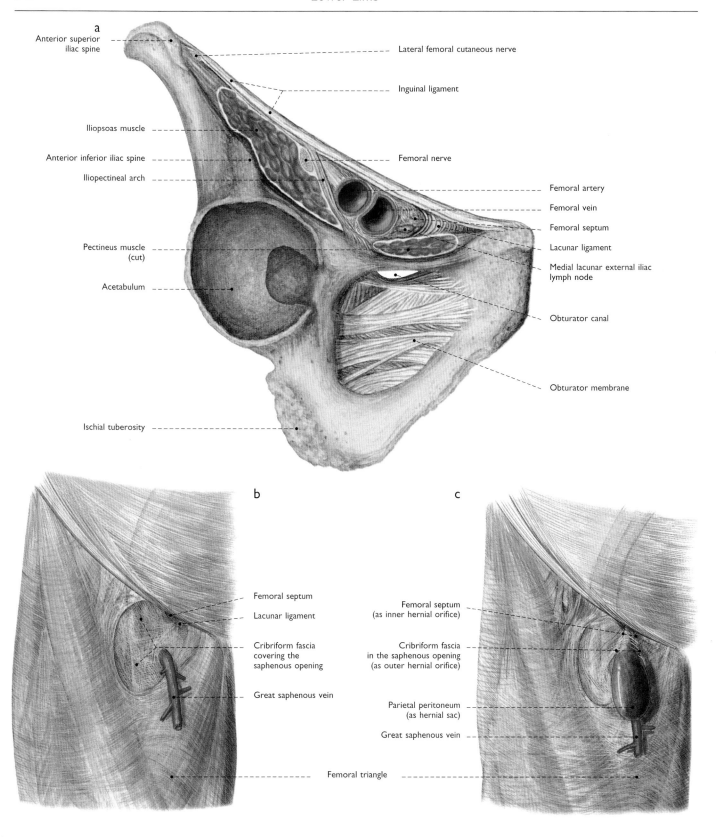

a

Anterior superior iliac spine

Lateral femoral cutaneous nerve

Inguinal ligament

Iliopsoas muscle

Anterior inferior iliac spine

Iliopectineal arch

Femoral nerve

Femoral artery

Femoral vein

Femoral septum

Pectineus muscle (cut)

Lacunar ligament

Medial lacunar external iliac lymph node

Acetabulum

Obturator canal

Obturator membrane

Ischial tuberosity

b

Femoral septum

Lacunar ligament

Cribriform fascia covering the saphenous opening

Great saphenous vein

Femoral triangle

c

Femoral septum (as inner hernial orifice)

Cribriform fascia in the saphenous opening (as outer hernial orifice)

Parietal peritoneum (as hernial sac)

Great saphenous vein

249 Inguinal region and femoral triangle

a Structures passing posterior to the inguinal ligament (60%)
(according to von Lanz and Wachsmuth, 1972),
inferior (distal) aspect

b, c Femoral triangle, saphenous opening, and femoral hernia (30%),
ventral aspect

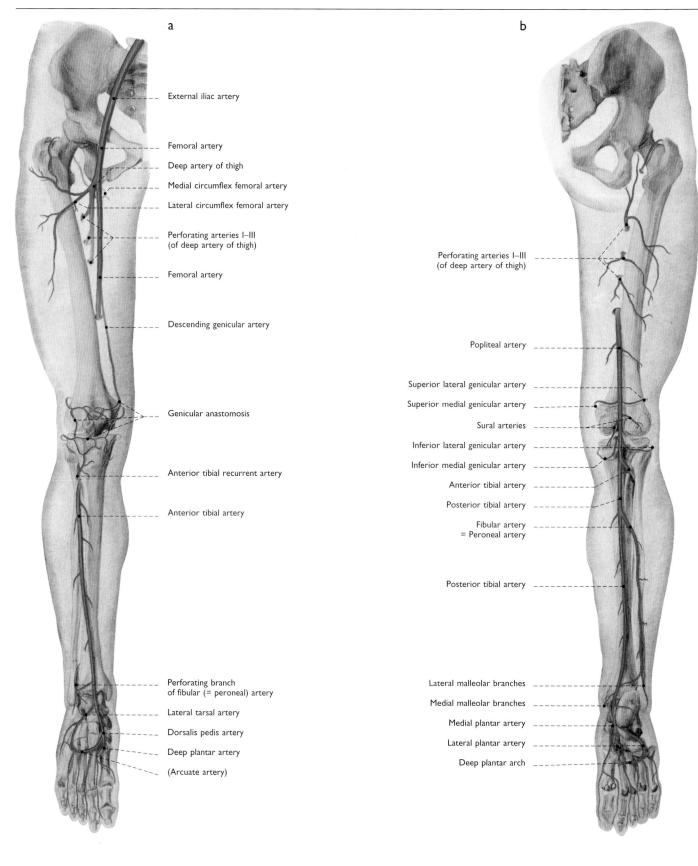

a

b

External iliac artery

Femoral artery

Deep artery of thigh

Medial circumflex femoral artery

Lateral circumflex femoral artery

Perforating arteries I–III
(of deep artery of thigh)

Femoral artery

Descending genicular artery

Genicular anastomosis

Anterior tibial recurrent artery

Anterior tibial artery

Perforating branch
of fibular (= peroneal) artery

Lateral tarsal artery

Dorsalis pedis artery

Deep plantar artery

(Arcuate artery)

Perforating arteries I–III
(of deep artery of thigh)

Popliteal artery

Superior lateral genicular artery

Superior medial genicular artery

Sural arteries

Inferior lateral genicular artery

Inferior medial genicular artery

Anterior tibial artery

Posterior tibial artery

Fibular artery
= Peroneal artery

Posterior tibial artery

Lateral malleolar branches

Medial malleolar branches

Medial plantar artery

Lateral plantar artery

Deep plantar arch

250 Arteries of the right lower limb (20%)

Schematic representations
a Ventral aspect
b Dorsal aspect

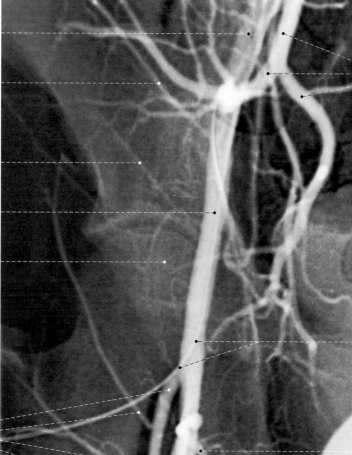
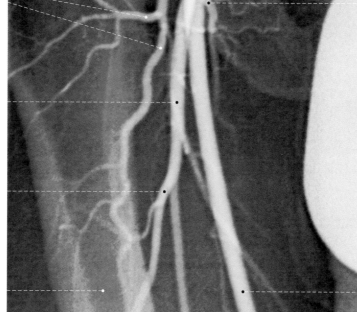

External iliac artery

Deep circumflex iliac artery

Superficial circumflex iliac artery

Femoral artery

Head of femur

Lateral circumflex femoral artery
Ascending branch –
Transverse branch –
Descending branch –

Deep artery of thigh

1st perforating artery
(of deep artery of thigh)

Body of femur

Internal iliac artery
– ⟨Posterior trunk⟩
– ⟨Anterior trunk⟩

(Catheter introduced
into the femoral artery)

Medial circumflex femoral artery

Femoral artery

251 Arteries of the right lower limb (80%)
Anteroposterior arteriogram of pelvic and femoral arteries

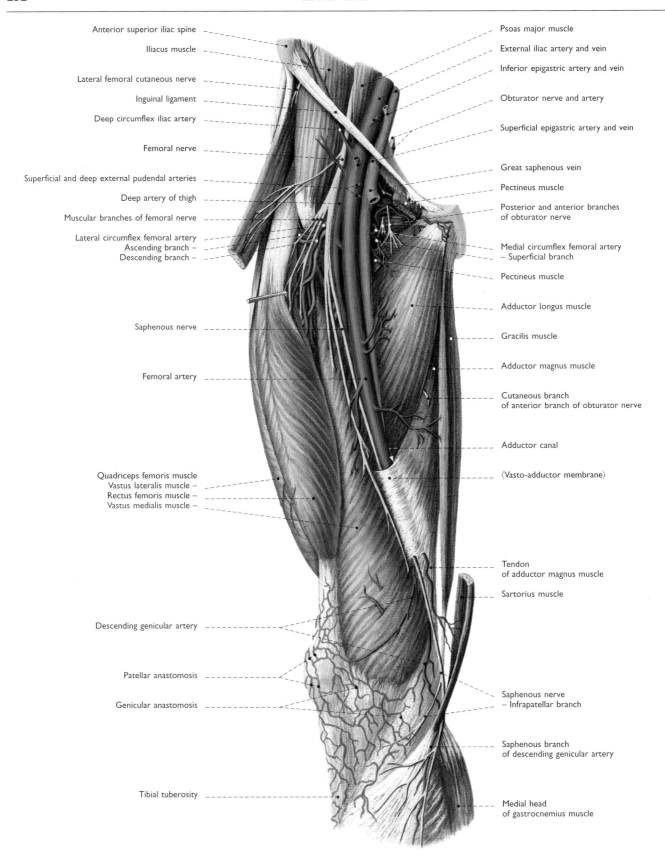

Anterior superior iliac spine

Iliacus muscle

Lateral femoral cutaneous nerve

Inguinal ligament

Deep circumflex iliac artery

Femoral nerve

Superficial and deep external pudendal arteries

Deep artery of thigh

Muscular branches of femoral nerve

Lateral circumflex femoral artery
Ascending branch –
Descending branch –

Saphenous nerve

Femoral artery

Quadriceps femoris muscle
Vastus lateralis muscle –
Rectus femoris muscle –
Vastus medialis muscle –

Descending genicular artery

Patellar anastomosis

Genicular anastomosis

Tibial tuberosity

Psoas major muscle

External iliac artery and vein

Inferior epigastric artery and vein

Obturator nerve and artery

Superficial epigastric artery and vein

Great saphenous vein

Pectineus muscle

Posterior and anterior branches
of obturator nerve

Medial circumflex femoral artery
– Superficial branch

Pectineus muscle

Adductor longus muscle

Gracilis muscle

Adductor magnus muscle

Cutaneous branch
of anterior branch of obturator nerve

Adductor canal

⟨Vasto-adductor membrane⟩

Tendon
of adductor magnus muscle

Sartorius muscle

Saphenous nerve
– Infrapatellar branch

Saphenous branch
of descending genicular artery

Medial head
of gastrocnemius muscle

**252   Blood vessels and nerves of the right thigh
and knee** (30%)
The sartorius and pectineus muscles were partially removed.
Ventral aspect

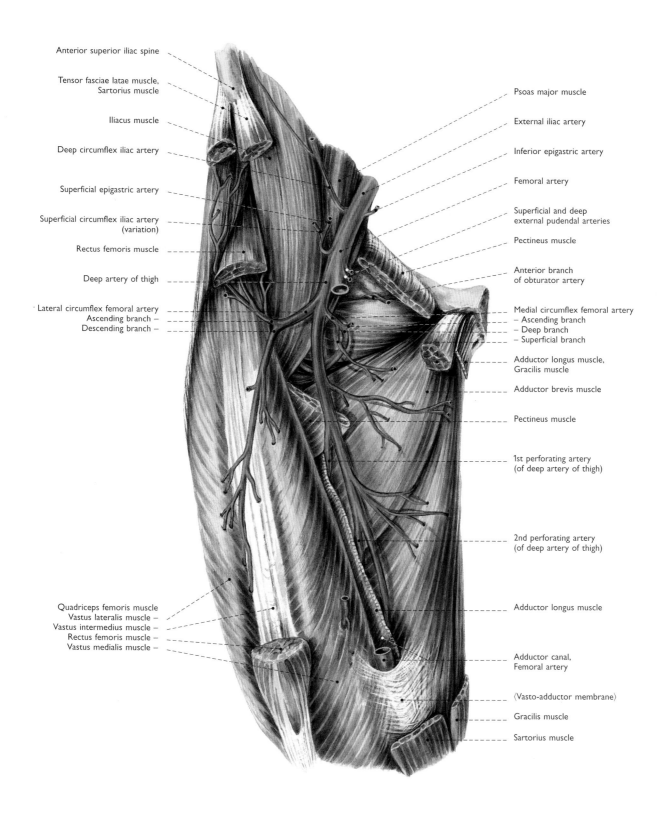

Anterior superior iliac spine

Tensor fasciae latae muscle,
Sartorius muscle

Iliacus muscle

Deep circumflex iliac artery

Superficial epigastric artery

Superficial circumflex iliac artery
(variation)

Rectus femoris muscle

Deep artery of thigh

Lateral circumflex femoral artery
Ascending branch —
Descending branch —

Quadriceps femoris muscle
Vastus lateralis muscle —
Vastus intermedius muscle —
Rectus femoris muscle —
Vastus medialis muscle —

Psoas major muscle

External iliac artery

Inferior epigastric artery

Femoral artery

Superficial and deep
external pudendal arteries

Pectineus muscle

Anterior branch
of obturator artery

Medial circumflex femoral artery
— Ascending branch
— Deep branch
— Superficial branch

Adductor longus muscle,
Gracilis muscle

Adductor brevis muscle

Pectineus muscle

1st perforating artery
(of deep artery of thigh)

2nd perforating artery
(of deep artery of thigh)

Adductor longus muscle

Adductor canal,
Femoral artery

〈Vasto-adductor membrane〉

Gracilis muscle

Sartorius muscle

**253 Deep artery of thigh and its branches
in the right thigh** (40%)
The superficial muscles were partially removed.
Ventral aspect

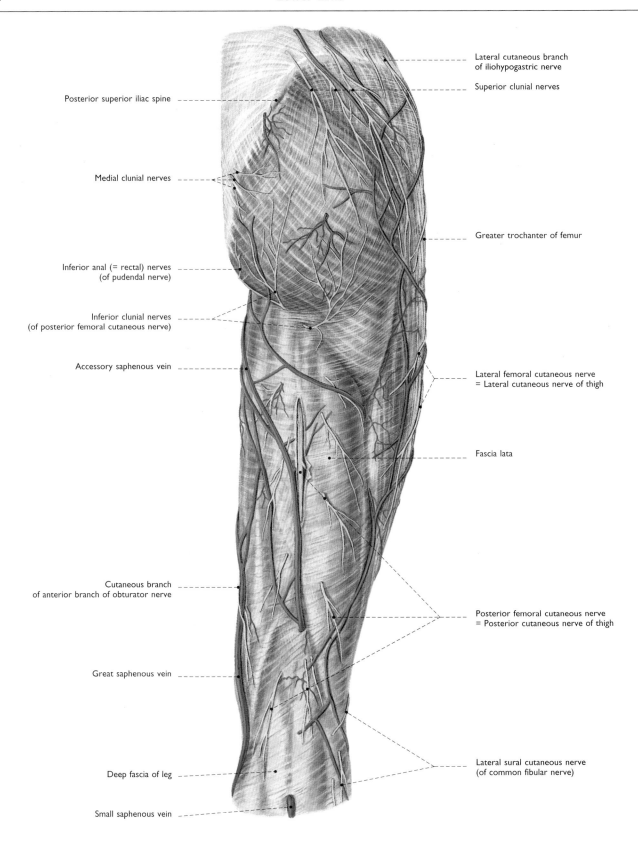

Lateral cutaneous branch
of iliohypogastric nerve

Superior clunial nerves

Posterior superior iliac spine

Medial clunial nerves

Greater trochanter of femur

Inferior anal (= rectal) nerves
(of pudendal nerve)

Inferior clunial nerves
(of posterior femoral cutaneous nerve)

Accessory saphenous vein

Lateral femoral cutaneous nerve
= Lateral cutaneous nerve of thigh

Fascia lata

Cutaneous branch
of anterior branch of obturator nerve

Posterior femoral cutaneous nerve
= Posterior cutaneous nerve of thigh

Great saphenous vein

Deep fascia of leg

Lateral sural cutaneous nerve
(of common fibular nerve)

Small saphenous vein

**254 Subcutaneous blood vessels and nerves
of the gluteal region, thigh, and popliteal fossa
of the right side** (30%)
Dorsal aspect

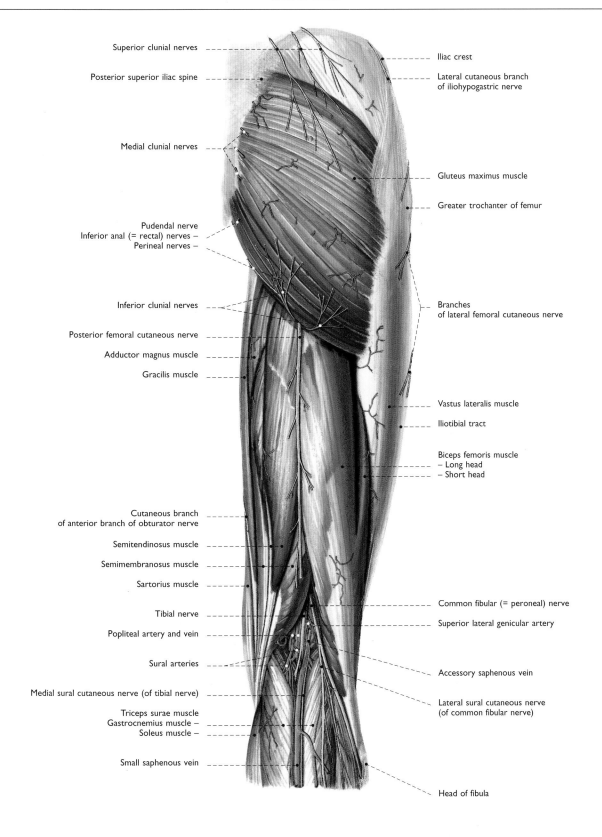

Superior clunial nerves

Posterior superior iliac spine

Medial clunial nerves

Pudendal nerve
Inferior anal (= rectal) nerves –
Perineal nerves –

Inferior clunial nerves

Posterior femoral cutaneous nerve

Adductor magnus muscle

Gracilis muscle

Cutaneous branch
of anterior branch of obturator nerve

Semitendinosus muscle

Semimembranosus muscle

Sartorius muscle

Tibial nerve

Popliteal artery and vein

Sural arteries

Medial sural cutaneous nerve (of tibial nerve)

Triceps surae muscle
Gastrocnemius muscle –
Soleus muscle –

Small saphenous vein

Iliac crest

Lateral cutaneous branch
of iliohypogastric nerve

Gluteus maximus muscle

Greater trochanter of femur

Branches
of lateral femoral cutaneous nerve

Vastus lateralis muscle

Iliotibial tract

Biceps femoris muscle
– Long head
– Short head

Common fibular (= peroneal) nerve

Superior lateral genicular artery

Accessory saphenous vein

Lateral sural cutaneous nerve
(of common fibular nerve)

Head of fibula

**255 Blood vessels and nerves of the gluteal region,
thigh, and popliteal fossa of the right side** (30%)
The fasciae of the lower limb were removed.

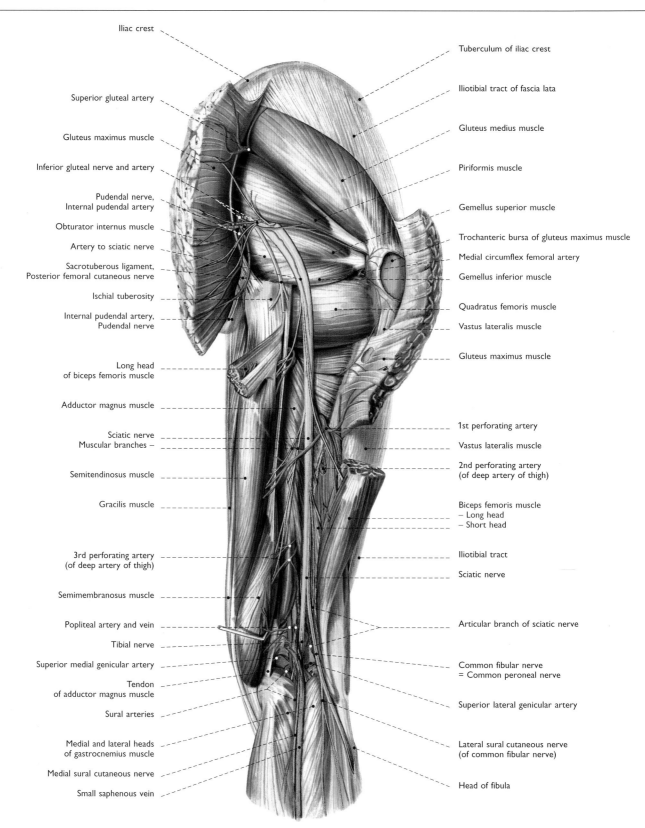

Iliac crest

Superior gluteal artery

Gluteus maximus muscle

Inferior gluteal nerve and artery

Pudendal nerve,
Internal pudendal artery

Obturator internus muscle

Artery to sciatic nerve

Sacrotuberous ligament,
Posterior femoral cutaneous nerve

Ischial tuberosity

Internal pudendal artery,
Pudendal nerve

Long head
of biceps femoris muscle

Adductor magnus muscle

Sciatic nerve
Muscular branches

Semitendinosus muscle

Gracilis muscle

3rd perforating artery
(of deep artery of thigh)

Semimembranosus muscle

Popliteal artery and vein

Tibial nerve

Superior medial genicular artery

Tendon
of adductor magnus muscle

Sural arteries

Medial and lateral heads
of gastrocnemius muscle

Medial sural cutaneous nerve

Small saphenous vein

Tuberculum of iliac crest

Iliotibial tract of fascia lata

Gluteus medius muscle

Piriformis muscle

Gemellus superior muscle

Trochanteric bursa of gluteus maximus muscle

Medial circumflex femoral artery

Gemellus inferior muscle

Quadratus femoris muscle

Vastus lateralis muscle

Gluteus maximus muscle

1st perforating artery

Vastus lateralis muscle

2nd perforating artery
(of deep artery of thigh)

Biceps femoris muscle
– Long head
– Short head

Iliotibial tract

Sciatic nerve

Articular branch of sciatic nerve

Common fibular nerve
= Common peroneal nerve

Superior lateral genicular artery

Lateral sural cutaneous nerve
(of common fibular nerve)

Head of fibula

**256 Blood vessels and nerves of the gluteal region,
thigh, and popliteal fossa of the right side** (30%)
The gluteus maximus muscle and the long head
of the biceps femoris muscle were divided. Dorsal aspect

a

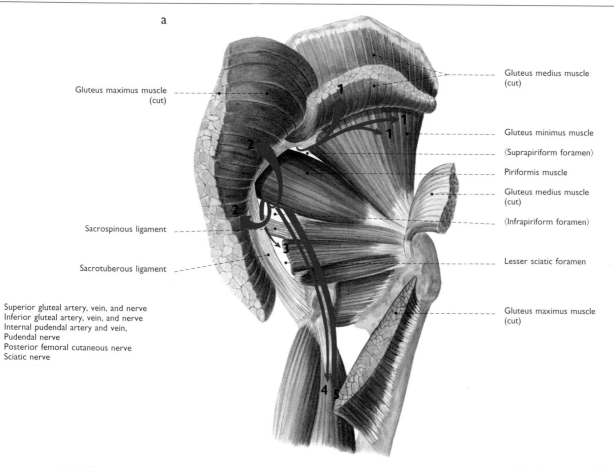

Gluteus maximus muscle (cut)

Gluteus medius muscle (cut)

Gluteus minimus muscle

⟨Suprapiriform foramen⟩

Piriformis muscle

Gluteus medius muscle (cut)

⟨Infrapiriform foramen⟩

Sacrospinous ligament

Lesser sciatic foramen

Sacrotuberous ligament

Gluteus maximus muscle (cut)

1 Superior gluteal artery, vein, and nerve
2 Inferior gluteal artery, vein, and nerve
3 Internal pudendal artery and vein,
   Pudendal nerve
4 Posterior femoral cutaneous nerve
5 Sciatic nerve

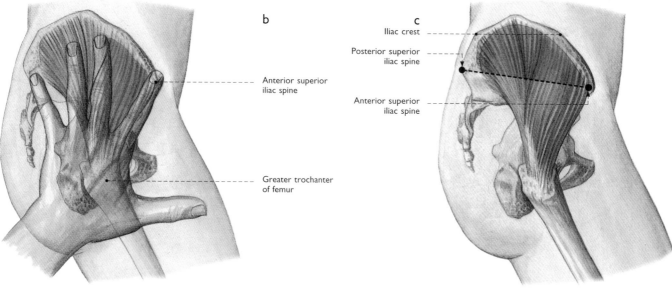

b

Anterior superior iliac spine

Greater trochanter of femur

c

Iliac crest

Posterior superior iliac spine

Anterior superior iliac spine

257 Gluteal region and intragluteal injection

a   The gluteus maximus and medius muscles were divided and retracted.
    The arteries and nerves passing through the greater sciatic foramen
    above and below the piriformis muscle are given by arrows (35%)
    (according to von Lanz and Wachsmuth, 1972). Dorsal aspect

b, c Intragluteal injection according to von Hochstetter (b) and
    von Lanz and Wachsmuth (c). The injection areas are indicated
    by red color (20%). Lateral aspect

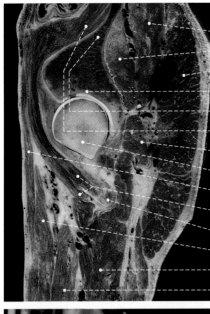

a

Gluteus medius muscle

Gluteus minimus muscle

Gluteus maximus muscle

Acetabulum

Ilium

Iliacus muscle

Piriformis muscle

Head of femur

Sartorius muscle

Iliopsoas muscle

Lesser trochanter of femur

Rectus femoris muscle

Adductor magnus muscle

Vastus medialis muscle

b

Gluteus medius muscle

Gluteus minimus muscle

Gluteus maximus muscle

Sartorius muscle

Greater trochanter of femur

Quadriceps femoris muscle
Rectus femoris muscle –
Vstus intermedius muscle –

Body of femur

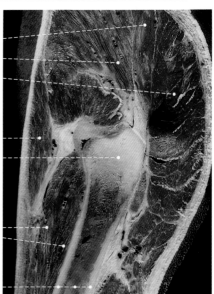

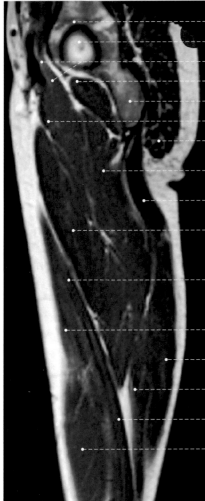

c

Acetabulum

Head of femur

Iliopsoas muscle

Obturator externus muscle

Ischial tuberosity

Pectineus muscle

Gluteus maximus muscle

Adductor magnus muscle

Semitendinosus muscle

Adductor longus muscle

Sartorius muscle

Rectus femoris muscle

Semitendinosus muscle

Semimembranosus muscle

Sartorius muscle

Vastus medialis muscle

d

Sartorius muscle

Greater trochanter of femur

Quadriceps femoris muscle
Rectus femoris muscle –
Vastus intermedius muscle –

Gluteus maximus muscle

Body of femur

Adductor magnus muscle

Long head
of biceps femoris muscle

Tendon
of quadriceps femoris muscle

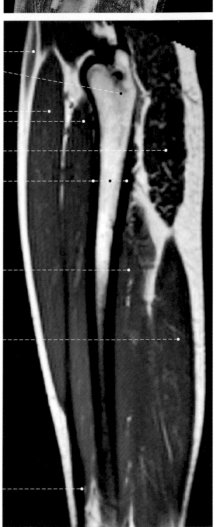

258 Thigh (30%)

a–d Sagittal sections through the head of femur (a, c) and, more laterally,
through the greater trochanter and the body of femur (b, d)

a, b Anatomical sections

c, d Magnetic resonance images (MRI, T$_1$-weighted)

a

Obturator externus muscle

Pectineus muscle

Adductor brevis muscle

Gracilis muscle

Quadriceps femoris muscle

Adductor magnus muscle

Adductor longus muscle

Femoral artery and vein

Sartorius muscle

Body of femur

Pubis

Tensor fasciae latae muscle

Labium majus

Femoral artery and vein

Iliotibial tract

Quadriceps femoris muscle
– Vastus lateralis muscle
– Rectus femoris muscle
– Vastus intermedius muscle
– Vastus medialis muscle

Femur
– Medial condyle
– Lateral condyle

b

Pectineus muscle

Adductor brevis muscle

Gracilis muscle

Adductor longus muscle

Sartorius muscle

Obturator externus muscle

Pubis

Crus of penis

Bulb of penis

Femoral vein and artery

Quadriceps femoris muscle
– Vastus lateralis muscle
– Rectus femoris muscle
– Vastus intermedius muscle
– Vastus medialis muscle

Iliotibial tract

Tendon
of quadriceps femoris muscle

Patella

259 Thigh (20%)

a, b   Coronal sections through the ventral parts of the thighs,
        ventral aspect
a   Anatomical section of a female
b   Magnetic resonance image (MRI, T$_1$-weighted) of a male

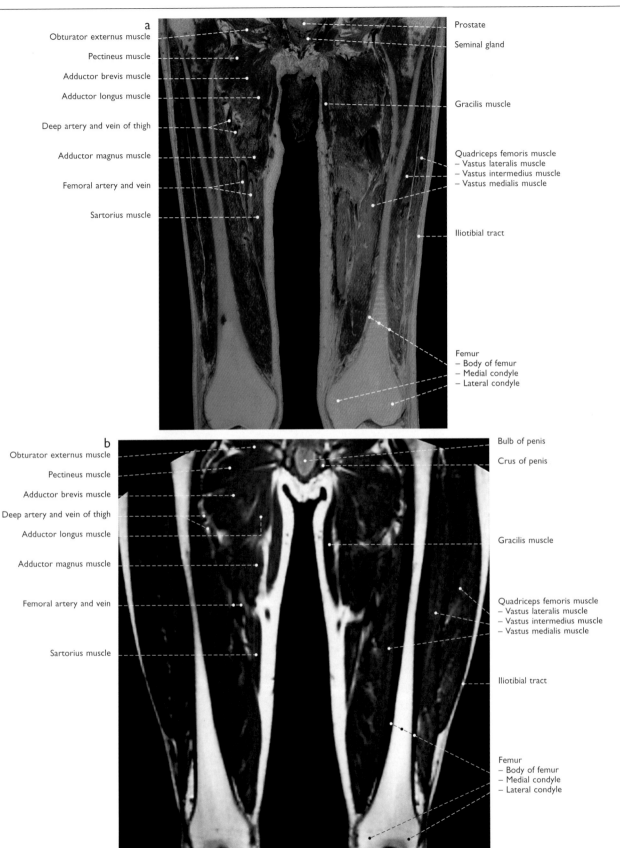

a

Obturator externus muscle
Pectineus muscle
Adductor brevis muscle
Adductor longus muscle
Deep artery and vein of thigh
Adductor magnus muscle
Femoral artery and vein
Sartorius muscle

Prostate
Seminal gland

Gracilis muscle

Quadriceps femoris muscle
– Vastus lateralis muscle
– Vastus intermedius muscle
– Vastus medialis muscle

Iliotibial tract

Femur
– Body of femur
– Medial condyle
– Lateral condyle

b

Obturator externus muscle
Pectineus muscle
Adductor brevis muscle
Deep artery and vein of thigh
Adductor longus muscle
Adductor magnus muscle
Femoral artery and vein
Sartorius muscle

Bulb of penis
Crus of penis

Gracilis muscle

Quadriceps femoris muscle
– Vastus lateralis muscle
– Vastus intermedius muscle
– Vastus medialis muscle

Iliotibial tract

Femur
– Body of femur
– Medial condyle
– Lateral condyle

260 Thigh (20%)

a, b Coronal sections through the middle parts
of the thighs of a male, ventral aspect
a Anatomical section
b Magnetic resonance image (MRI, T$_1$-weighted)

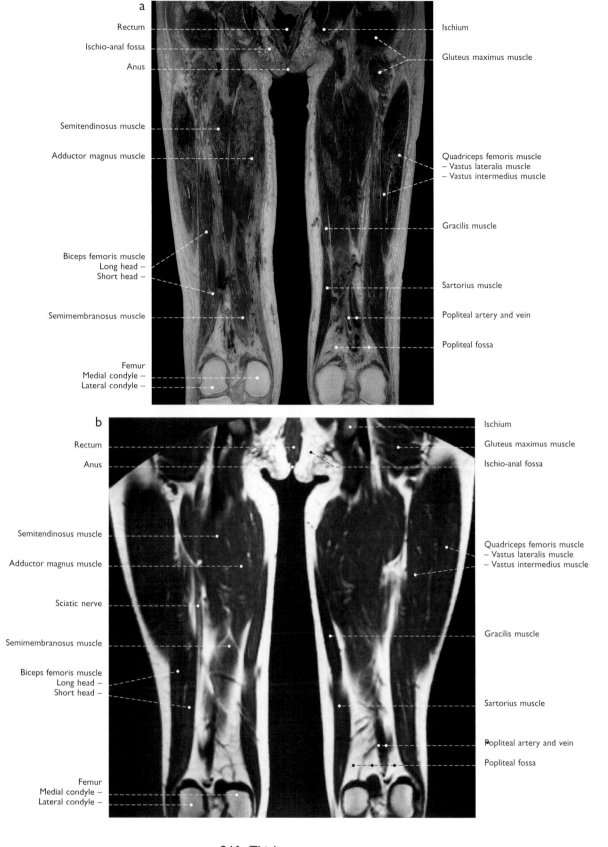

a

Rectum
Ischio-anal fossa
Anus

Semitendinosus muscle

Adductor magnus muscle

Biceps femoris muscle
Long head –
Short head –

Semimembranosus muscle

Femur
Medial condyle –
Lateral condyle –

Ischium
Gluteus maximus muscle

Quadriceps femoris muscle
– Vastus lateralis muscle
– Vastus intermedius muscle

Gracilis muscle

Sartorius muscle

Popliteal artery and vein

Popliteal fossa

b

Rectum
Anus

Semitendinosus muscle

Adductor magnus muscle

Sciatic nerve

Semimembranosus muscle

Biceps femoris muscle
Long head –
Short head –

Femur
Medial condyle –
Lateral condyle –

Ischium
Gluteus maximus muscle
Ischio-anal fossa

Quadriceps femoris muscle
– Vastus lateralis muscle
– Vastus intermedius muscle

Gracilis muscle

Sartorius muscle

Popliteal artery and vein
Popliteal fossa

261 Thigh (20%)

a, b Coronal sections through the dorsal parts
of the thighs of a male, ventral aspect
a Anatomical section
b Magnetic resonance image (MRI, T$_1$-weighted)

a

Quadriceps femoris muscle
Rectus femoris muscle –
Vastus intermedius muscle –
Vastus lateralis muscle –
Vastus medialis muscle –

Femur

Perforating artery and veins
(of deep artery and vein of thigh)

Vastus lateralis muscle

Sciatic nerve

Gluteus maximus muscle

Sartorius muscle

Great saphenous vein

Adductor longus muscle

Femoral artery and vein

Gracilis muscle

Deep artery and vein of thigh

Adductor brevis muscle

Adductor magnus muscle

Tendon
of semimembranosus muscle

Semitendinosus muscle

Long head
of biceps femoris muscle

b

Quadriceps femoris muscle
Rectus femoris muscle –
Vastus intermedius muscle –
Vastus lateralis muscle –
Vastus medialis muscle –

Femur

Vastus lateralis muscle

Sciatic nerve

Gluteus maximus muscle

Sartorius muscle

Great saphenous vein

Adductor longus muscle

Femoral artery and vein

Gracilis muscle

Deep artery and vein of thigh

Adductor brevis muscle

Adductor magnus muscle

Tendon
of semimembranosus muscle

Semitendinosus muscle

Long head
of biceps femoris muscle

262 Right thigh (50%)

Transverse sections through the proximal thigh at the transition
from the gluteal to the femoral region, inferior (distal) aspect
a   Anatomical section
b   Magnetic resonance image (MRI, T$_1$-weighted)

a

Quadriceps femoris muscle
Rectus femoris muscle –
Vastus medialis muscle –
Vastus intermedius muscle –
Vastus lateralis muscle –

Femur

Perforating vein and artery
(of deep vein and artery of thigh)

Biceps femoris muscle
Short head –
Long head –

Sartorius muscle

Femoral artery and vein,
Saphenous nerve

Great saphenous vein

Adductor longus muscle

Gracilis muscle

Adductor magnus muscle

Common fibular nerve,
Tibial nerve

Semimembranosus muscle

Semitendinosus muscle

b

Quadriceps femoris muscle
Rectus femoris muscle –
Vastus medialis muscle –
Vastus intermedius muscle –
Vastus lateralis muscle –

Femur

Perforating vein and artery
(of deep vein and artery of thigh)

Biceps femoris muscle
Short head –
Long head –

Sartorius muscle

Femoral artery and vein,
Saphenous nerve

Great saphenous vein

Adductor longus muscle

Gracilis muscle

Adductor magnus muscle

Common fibular nerve,
Tibial nerve

Semimembranosus muscle

Semitendinosus muscle

263 Right thigh (60%)

Transverse sections through the proximal third of the thigh,
inferior (distal) aspect
a Anatomical section
b Magnetic resonance image (MRI, T_1-weighted)

a

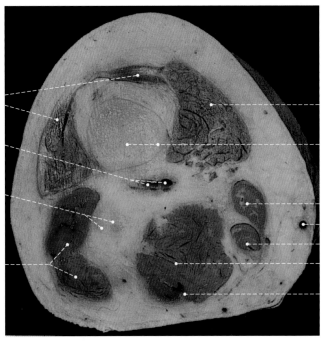

Quadriceps femoris muscle
Tendons
of rectus femoris and
vastus intermedius muscles −
Vastus lateralis muscle −

Popliteal artery and vein

Tibial nerve,
Common fibular nerve

Biceps femoris muscle

Quadriceps femoris muscle
− Vastus medialis muscle

Femur

Sartorius muscle

Great saphenous vein

Gracilis muscle

Semimembranosus muscle

Tendon of semitendinosus muscle

b

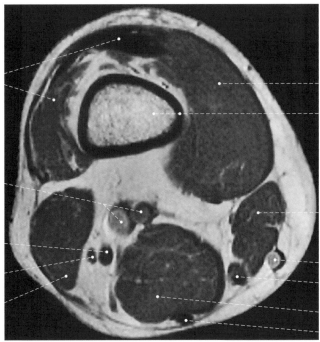

Quadriceps femoris muscle
Tendons
of rectus femoris and
vastus intermedius muscles −
Vastus lateralis muscle −

Popliteal artery and vein

Tibial nerve

Common fibular nerve

Biceps femoris muscle

Quadriceps femoris muscle
− Vastus medialis muscle

Femur

Sartorius muscle

Great saphenous vein

Tendon of gracilis muscle

Semimembranosus muscle

Tendon of semitendinosus muscle

264 Right thigh (60%)

Transverse sections through the distal third of the thigh,
inferior (distal) aspect
a Anatomical section
b Magnetic resonance image (MRI, T$_1$-weighted)

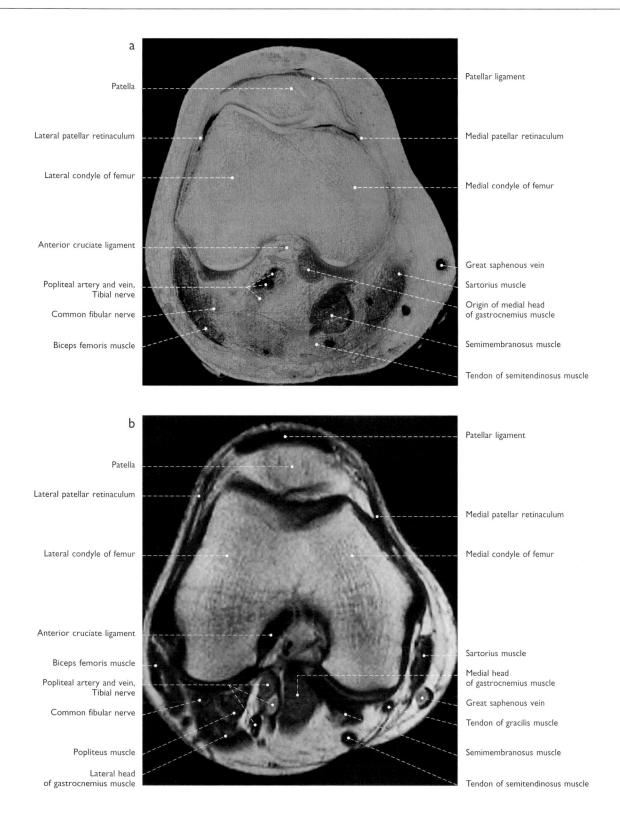

a

Patella

Lateral patellar retinaculum

Lateral condyle of femur

Anterior cruciate ligament

Popliteal artery and vein,
Tibial nerve

Common fibular nerve

Biceps femoris muscle

Patellar ligament

Medial patellar retinaculum

Medial condyle of femur

Great saphenous vein

Sartorius muscle

Origin of medial head
of gastrocnemius muscle

Semimembranosus muscle

Tendon of semitendinosus muscle

b

Patella

Lateral patellar retinaculum

Lateral condyle of femur

Anterior cruciate ligament

Biceps femoris muscle

Popliteal artery and vein,
Tibial nerve

Common fibular nerve

Popliteus muscle

Lateral head
of gastrocnemius muscle

Patellar ligament

Medial patellar retinaculum

Medial condyle of femur

Sartorius muscle

Medial head
of gastrocnemius muscle

Great saphenous vein

Tendon of gracilis muscle

Semimembranosus muscle

Tendon of semitendinosus muscle

265 Right thigh (60%)

Transverse sections through the proximal parts of the knee joint,
inferior (distal) aspect
a Anatomical section
b Magnetic resonance image (MRI, T_1-weighted)

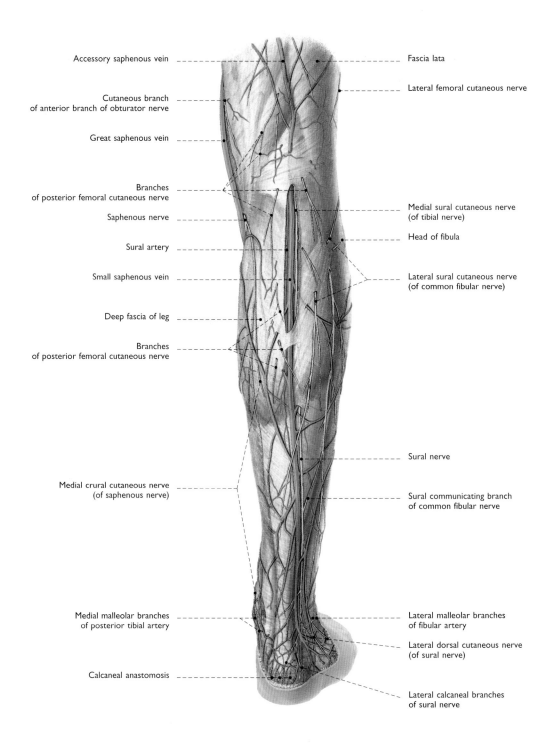

Accessory saphenous vein

Cutaneous branch
of anterior branch of obturator nerve

Great saphenous vein

Branches
of posterior femoral cutaneous nerve

Saphenous nerve

Sural artery

Small saphenous vein

Deep fascia of leg

Branches
of posterior femoral cutaneous nerve

Medial crural cutaneous nerve
(of saphenous nerve)

Medial malleolar branches
of posterior tibial artery

Calcaneal anastomosis

Fascia lata

Lateral femoral cutaneous nerve

Medial sural cutaneous nerve
(of tibial nerve)

Head of fibula

Lateral sural cutaneous nerve
(of common fibular nerve)

Sural nerve

Sural communicating branch
of common fibular nerve

Lateral malleolar branches
of fibular artery

Lateral dorsal cutaneous nerve
(of sural nerve)

Lateral calcaneal branches
of sural nerve

**266 Subcutaneous blood vessels and nerves
of the popliteal fossa and the leg
of the right side** (30%)
Dorsal aspect

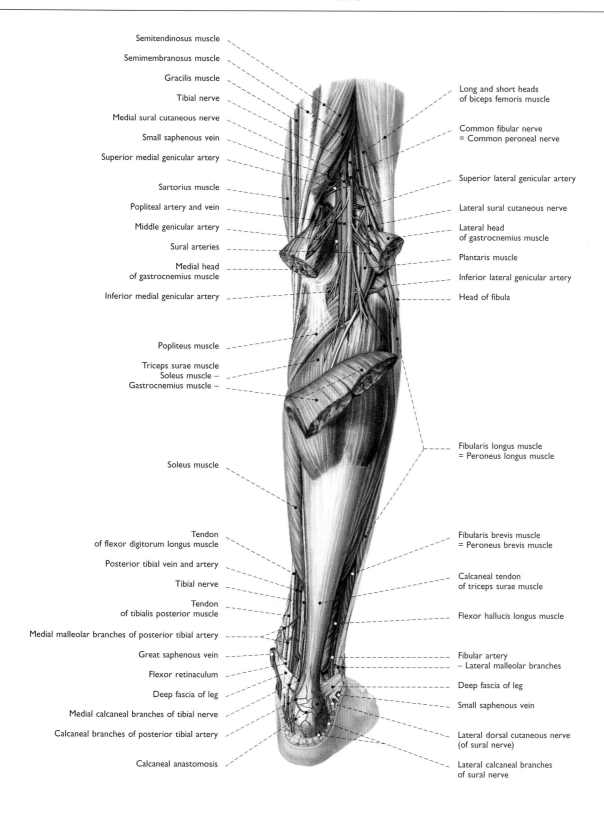

Semitendinosus muscle

Semimembranosus muscle

Gracilis muscle

Tibial nerve

Medial sural cutaneous nerve

Small saphenous vein

Superior medial genicular artery

Sartorius muscle

Popliteal artery and vein

Middle genicular artery

Sural arteries

Medial head
of gastrocnemius muscle

Inferior medial genicular artery

Popliteus muscle

Triceps surae muscle
Soleus muscle –
Gastrocnemius muscle –

Soleus muscle

Tendon
of flexor digitorum longus muscle

Posterior tibial vein and artery

Tibial nerve

Tendon
of tibialis posterior muscle

Medial malleolar branches of posterior tibial artery

Great saphenous vein

Flexor retinaculum

Deep fascia of leg

Medial calcaneal branches of tibial nerve

Calcaneal branches of posterior tibial artery

Calcaneal anastomosis

Long and short heads
of biceps femoris muscle

Common fibular nerve
= Common peroneal nerve

Superior lateral genicular artery

Lateral sural cutaneous nerve

Lateral head
of gastrocnemius muscle

Plantaris muscle

Inferior lateral genicular artery

Head of fibula

Fibularis longus muscle
= Peroneus longus muscle

Fibularis brevis muscle
= Peroneus brevis muscle

Calcaneal tendon
of triceps surae muscle

Flexor hallucis longus muscle

Fibular artery
– Lateral malleolar branches

Deep fascia of leg

Small saphenous vein

Lateral dorsal cutaneous nerve
(of sural nerve)

Lateral calcaneal branches
of sural nerve

**267 Blood vessels and nerves
of the popliteal fossa and the leg
of the right side** (30%)
The gastrocnemius muscle was divided. Dorsal aspect

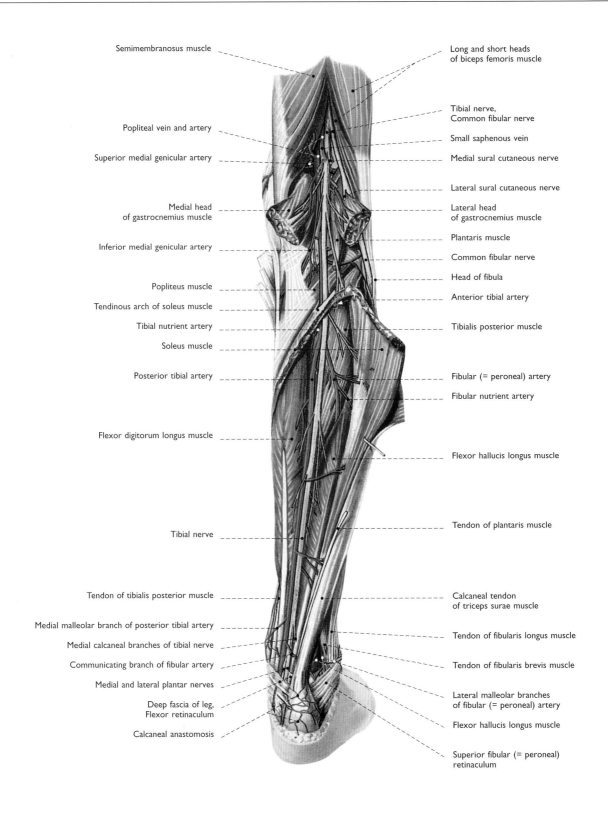

Semimembranosus muscle

Popliteal vein and artery

Superior medial genicular artery

Medial head
of gastrocnemius muscle

Inferior medial genicular artery

Popliteus muscle

Tendinous arch of soleus muscle

Tibial nutrient artery

Soleus muscle

Posterior tibial artery

Flexor digitorum longus muscle

Tibial nerve

Tendon of tibialis posterior muscle

Medial malleolar branch of posterior tibial artery

Medial calcaneal branches of tibial nerve

Communicating branch of fibular artery

Medial and lateral plantar nerves

Deep fascia of leg,
Flexor retinaculum

Calcaneal anastomosis

Long and short heads
of biceps femoris muscle

Tibial nerve,
Common fibular nerve

Small saphenous vein

Medial sural cutaneous nerve

Lateral sural cutaneous nerve

Lateral head
of gastrocnemius muscle

Plantaris muscle

Common fibular nerve

Head of fibula

Anterior tibial artery

Tibialis posterior muscle

Fibular (= peroneal) artery

Fibular nutrient artery

Flexor hallucis longus muscle

Tendon of plantaris muscle

Calcaneal tendon
of triceps surae muscle

Tendon of fibularis longus muscle

Tendon of fibularis brevis muscle

Lateral malleolar branches
of fibular (= peroneal) artery

Flexor hallucis longus muscle

Superior fibular (= peroneal)
retinaculum

**268 Blood vessels and nerves
of the popliteal fossa and the leg
of the right side** (30%)
The gastrocnemius and soleus muscles were divided,
the deep veins removed. Dorsal aspect

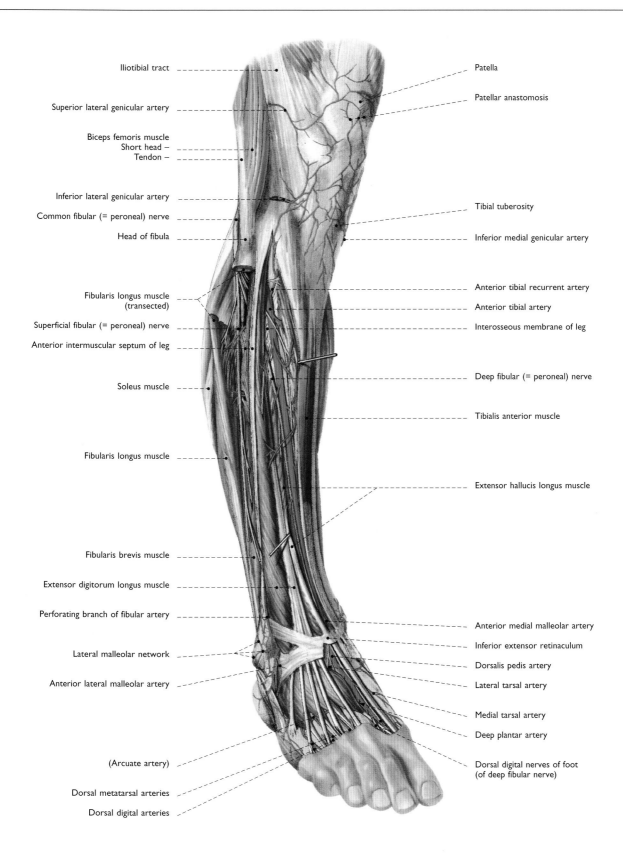

Iliotibial tract

Superior lateral genicular artery

Biceps femoris muscle
Short head –
Tendon –

Inferior lateral genicular artery

Common fibular (= peroneal) nerve

Head of fibula

Fibularis longus muscle
(transected)

Superficial fibular (= peroneal) nerve

Anterior intermuscular septum of leg

Soleus muscle

Fibularis longus muscle

Fibularis brevis muscle

Extensor digitorum longus muscle

Perforating branch of fibular artery

Lateral malleolar network

Anterior lateral malleolar artery

(Arcuate artery)

Dorsal metatarsal arteries

Dorsal digital arteries

Patella

Patellar anastomosis

Tibial tuberosity

Inferior medial genicular artery

Anterior tibial recurrent artery

Anterior tibial artery

Interosseous membrane of leg

Deep fibular (= peroneal) nerve

Tibialis anterior muscle

Extensor hallucis longus muscle

Anterior medial malleolar artery

Inferior extensor retinaculum

Dorsalis pedis artery

Lateral tarsal artery

Medial tarsal artery

Deep plantar artery

Dorsal digital nerves of foot
(of deep fibular nerve)

271 Arteries and nerves of the right leg and foot (30%)
The deep veins were removed. Ventrolateral aspect

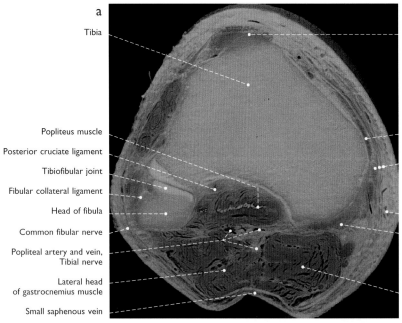

a

Tibia — Patellar ligament

Popliteus muscle — Tibial collateral ligament

Posterior cruciate ligament —

Tibiofibular joint — Tendons of semitendinosus, gracilis, and sartorius muscles, ⟨Pes anserinus⟩

Fibular collateral ligament —

Head of fibula — Great saphenous vein

Common fibular nerve — Tendon of semimembranosus muscle

Popliteal artery and vein, Tibial nerve —

Lateral head of gastrocnemius muscle —

Small saphenous vein — Medial head of gastrocnemius muscle

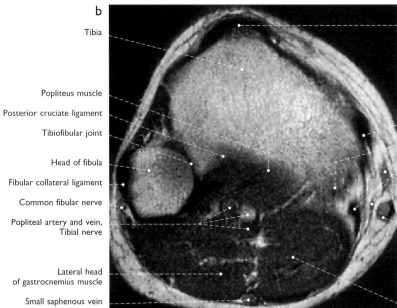

b

Tibia — Patellar ligament

Popliteus muscle —

Posterior cruciate ligament — Tibial collateral ligament

Tibiofibular joint — Tendon of semimembranosus muscle

Head of fibula — Tendons of sartorius, semitendinosus, and gracilis muscles, ⟨Pes anserinus⟩

Fibular collateral ligament —

Common fibular nerve — Great saphenous vein

Popliteal artery and vein, Tibial nerve —

Lateral head of gastrocnemius muscle —

Small saphenous vein — Medial head of gastrocnemius muscle

272 Right leg (70%)

Transverse sections through the proximal leg at the level
of the superior tibiofibular joint, inferior (distal) aspect

a   Anatomical section
b   Magnetic resonance image (MRI, T$_1$-weighted)

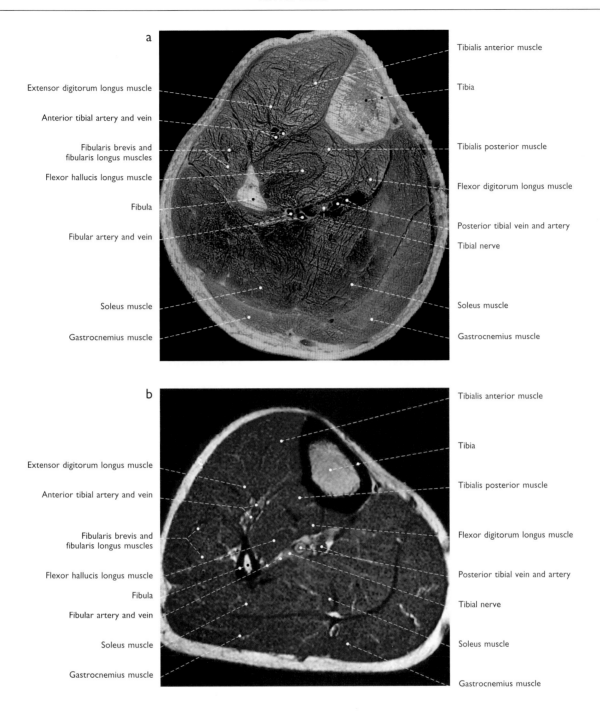

a

Extensor digitorum longus muscle

Anterior tibial artery and vein

Fibularis brevis and
fibularis longus muscles

Flexor hallucis longus muscle

Fibula

Fibular artery and vein

Soleus muscle

Gastrocnemius muscle

Tibialis anterior muscle

Tibia

Tibialis posterior muscle

Flexor digitorum longus muscle

Posterior tibial vein and artery

Tibial nerve

Soleus muscle

Gastrocnemius muscle

b

Extensor digitorum longus muscle

Anterior tibial artery and vein

Fibularis brevis and
fibularis longus muscles

Flexor hallucis longus muscle

Fibula

Fibular artery and vein

Soleus muscle

Gastrocnemius muscle

Tibialis anterior muscle

Tibia

Tibialis posterior muscle

Flexor digitorum longus muscle

Posterior tibial vein and artery

Tibial nerve

Soleus muscle

Gastrocnemius muscle

273 Right leg (70%)
Transverse sections through the proximal third of the leg,
inferior (distal) aspect
a Anatomical section
b Magnetic resonance image (MRI, T$_1$-weighted)

a

Extensor hallucis longus muscle

Extensor digitorum longus muscle

Fibularis brevis and fibularis longus muscles

Fibula

Fibular artery and vein

Flexor hallucis longus muscle

Soleus muscle

Small saphenous vein

Tibialis anterior muscle

Tibia

Anterior tibial artery and vein, Deep fibular nerve

Tibialis posterior muscle

Flexor digitorum longus muscle

Posterior tibial artery and vein, Tibial nerve

Soleus muscle

Gastrocnemius muscle

b

Extensor hallucis longus muscle

Extensor digitorum longus muscle

Fibularis brevis muscle

Fibula

Fibular artery and vein

Flexor hallucis longus muscle

Fibularis longus muscle

Soleus muscle

Tibialis anterior muscle

Tibia

Anterior tibial artery and vein, Deep fibular nerve

Great saphenous vein

Tibialis posterior muscle

Flexor digitorum longus muscle

Posterior tibial artery and vein, Tibial nerve

Soleus muscle

Gastrocnemius muscle

Small saphenous vein

274 Right leg (75%)

Transverse sections through the middle third of the leg, inferior (distal) aspect
a Anatomical section
b Magnetic resonance image (MRI, T$_1$-weighted)

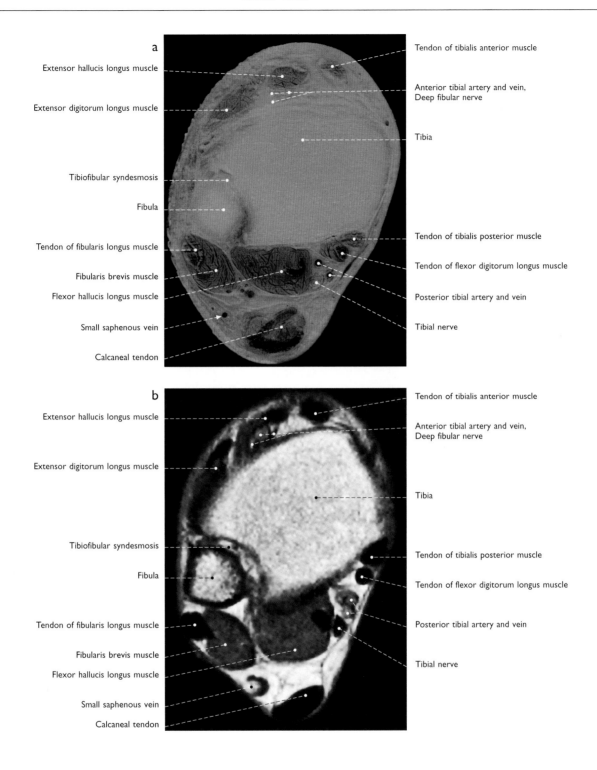

a

Extensor hallucis longus muscle

Extensor digitorum longus muscle

Tibiofibular syndesmosis

Fibula

Tendon of fibularis longus muscle

Fibularis brevis muscle

Flexor hallucis longus muscle

Small saphenous vein

Calcaneal tendon

Tendon of tibialis anterior muscle

Anterior tibial artery and vein,
Deep fibular nerve

Tibia

Tendon of tibialis posterior muscle

Tendon of flexor digitorum longus muscle

Posterior tibial artery and vein

Tibial nerve

b

Extensor hallucis longus muscle

Extensor digitorum longus muscle

Tibiofibular syndesmosis

Fibula

Tendon of fibularis longus muscle

Fibularis brevis muscle

Flexor hallucis longus muscle

Small saphenous vein

Calcaneal tendon

Tendon of tibialis anterior muscle

Anterior tibial artery and vein,
Deep fibular nerve

Tibia

Tendon of tibialis posterior muscle

Tendon of flexor digitorum longus muscle

Posterior tibial artery and vein

Tibial nerve

275 Right leg (75%)

Transverse sections through the distal leg at the level
of the inferior tibiofibular joint (= tibiofibular syndesmosis),
inferior (distal) aspect

a Anatomical section
b Magnetic resonance image (MRI, T$_1$-weighted)

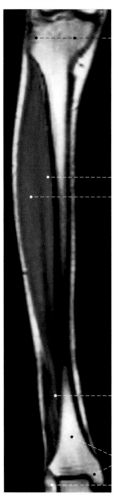

a

Lateral and medial
condyles of tibia

Tibialis anterior muscle

Extensor digitorum
longus muscle

Extensor hallucis
longus muscle

Tibia
– Body of tibia
– Medial malleolus

Lateral malleolus
of fibula

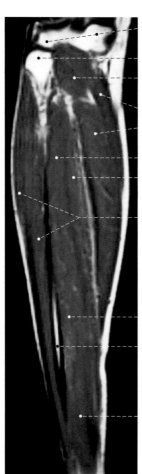

b

Lateral and medial
condyles of tibia

Head of fibula

Popliteus muscle

Triceps surae muscle
– Medial head
of gastrocnemius muscle
– Soleus muscle

Tibialis posterior muscle

Flexor digitorum
longus muscle

Fibularis longus
and fibularis brevis
muscles

Flexor hallucis
longus muscle

Fibula

Flexor hallucis
longus muscle

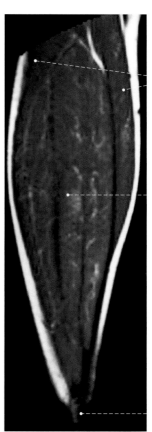

c

Gastrocnemius
muscle
– Lateral head
– Medial head

Soleus muscle

Calcaneal tendon
of triceps surae
muscle

276 Right leg (30%)

a–c Coronal magnetic resonance images (MRI, T_1-weighted)
through the
a ventral part
b middle part
c dorsal part
of the leg, ventral aspect

a

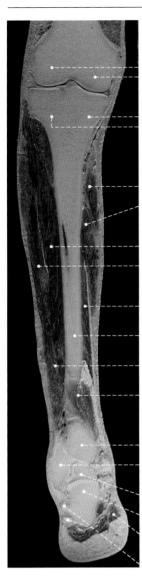

Femur
– Lateral condyle
– Medial condyle

Tibia
– Medial condyle
– Lateral condyle

Triceps surae muscle
– Medial head
  of gastrocnemius m.
– Soleus muscle

Tibialis anterior muscle

Extensor digitorum
longus muscle

Flexor digitorum
longus muscle

Body of tibia

Extensor hallucis
longus muscle

Flexor hallucis
longus muscle

Tibia

Lateral malleolus
of fibula

Talus

Calcaneus

Abductor hallucis
muscle

Tendons
of fibularis brevis
and fibularis longus
muscles

b

Lateral head
of gastrocnemius muscle

Medial condyle
of femur

Medial condyle
of tibia

Popliteus muscle

Posterior tibial a., vv.,
Tibial nerve

Head of fibula

Soleus muscle

Fibularis longus m.

Tibialis posterior m.

Flexor digitorum
longus muscle

Body of fibula

Fibularis brevis muscle

Flexor hallucis longus
muscle

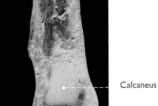

Calcaneus

c

Sartorius muscle

Small saphenous vein

Gastrocnemius muscle
– Medial head
– Lateral head

Soleus muscle

Calcaneal tendon
of triceps surae muscle

Calcaneus

277 **Right leg** (30%)

a–c Coronal anatomical sections
     through the
a   ventral part
b   middle part
c   dorsal part
     of the leg, ventral aspect

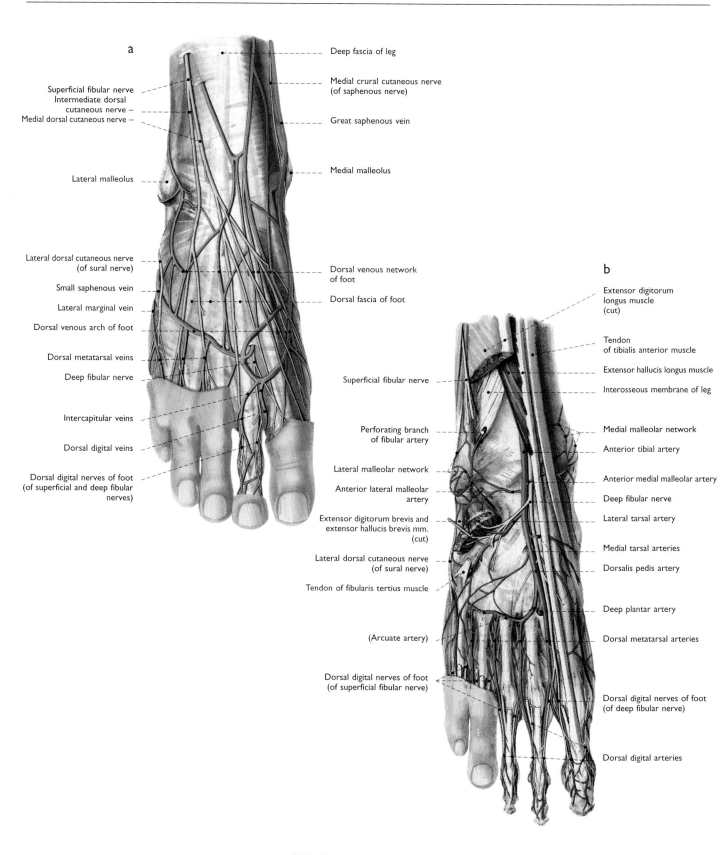

a

Superficial fibular nerve
Intermediate dorsal
cutaneous nerve –
Medial dorsal cutaneous nerve –

Lateral malleolus

Lateral dorsal cutaneous nerve
(of sural nerve)

Small saphenous vein

Lateral marginal vein

Dorsal venous arch of foot

Dorsal metatarsal veins

Deep fibular nerve

Intercapitular veins

Dorsal digital veins

Dorsal digital nerves of foot
(of superficial and deep fibular
nerves)

Deep fascia of leg

Medial crural cutaneous nerve
(of saphenous nerve)

Great saphenous vein

Medial malleolus

Dorsal venous network
of foot

Dorsal fascia of foot

b

Extensor digitorum
longus muscle
(cut)

Tendon
of tibialis anterior muscle

Extensor hallucis longus muscle

Interosseous membrane of leg

Superficial fibular nerve

Perforating branch
of fibular artery

Lateral malleolar network

Anterior lateral malleolar
artery

Extensor digitorum brevis and
extensor hallucis brevis mm.
(cut)

Lateral dorsal cutaneous nerve
(of sural nerve)

Tendon of fibularis tertius muscle

(Arcuate artery)

Dorsal digital nerves of foot
(of superficial fibular nerve)

Medial malleolar network

Anterior tibial artery

Anterior medial malleolar artery

Deep fibular nerve

Lateral tarsal artery

Medial tarsal arteries

Dorsalis pedis artery

Deep plantar artery

Dorsal metatarsal arteries

Dorsal digital nerves of foot
(of deep fibular nerve)

Dorsal digital arteries

**278 Blood vessels and nerves of the dorsum
of the right foot** (50%)
Ventral aspect
a Subcutaneous veins and nerves
b Arteries and nerves after removal of the dorsal fascia of foot

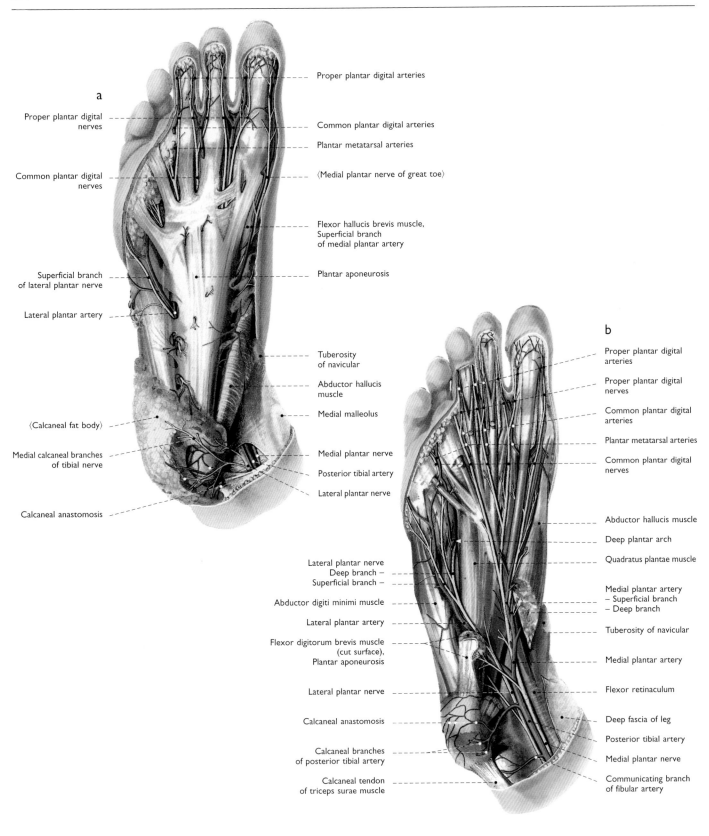

a

Proper plantar digital arteries

Proper plantar digital nerves

Common plantar digital arteries

Plantar metatarsal arteries

Common plantar digital nerves

⟨Medial plantar nerve of great toe⟩

Flexor hallucis brevis muscle, Superficial branch of medial plantar artery

Superficial branch of lateral plantar nerve

Plantar aponeurosis

Lateral plantar artery

Tuberosity of navicular

Abductor hallucis muscle

Medial malleolus

⟨Calcaneal fat body⟩

Medial calcaneal branches of tibial nerve

Medial plantar nerve

Posterior tibial artery

Lateral plantar nerve

Calcaneal anastomosis

b

Proper plantar digital arteries

Proper plantar digital nerves

Common plantar digital arteries

Plantar metatarsal arteries

Common plantar digital nerves

Abductor hallucis muscle

Deep plantar arch

Quadratus plantae muscle

Medial plantar artery – Superficial branch – Deep branch

Lateral plantar nerve
Deep branch –
Superficial branch –

Abductor digiti minimi muscle

Lateral plantar artery

Tuberosity of navicular

Flexor digitorum brevis muscle (cut surface), Plantar aponeurosis

Medial plantar artery

Lateral plantar nerve

Flexor retinaculum

Calcaneal anastomosis

Deep fascia of leg

Calcaneal branches of posterior tibial artery

Posterior tibial artery

Medial plantar nerve

Calcaneal tendon of triceps surae muscle

Communicating branch of fibular artery

279 Arteries and nerves of the sole of the right foot (50%)

Plantar aspect
a Superficial layer
b The abductor hallucis muscle and the short flexor muscle of toes were partially removed.

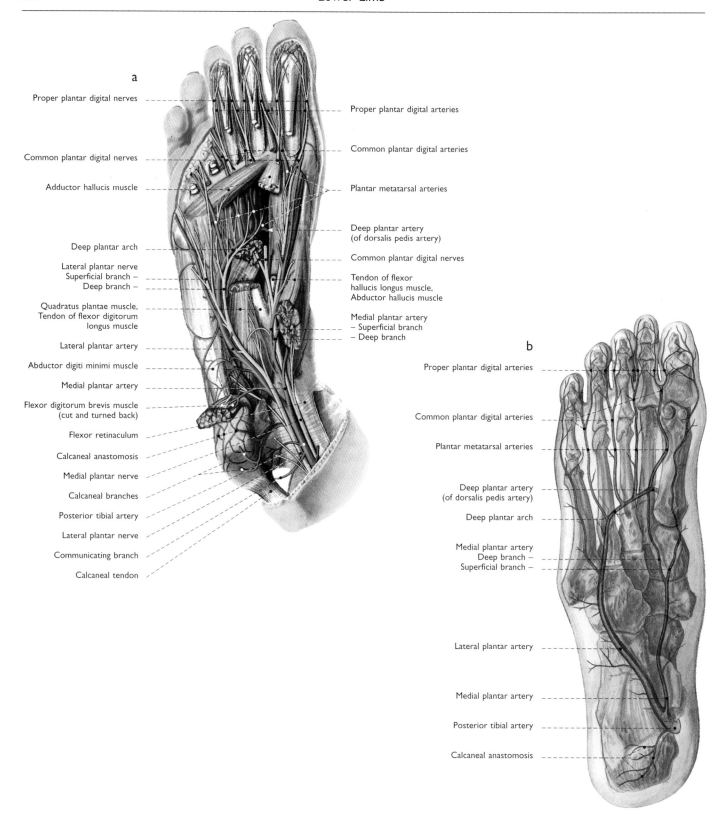

a

Proper plantar digital nerves

Common plantar digital nerves

Adductor hallucis muscle

Deep plantar arch

Lateral plantar nerve
Superficial branch –
Deep branch –

Quadratus plantae muscle,
Tendon of flexor digitorum
longus muscle

Lateral plantar artery

Abductor digiti minimi muscle

Medial plantar artery

Flexor digitorum brevis muscle
(cut and turned back)

Flexor retinaculum

Calcaneal anastomosis

Medial plantar nerve

Calcaneal branches

Posterior tibial artery

Lateral plantar nerve

Communicating branch

Calcaneal tendon

Proper plantar digital arteries

Common plantar digital arteries

Plantar metatarsal arteries

Deep plantar artery
(of dorsalis pedis artery)

Common plantar digital nerves

Tendon of flexor
hallucis longus muscle,
Abductor hallucis muscle

Medial plantar artery
– Superficial branch
– Deep branch

b

Proper plantar digital arteries

Common plantar digital arteries

Plantar metatarsal arteries

Deep plantar artery
(of dorsalis pedis artery)

Deep plantar arch

Medial plantar artery
Deep branch –
Superficial branch –

Lateral plantar artery

Medial plantar artery

Posterior tibial artery

Calcaneal anastomosis

**280 Arteries and nerves of the sole
of the right foot** (50%)

Plantar aspect
a The oblique head of the abductor hallucis muscle and
the short flexor muscle of toes were partially removed.
b Arteries of the sole of the right foot, schematic representation

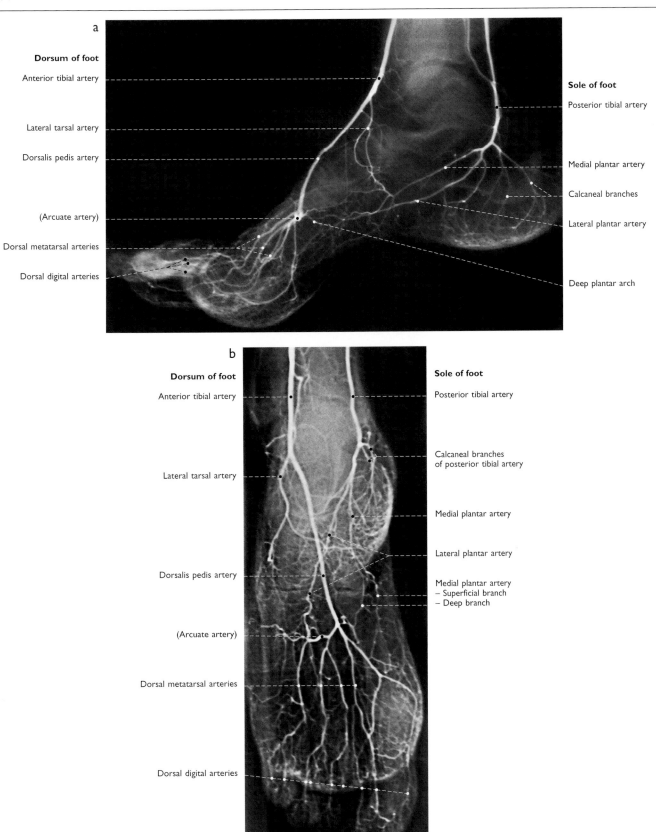

a

Dorsum of foot

Anterior tibial artery

Lateral tarsal artery

Dorsalis pedis artery

(Arcuate artery)

Dorsal metatarsal arteries

Dorsal digital arteries

Sole of foot

Posterior tibial artery

Medial plantar artery

Calcaneal branches

Lateral plantar artery

Deep plantar arch

b

Dorsum of foot

Anterior tibial artery

Lateral tarsal artery

Dorsalis pedis artery

(Arcuate artery)

Dorsal metatarsal arteries

Dorsal digital arteries

Sole of foot

Posterior tibial artery

Calcaneal branches
of posterior tibial artery

Medial plantar artery

Lateral plantar artery

Medial plantar artery
– Superficial branch
– Deep branch

281 Arteries of the right foot (45%)

a Lateromedial arteriogram
b Dorsoplantar (anteroposterior) arteriogram
of the arteries of the right foot

Subject Index

Volume numbering is given in bold print, followed by page numbers.
Adjectives generally precede nouns (as in the index of the Terminologia Anatomica).
Brackets in the text of illustrations were omitted in the subject index.

A

A1 segment of anterior cerebral artery →
Precommunicating part of anterior cerebral
artery
A2 segment of anterior cerebral artery →
Postcommunicating part of anterior cerebral
artery
Abdomen **1**: 2, 62, 75; **2**: 154–155, 162, 167,
172, 182, 190–193, 196–207, 218–225,
227–229
Abdominal aorta **1**: 12–14; **2**: 105, 107, 155,
162, 171, 182, 186, 189, 196, 199, 202–203,
206–208, 211, 213–215, 218–224, 228–230,
234, 243
– aortic nerve plexus **1**: 25; **2**: 248–249
– cavity **2**: 171
– lymph nodes **1**: 15
– organs **1**: 170–172, 190–193
– ostium of uterine tube **2**: 239–240
– part of esophagus **2**: 105, 174–175, 206–207
– – – pectoralis major muscle **1**: 63–65
– – – thoracic duct **1**: 15
– – – ureter **2**: 216
– viscera **1**: 18–21; **2**: 170–172, 190–193
– wall **1**: 54
Abducens nerve [VI] → Abducent nerve [VI]
Abducent nerve [VI] **1**: 22; **2**: 291–295, 298,
306, 309, 311, 378–382
Abduction **1**: 5
Abductor digiti minimi muscle of foot **1**: 208,
211, 214, 232, 236–238, 240, 279–280
– – – – – hand **1**: 103, 121–125, 127–128, 130,
165–166
– hallucis muscle **1**: 208, 214–215, 231,
236–238, 240–241, 277, 279–280
– pollicis brevis muscle **1**: 103, 116, 121–122,
124, 128, 130, 152, 162, 166
– – longus muscle **1**: 114–119, 121–122, 124,
128, 130, 152–154, 157–159, 162, 165
Aberrant ductules of epididymis **2**: 270
Accessory cephalic vein **1**: 150
– hemi-azygos vein **1**: 14; **2**: 163
– hepatic ducts **2**: 187
– lacrimal gland **2**: 366
– nasal cartilages **2**: 54
– nerve [XI] **1**: 22, 51, 60, 68, 112; **2**: 32, 37,
92–93, 96, 98–100, 149, 284, 289, 291–292,
294–295, 306, 311, 340
– pancreatic duct **2**: 188
– parotid gland **2**: 44
– process of lumbar vertebra **1**: 33
– renal arteries **2**: 162, 214–215
– saphenous vein **1**: 245, 248, 254–255, 266;
2: 228
Acetabular branch of obturator artery **1**: 193
– fossa **1**: 172–173, 176, 190–191, 193–194;
2: 195, 257–259
– index **1**: 177
– labrum **1**: 193

Acetabular
– margin **1**: 172, 175–176, 193
– notch **1**: 172, 176
Acetabulum **1**: 172, 175–177, 190–191, 193,
249, 258; **2**: 205, 250, 252, 254
Acoustic areas of cerebral cortex **2**: 319
– radiation **2**: 332, 350
Acromial anastomosis of thoraco-acromial
artery **1**: 135, 142; **2**: 91–92
– angle **1**: 84–85
– branch of thoraco-acromial artery **2**: 93, 98
– end of clavicle **1**: 84, 95, 97, 142–143
– facet of clavicle **1**: 84
– part of deltoid muscle **1**: 108
Acromioclavicular joint **1**: 82–83, 95–96, 111
– ligament **1**: 9, 95–96, 108
Acromion **1**: 53, 63–64, 84–85, 87, 95–97, 105,
108, 136, 142–143, 149
Adduction **1**: 5
Adductor brevis muscle **1**: 220, 227–229, 253,
259–260, 262
– canal **1**: 219, 252–253
– hallucis muscle **1**: 238, 240, 280
– hiatus **1**: 220
– longus muscle **1**: 219–221, 227–229, 252–253,
258–260, 262–263; **2**: 228
– magnus muscle **1**: 195, 219–224, 227–229,
233, 252, 255–256, 258–263; **2**: 253, 255
– minimus muscle **1**: 220, 223–224, 227–228
– pollicis muscle **1**: 121–124, 126, 128, 130, 162,
166–167
– tubercle of femur **1**: 179–180
Adductors of thigh → Medial muscles of thigh
Adenohypophysis **2**: 293, 307, 328
Aditus to mastoid antrum **2**: 396
Adrenal gland → Suprarenal gland
Adult peritoneal cavity **2**: 170
Afferent nerve fiber(s) **1**: 23
Affluent blood pathway of left ventricle of heart
2: 133
Agger nasi **2**: 55
Ala of crista galli **2**: 22
– – ilium **1**: 173–176, 191, 205, 220, 225, 252,
254
– – nose **2**: 44
– – sacrum **1**: 34–35
– – vomer **2**: 23
Alar folds of infrapatellar synovial fold **1**: 198,
200
– ligament(s) **1**: 50
– part of nasalis muscle **2**: 30
Alimentary system **1**: 16; **2**: 52–53
Alveolar arch of mandible **2**: 25
– – – maxilla **2**: 24
– foramina of maxilla **2**: 24
– margin of maxilla **2**: 24
– part of mandible **2**: 25, 41
– process of maxilla **2**: 24, 58–59, 369
– yokes of mandible **2**: 25
– – – maxilla **2**: 4, 24
Alveoli of lung **2**: 115

Alveus of hippocampus **2**: 324, 326, 340, 348
Ambient cistern → Cisterna ambiens
– gyrus **2**: 315, 317, 324, 334, 338
Amnion **2**: 243
Amniotic cavity **2**: 242
Ampulla of ductus deferens **1**: 17, 77;
2: 236–237
– – duodenum **2**: 174–176, 194
– – lacrimal canaliculus **2**: 365
– – uterine tube **1**: 17; **2**: 239–240
Ampullary bony limbs **2**: 401
– renal pelvis **2**: 216
Amygdaloid body **2**: 325, 330–331, 338, 344
– complex → Amygdaloid body
Anal canal **1**: 16–17, 19; **2**: 179, 232–233, 237,
243, 253, 255, 265–267
– columns **2**: 179, 251
– hiatus of pelvic diaphragm **2**: 264–265
– pecten **2**: 179
– sinuses **2**: 179
– valves **2**: 179
Anastomotic branch of middle meningeal artery
with lacrimal artery **2**: 77
Anatomical conjugate **1**: 178
– neck of humerus **1**: 86
– snuffbox **1**: 105, 125
Anconeus muscle **1**: 101, 105, 109, 113,
117–119, 142–143, 154, 156
Angle of mandible **2**: 5, 7, 25, 31
– – mouth **2**: 38, 44
– – rib **1**: 42, 44
Angular artery **2**: 76, 85–87, 383
– gyrus **2**: 297, 316
– incisure of stomach **2**: 173–176, 194
– vein **2**: 80, 383
Ankle bone → Talus
– joint **1**: 170–171, 188, 206, 208–214, 234
Annular → Anular
Annulus → Anulus
Anococcygeal body **2**: 230, 265–266, 279
– ligament → Anococcygeal body
– nerve(s) **2**: 279
Anocutaneous line **2**: 179
Anomalous tubercle of tooth **2**: 39
Anorectal flexure of anal canal **2**: 232
– junction **2**: 179
Ansa cervicalis **1**: 112; **2**: 34–35, 87, 93–94,
97–100
– subclavia **2**: 96, 100, 167
Antebrachial fascia **1**: 106–109, 114–115,
119–120, 135–136, 141, 150–152, 160
Anterior **1**: 5
– abdominal wall **1**: 63–67, 75, 77, 79; **2**: 238,
272–273
– ampullary bony limb **2**: 401
– – nerve **2**: 405
– arch of atlas **1**: 30, 36–37, 40, 51, 60; **2**: 37,
52, 294, 302
– articular facet of dens axis **1**: 30
– atlanto-axial membrane **1**: 49, 51
– atlanto-occipital membrane **1**: 49, 51; **2**: 294

Anterior
- auricular branch(es) of superficial temporal artery **2**: 98
- axillary fold **1**: 62
- – line **1**: 4
- – lymph nodes → Pectoral axillary lymph nodes
- basal segment of left lung [S VIII] **2**: 117
- – – – right lung [S VIII] **2**: 116
- – segmental bronchus of left lung [B VIII] **2**: 108–109, 114
- – – – – right lung [B VIII] **2**: 108–109, 114, 120–121
- belly of digastric muscle **2**: 32, 34, 36, 44–45, 47–48, 98–99
- bony ampulla **2**: 401–402
- border of fibula **1**: 182–183
- – – – lung **2**: 111–112
- – – radius **1**: 88
- – – testis **2**: 270
- – – tibia **1**: 182–183, 216, 230
- – – ulna **1**: 89
- branch(es) of great auricular nerve **2**: 82, 91–92
- – – inferior pancreaticoduodenal artery **2**: 198
- – – medial antebrachial cutaneous nerve **1**: 132, 136, 151
- – – obturator artery **1**: 193, 253
- – – – nerve **1**: 242–243, 248, 252, 254–255, 266
- – – renal artery **2**: 218
- – – ulnar recurrent artery **1**: 153
- cardiac vein(s) → Anterior vein(s) of right ventricle
- cerebral artery **2**: 292, 298–302, 347, 349, 351, 354–358
- – veins **2**: 300
- cervical region **1**: 4; **2**: 99
- chamber of eyeball **2**: 374–375, 384–385
- choroidal artery **2**: 300
- ciliary artery(-ies) **2**: 371–373
- – vein(s) **2**: 373
- circumflex humeral artery **1**: 138–141, 143
- clinoid process **2**: 7, 10, 19, 293, 301, 368, 378, 380
- commissure of diencephalon **2**: 307, 317, 320, 324, 328, 330, 333–335, 338–339, 344, 350
- – – labia majora **2**: 269
- communicating artery **2**: 292, 298–299, 301, 351
- conjunctival artery(-ies) **2**: 372–373
- – vein(s) **2**: 373
- corticospinal tract **2**: 288
- cranial fossa **2**: 10, 56, 60, 291, 362, 369, 394
- cruciate ligament **1**: 196, 198–204, 265
- cusp of mitral valve **2**: 133–135, 140
- – – tricuspid valve **2**: 132, 135
- cutaneous branch(es) of femoral nerve **1**: 78, 242, 248, 270; **2**: 227–228
- – – – iliohypogastric nerve **1**: 242
- – – – intercostal nerves **1**: 23, 78, 132; **2**: 93
- deep temporal artery **2**: 76
- ethmoidal artery **2**: 77, 88, 90, 380–382
- – cells **2**: 60, 62, 336, 358–359, 365, 369, 380, 385–386
- – foramen **2**: 21, 367–368
- – nerve **2**: 82–86, 88, 90, 381–383
- – vein **2**: 381
- extremity of spleen **2**: 189
- facet on talus for calcaneus **1**: 187, 207
- fold of malleus **2**: 391–392, 398

Anterior
- fontanelle **2**: 17
- funiculus of spinal cord **2**: 288, 340
- gastric branches of anterior vagal trunk **2**: 167, 248
- gluteal line of ilium **1**: 176
- horn of lateral meniscus **1**: 201
- – – – ventricle → Frontal horn of lateral ventricle
- – – – medial meniscus **1**: 201
- – – – spinal cord **1**: 23, 79; **2**: 288
- hypothalamic nucleus **2**: 328
- inferior cerebellar artery **2**: 292, 298–299, 302
- – fissure of cerebellum → Intrabiventral fissure of cerebellum
- – iliac spine **1**: 172–174, 176, 191–192, 249
- – segmental artery of kidney **2**: 212, 214
- intercavernous sinus → Intercavernous sinus(es)
- intercondylar area **1**: 182
- intercostal branches of internal thoracic artery **1**: 75–76
- – – – – – vein **1**: 75
- intermuscular septum of leg **1**: 271
- internal vertebral venous plexus **2**: 285, 287
- interosseous artery **1**: 138, 153–155, 157
- – nerve **1**: 153
- – veins **1**: 157
- interpositus nucleus **2**: 309
- interventricular branch of left coronary artery **2**: 124, 129, 132, 135, 141–142, 144, 147–148
- – sulcus **2**: 124, 132, 134, 141, 145
- – vein **2**: 129, 132, 142
- jugular vein **2**: 33, 74–75, 91, 97–98, 122, 149
- labial nerve(s) **2**: 280
- lacrimal crest of maxilla **2**: 24, 367–368
- lateral malleolar artery **1**: 271, 278
- – nasal branches of anterior ethmoidal artery **2**: 77, 88
- – segment of liver [VI] **2**: 184
- layer of rectus sheath **1**: 63–65
- – – thoracolumbar fascia **1**: 54–55
- ligament of fibular head **1**: 195–196, 205
- limb of internal capsule **2**: 332–334, 337, 348, 350, 355–356
- – – stapes **2**: 397
- lobe of pituitary gland → Adenohypophysis
- longitudinal ligament **1**: 37, 39, 46–49, 51, 190
- medial malleolar artery **1**: 271, 278
- – segment of liver [V] **2**: 184
- median fissure of medulla oblongata **2**: 306
- – – – spinal cord **2**: 285, 288, 340
- – line **1**: 4
- mediastinum **2**: 104
- membranous ampulla **2**: 405
- meningeal branch of anterior ethmoidal artery **2**: 77, 90
- meniscofemoral ligament **1**: 200
- muscles of thigh **1**: 219
- nasal spine of maxilla **2**: 4, 6, 12, 23–24, 56–57
- notch of auricle **2**: 390
- nuclei of thalamus **2**: 325–327, 331, 340, 344
- palpebral margin **2**: 364, 366
- papillary muscle of left ventricle of heart **2**: 133–134, 137, 140, 145
- – – – right ventricle of heart **2**: 132
- para-olfactory sulcus **2**: 304, 317
- paraventricular nucleus of thalamus **2**: 331
- part of cerebral peduncle → Cerebral crus
- – – diaphragmatic surface of liver **2**: 180

Anterior part of
- – – dorsum of tongue → Anterior part of tongue
- – – medial palpebral ligament **2**: 365
- – – tongue **2**: 101
- – – vaginal fornix **2**: 240
- pectoral cutaneous branches of intercostal nerves **1**: 23
- perforated substance **2**: 306, 315, 324–325, 331, 335
- petroclinoid fold **2**: 291, 293
- pharyngeal wall **2**: 101
- pillar of fauces → Palatoglossal arch
- pole of eyeball **2**: 374
- – – lens **2**: 374, 377
- process of malleus **2**: 397
- quadrangular lobule of cerebellum **2**: 308
- ramus(-i) of cervical nerves **2**: 94, 284, 286
- – – lateral cerebral sulcus **2**: 316
- – – lumbar nerves **2**: 226
- – – sacral nerves **2**: 284
- – – spinal nerve **1**: 23, 79; **2**: 284–286
- – – thoracic nerves → Intercostal nerves
- recess of tympanic membrane **2**: 398
- region of arm **1**: 4
- – – elbow **1**: 106, 137, 140–141, 151
- – – forearm **1**: 151
- – – thigh **1**: 4
- right ventricular branch(es) of right coronary artery **2**: 124, 135, 142, 144, 146
- root of ansa cervicalis → Superior root of ansa cervicalis
- – – cervical nerve **2**: 95, 166, 288–289, 306
- – – sacral nerve **2**: 232
- – – spinal nerve **1**: 23; **2**: 95, 166, 285–286, 288–289, 306
- – – thoracic nerve **2**: 166, 286
- rootlets of cervical nerve **2**: 311
- – – spinal nerve **1**: 23; **2**: 285, 288, 311
- sacral foramina **1**: 34, 38, 172, 174
- sacro-iliac ligament **1**: 190–191
- scalene muscle **1**: 68; **2**: 33–37, 72, 75, 92–93, 96, 98, 149, 165
- scrotal nerves **1**: 78, 248
- segment of left lung [S III] **2**: 117
- – – right lung [S III] **2**: 116
- segmental bronchus of left lung [B III] **2**: 108–109, 114
- – – – right lung [B III] **2**: 108–109, 114, 120–121
- semicircular canal **2**: 396, 398–402, 407
- – duct **2**: 399, 405, 407
- semilunar cusp of pulmonary valve **2**: 132, 135
- septal branches of anterior ethmoidal artery **2**: 90
- spinal artery **2**: 285–286, 295, 298
- – veins **2**: 285–286
- spinocerebellar tract **2**: 288
- spinothalamic tract **2**: 288
- sternoclavicular ligament **1**: 45
- superior iliac spine **1**: 62–65, 172–176, 191–193, 216, 218–220, 226, 248–249, 252–253, 257; **2**: 228
- – pancreaticoduodenal artery **2**: 198, 200, 203, 219
- – segmental artery of kidney **2**: 212, 214
- surface of cornea **2**: 374
- – – eyelid **2**: 366
- – – kidney **2**: 208, 218
- – – lens **2**: 374, 377
- – – maxilla **2**: 24
- – – patella **1**: 181

Anterior surface of
– – – petrous part of temporal bone **2**: 20
– – – prostate **2**: 237
– – – radius **1**: 88
– – – ulna **1**: 89
– talar articular surface of calcaneus **1**: 187, 207
– talofibular ligament **1**: 206
– tegmental nuclei of midbrain **2**: 328
– temporal branch of middle cerebral artery **2**: 302
– thalamic radiation **2**: 332–333
– tibial artery **1**: 250, 268–269, 271, 273–275, 278, 281
– – recurrent artery **1**: 250, 271
– – vein(s) **1**: 247, 273–275
– tibiofibular ligament **1**: 205–206
– tibiotalar part of medial ligament of ankle joint **1**: 212
– triangle → Anterior cervical region
– tubercle of atlas **1**: 30, 50; **2**: 37
– – – cervical vertebra **1**: 30–31; **2**: 33
– tympanic artery **2**: 77, 87–89
– vagal trunk **1**: 25; **2**: 167, 248–249
– vein(s) of right ventricle of heart **2**: 135, 142
– – – septum pellucidum **2**: 300, 322, 337
– vertebral muscles **2**: 37
– wall of vagina **2**: 240, 245
– white commissure of spinal cord **2**: 288
Anterolateral central arteries **2**: 298, 300, 338
– fontanelle → Sphenoidal fontanelle
– spinal artery **2**: 298
– sulcus of medulla oblongata **2**: 306
– – – spinal cord **1**: 23; **2**: 285, 288, 311, 340
– surface of arytenoid cartilage **2**: 64
– – – humerus **1**: 86
Anteromedial central artery **2**: 300
– frontal branch of callosomarginal artery **2**: 299
– nucleus of spinal cord **2**: 288
– surface of humerus **1**: 86
Antihelix **2**: 390
Antitragus **2**: 390
Anular ligament(s) of radius **1**: 98–99
– – – trachea **2**: 47, 50, 65–66, 70, 108–109
– part of fibrous sheaths of digits of hand **1**: 121
– – – – – – toes **1**: 238
Anulus fibrosus of intervertebral disc **1**: 39, 47–48
Anus **1**: 17, 261; **2**: 232, 251, 253, 255, 269, 278
Aorta **2**: 78–79, 96–97, 104–107, 110, 118, 122–135, 137, 139–144, 146–147, 149, 154–155, 157–162, 164–165, 171–172, 182, 196–199, 202–203, 206–208, 211, 213–215, 218–224, 228–230, 234, 243
Aortic arch → Arch of aorta
– bifurcation **1**: 14; **2**: 162, 218–219, 229, 234, 238
– bulb **1**: 14; **2**: 130, 161–162
– hiatus **1**: 69; **2**: 199
– orifice **2**: 141
– sinus **2**: 133
– valve **2**: 104, 128–130, 133–138, 141
Aorticorenal ganglia **2**: 167
Apex of arytenoid cartilage **2**: 64, 69
– – bladder **2**: 235, 238, 245
– – dens axis **1**: 30
– – head of fibula **1**: 182–183
– – heart **2**: 124–125, 132–133, 141–142, 159
– – lung **2**: 72, 111–112, 114, 126, 153
– – nose **2**: 44
– – patella **1**: 181
– – petrous part of temporal bone **2**: 20, 352, 359, 399

Apex of
– – posterior horn of spinal cord **2**: 288
– – prostate **2**: 235–237
– – sacrum **1**: 34–35
– – tongue **2**: 38–39, 46
Apical axillary lymph nodes **1**: 72–73
– bursa of dens axis **1**: 51
– foramen of tooth **2**: 40
– ligament of dens axis **1**: 50–51; **2**: 294
– segment of right lung [S I] **2**: 116
– segmental artery of right lung **2**: 113
– – bronchus of right lung [B I] **2**: 108–109, 113–114, 120–121
Apicoposterior segment of left lung [S I + II] **2**: 117
– segmental bronchus of left lung [B I + II] **2**: 108–109, 114
Aponeurosis of external oblique muscle **1**: 64, 66; **2**: 274
– – trapezius muscle **1**: 53
Appendicular artery **2**: 202–203
– lymph node(s) **2**: 203
– vein **2**: 202
Appendix → Vermiform appendix
– of epididymis **2**: 270
– – testis **1**: 17; **2**: 270, 274
Aqueduct of midbrain **2**: 304–305, 315, 320–321, 324, 328, 335, 340, 350–353, 357–358, 361
Arachnoid granulations **2**: 295–297, 321
– mater **2**: 285–286, 295, 321, 405
Arch of aorta **1**: 12–14, 18–19, 43; **2**: 78–79, 97, 104–107, 110, 118, 122–131, 139, 142–144, 154–155, 161–162, 164–165, 172
– – cricoid cartilage **2**: 52, 64–66, 68, 70, 108
– – thoracic duct **1**: 15, 76; **2**: 149, 163
Arcuate artery of foot **1**: 250, 271, 278, 281
– crest of arytenoid cartilage **2**: 64
– eminence **2**: 10, 291, 396
– fasciculus → Superior longitudinal fasciculus
– fibers of telencephalon **2**: 333
– line of ilium **1**: 176, 191; **2**: 244, 264
– – – rectus sheath **1**: 65
– nucleus of hypothalamus **2**: 328
– popliteal ligament **1**: 195, 233–234
– pubic ligament → Inferior pubic ligament
Areas of cerebral cortex **2**: 318–319
Areola **1**: 70–71
Areolar glands **1**: 70
– venous plexus **1**: 75
Arm **1**: 2, 105–111, 135–137, 139–149
Arterial circle of cerebrum **2**: 292
– grooves on calvaria → Grooves for meningeal arteries
Arteriovenous anastomoses of penis **2**: 277
Artery(-ies) of abdomen **2**: 196–198, 202, 218–219, 229
– – anterior abdominal wall **1**: 77
– – – region of elbow **1**: 140–141
– – arm **1**: 139–143
– – axilla **2**: 93, 149
– – brain **2**: 298–302
– – bulb of penis **2**: 267
– – central sulcus **2**: 297–298
– – dorsal body wall **2**: 162
– – dorsum of foot **1**: 278
– – – – hand **1**: 165
– – eyeball **2**: 372–373
– – face **2**: 86–90
– – female pelvis **2**: 245
– – fingers **1**: 165
– – foot **1**: 271, 278–281

Artery(-ies) of
– – forearm **1**: 152–155
– – gluteal region **1**: 255–257
– – hand **1**: 160–163, 165
– – head **2**: 78–79, 86–90
– – heart **2**: 142–148
– – hypophysis **2**: 301
– – kidney **2**: 214
– – large intestine **2**: 202
– – larynx **2**: 101
– – leg **1**: 267–268, 271
– – lower limb **1**: 250–251, 269
– – male pelvis **2**: 234, 244
– – mediastinum **2**: 149, 165
– – mesentery **2**: 203
– – neck **2**: 78–79, 93, 97–99, 118, 149, 165
– – ovary **2**: 241
– – palm of hand **1**: 160–162
– – penis **2**: 277
– – perineum **2**: 279–280
– – peripharyngeal space **2**: 100
– – pituitary gland **2**: 301
– – popliteal fossa **1**: 255–256, 267–269
– – postcentral sulcus **2**: 297
– – posterior abdominal wall **2**: 228
– – – region of elbow **1**: 142–143
– – precentral sulcus **2**: 297–298
– – pterygoid canal **2**: 88–89
– – rectum **2**: 230–231
– – retroperitoneal organs of upper abdomen **2**: 203
– – round ligament of uterus **2**: 245
– – sheath of optic nerve **2**: 373
– – shoulder **1**: 140, 142–143
– – skull **2**: 76–77
– – sole of foot **1**: 279–280
– – spinal cord **2**: 286
– – thigh **1**: 251–253, 255–256; **2**: 228
– – thorax **1**: 76; **2**: 93, 97, 118
– – thyroid gland **2**: 101
– – tongue **2**: 97
– – trunk **1**: 14
– – upper limb **1**: 138–139
– – uterine tube **2**: 241
– – uterus **2**: 241
– – ventral body wall **1**: 75
– – vertebral column **2**: 286
– to ductus deferens **2**: 234, 244, 274
– – sciatic nerve **1**: 256
– – tail of pancreas **2**: 188
Articular branch(es) of descending genicular artery **1**: 248, 269
– – – sciatic nerve **1**: 256
– capsule **1**: 10–11
– – of atlanto-occipital joint **1**: 49–50
– – – crico-arytenoid joint **2**: 65
– – – cricothyroid joint **2**: 65–67
– – – elbow joint **1**: 98, 116
– – – glenohumeral joint **1**: 95–96, 109–110
– – – hip joint **1**: 193, 220
– – – interphalangeal joint of hand **1**: 104
– – – knee joint **1**: 10, 195, 198–200
– – – lateral atlanto-axial joint **1**: 49–50
– – – temporomandibular joint **2**: 26, 31
– – – zygapophysial joint **1**: 48
– cartilage **1**: 10–11, 202–203
– cavity **1**: 10
– circumference of head of radius **1**: 88, 99
– – – – – ulna **1**: 89, 92, 94
– disc of distal radio-ulnar joint **1**: 104
– – – sternoclavicular joint **1**: 45
– – – temporomandibular joint **2**: 26, 31

Articular
– facet of head of fibula **1**: 183
– – – – radius **1**: 88, 99
– – – – rib **1**: 44
– – – incus **2**: 397
– – – inferior articular process of vertebra **1**: 30, 32–33, 46
– – – lateral malleolus **1**: 182–183, 214
– – – malleus **2**: 397
– – – medial malleolus **1**: 182–183, 205, 214
– – – stapes **2**: 397
– – – superior articular process of sacrum **1**: 34–35
– – – – – – vertebra **1**: 30–33, 42, 46–47; **2**: 286
– – – tubercle of rib **1**: 44
– – on triquetrum for pisiform **1**: 94
– surface of arytenoid cartilage **2**: 64
– – – mandibular fossa of temporal bone **2**: 20
– – – patella **1**: 181, 196, 198, 200
– – on calcaneus for cuboid **1**: 187
– tubercle of temporal bone **2**: 20, 26
Articularis genus muscle **1**: 195, 229
Articulations of auditory ossicles **2**: 397
Ary-epiglottic fold **2**: 50, 52, 101
– part of oblique arytenoid muscle **2**: 67
Arytenoid articular surface of cricoid cartilage **2**: 64
– cartilage **2**: 64–66, 68–69
Ascending aorta **1**: 12, 14; **2**: 78, 96, 104, 107, 122, 124, 128–130, 132–135, 137, 140, 142, 146–147, 149, 157–158, 161–162, 164–165, 167
– branch of lateral circumflex femoral artery **1**: 251–253
– cervical artery **2**: 79, 93, 100, 118, 149
– colon **1**: 16, 18–20; **2**: 171–172, 177–178, 190, 192, 194–196, 200, 202–207, 220, 223–224
– lumbar vein **2**: 287
– palatine artery **2**: 76–77, 99
– part of duodenum **2**: 188, 194, 206
– pharyngeal artery **2**: 76–77, 79, 99–100
– ramus of lateral cerebral sulcus **2**: 316
Association fibers of telencephalon **2**: 333
Athletic person **1**: 6; **2**: 153
Atlantic part of vertebral artery **1**: 60; **2**: 73, 79, 292, 302
Atlanto-axial joints **1**: 49–50
Atlanto-occipital joint **1**: 49–51; **2**: 72
Atlas [C I] **1**: 28, 30–31, 36–37, 40, 49–51, 55, 58–60; **2**: 7, 37, 52, 72–73, 79, 284, 289, 294, 302, 321, 408
Atonic stomach **2**: 174
Atrecial ovarian follicle **2**: 245
Atrial branches of left coronary artery **2**: 144
– – – right coronary artery **2**: 144
– myocardium **2**: 133
Atrioventricular bundle **2**: 135, 140
– nodal branch of right coronary artery **2**: 135, 144
– node **2**: 140
Atrium of middle meatus **2**: 55
Attachment lines of mesenteries **2**: 206
– of muscle(s) **1**: 10
– – – of soft palate to cranial base **2**: 395
Auditory ossicles **2**: 361, 397
– tube → Pharyngotympanic tube
Auricle **2**: 390, 408
Auricular branch of occipital artery **2**: 76
– – – posterior auricular artery **2**: 85, 91–92
– – – vagus nerve **2**: 82

Auricular
– cartilage **2**: 390–391
– surface of ilium **1**: 176
– – – sacrum **1**: 34–35
– tubercle **2**: 390
Auricularis anterior muscle **2**: 28–29
– posterior muscle **2**: 29–30, 91–92
– superior muscle **2**: 28–29, 366
Auriculotemporal nerve **2**: 82–87, 89, 98–99
Autonomic areas of nerves of lower limb **1**: 242–243
– – – – – upper limb **1**: 132–133
– division of peripheral nervous system → Autonomic nervous system
– innervation of eyeball **2**: 382
– nervous system **1**: 24–25; **2**: 95–96, 166–167, 231, 248–249
– – – in abdomen **2**: 167
– – – – lesser pelvis **2**: 231
– – – – neck **2**: 95–96
– – – – retroperitoneal space **2**: 248–249
– – – – thorax **2**: 95–96, 167
– part of peripheral nervous system → Autonomic nervous system
Axes **1**: 5
– of eyeball **2**: 374
Axilla **1**: 72–74, 144; **2**: 93
Axillary artery **1**: 138–141, 143, 148; **2**: 79, 93–94, 149
– fossa **1**: 149; **2**: 93
– lymph nodes **1**: 15, 73–74; **2**: 163
– lymphatic plexus **1**: 15; **2**: 163
– nerve **1**: 61, 78, 112–113, 132–135, 140–141, 143; **2**: 94
– recess of glenohumeral joint **1**: 95–97, 109
– region **2**: 149
– vein **1**: 73, 137, 148; **2**: 149, 163
Axis [C II] **1**: 30–31, 36–37, 40, 49–51, 55; **2**: 5, 7, 52, 72, 294, 408
– of pelvis **1**: 178
Azygos vein **1**: 14; **2**: 97, 122, 130, 132, 155–159, 161–165, 167, 222

B

Back **1**: 52–60
Bare area of diaphragmatic surface of liver **2**: 180–181, 206–207
Basal nuclei **2**: 329–331
Base of arytenoid cartilage **2**: 64
– – cochlea **2**: 401, 403, 406
– – lung **2**: 111–112
– – mandible **2**: 25, 41, 99
– – metacarpal bone **1**: 94, 103, 123, 129
– – metatarsal bone **1**: 186, 209–210
– – modiolus cochleae **2**: 403
– – nose **2**: 44
– – patella **1**: 181
– – phalanx of foot **1**: 186
– – – – hand **1**: 94
– – posterior horn of spinal cord **2**: 288
– – prostate **2**: 235–237
– – renal pyramid **2**: 212
– – sacrum **1**: 34–35, 172, 174; **2**: 264
– – skull **2**: 8–11, 16, 37, 293, 394–395, 400
– – stapes **2**: 397
Basicranium → Cranial base
Basilar artery **2**: 292, 295, 298–302, 352–353, 358–359, 361, 409
– lamina of spiral membrane → Basilar membrane of cochlear duct

Basilar
– membrane of cochlear duct **2**: 404
– part of occipital bone **1**: 37, 49; **2**: 8, 18, 49, 51, 290, 294
– sulcus of pons **2**: 309, 344
– venous plexus **1**: 51; **2**: 291, 293–294
Basilic vein **1**: 105, 136–137, 140, 146–147, 150–151, 164
Basivertebral veins **2**: 287
Belly of muscle **1**: 10
Biceps brachii muscle **1**: 62, 64, 95–99, 101, 105–112, 114–117, 140–149, 151–153, 156; **2**: 93
– femoris muscle **1**: 195, 199–200, 204, 217, 221–224, 226–227, 229, 232–235, 255–256, 258, 261–265, 267–268, 271
Bicipital aponeurosis **1**: 106, 114, 136, 140–141, 151–153
– groove → Intertubercular sulcus of humerus
Bicipitoradial bursa **1**: 116
Bifurcate ligament **1**: 206–207
Bile duct **2**: 181, 183, 186–188, 198–199, 223, 248
Biventral lobule of cerebellum **2**: 307–309
Body of bladder **2**: 232–233, 235, 245, 258–259
– – breast **1**: 70–71, 74
– – calcaneus **1**: 187
– – caudate nucleus **2**: 300, 322, 326, 329–332, 340–341, 344, 361
– – clavicle **1**: 84
– – clitoris **2**: 233, 260, 268
– – corpus callosum → Trunk of corpus callosum
– – epididymis **2**: 270–272
– – femur **1**: 177, 179–180, 197, 202–203, 247, 251, 258–260
– – fibula **1**: 182–183, 197, 205, 209, 214, 277
– – fornix **2**: 299–300, 304–305, 307, 322, 324–326, 340, 344, 346, 361
– – gallbladder **2**: 186
– – humerus **1**: 86–87, 90–91, 95–98, 100, 109–111, 145–146, 149
– – hyoid bone **2**: 27, 36, 47–48, 52, 65–66, 68, 70
– – ilium **1**: 175
– – incus **2**: 397–400
– – ischium **1**: 172, 175–176
– – lateral ventricle → Central part of lateral ventricle
– – mandible **1**: 36; **2**: 4–7, 25, 27, 41, 48
– – maxilla **2**: 4, 24, 48, 367–368
– – metacarpal bone **1**: 94
– – metatarsal bone **1**: 186
– – nail **1**: 11
– – pancreas **2**: 186, 188, 203, 206
– – penis **2**: 274–276, 278
– – phalanx of foot **1**: 186
– – – – hand **1**: 94
– – radius **1**: 88, 90–91, 99–100
– – rib **1**: 44
– – sphenoidal bone **2**: 19, 55, 63, 359, 368
– – sternum **1**: 40–41, 45; **2**: 107, 158–159, 161
– – stomach **2**: 154, 167, 173–176, 190–191, 194, 200, 222–223, 248
– – talus **1**: 187, 215
– – tibia **1**: 182–183, 197, 202, 205, 208–209, 214, 216, 230–231, 234, 241, 270, 276–277
– – ulna **1**: 89–91, 99–101
– – uterus **2**: 233, 238–239, 242, 252, 256–257, 260
– types **1**: 6

Bone(s) **1**: 7, 9
– marrow **1**: 10
– of foot **1**: 184–189, 206, 208–211, 240
– – hand **1**: 8, 92–94, 128
– – human body **1**: 2–3
– – lateral arch of foot **1**: 189
– – leg **1**: 182–183
– – medial arch of foot **1**: 189
Bony external acoustic meatus **2**: 391–392
– labyrinth **2**: 400–402
– – of newborn child **2**: 401
– nasal cavity **2**: 55–57, 369
– – septum **2**: 4, 23, 54, 58–59, 61, 365, 369
– palate **2**: 5, 7, 45, 55–57
– part of nasal septum **2**: 54
– union **1**: 9
Border(s) of lung lobes **2**: 152
– – lungs **2**: 152
– – oval fossa → Limbus fossae ovalis
– – pleura **2**: 152
Boyd's perforating veins **1**: 246
Brachial artery **1**: 138–143, 145–147, 152–153, 156; **2**: 149
– fascia **1**: 136, 151
– plexus **1**: 68, 72, 134, 140–141, 144; **2**: 35, 72, 75, 81, 92–96, 98, 165–167
– veins **1**: 137, 140, 145–147, 156
Brachialis muscle **1**: 101, 105–109, 111, 113–119, 140–143, 146–149, 152–154, 156
Brachiocephalic trunk **2**: 78–79, 96–97, 100, 104–107, 118, 122–125, 130, 139, 142–143, 149, 151, 156, 161–163, 165, 167
– vein **1**: 12, 14, 76, 137; **2**: 96–97, 104, 107, 122, 128–130, 149–151, 156, 162–164
Brachioradialis muscle **1**: 101, 105–109, 113–119, 140–143, 147–149, 151–154, 156
Brachium of inferior colliculus **2**: 310–311
– – superior colliculus **2**: 310–311, 335
Brachycephalic skull **2**: 2
Brain **1**: 22; **2**: 295–306, 336–362
Brainstem **2**: 289, 294, 303, 307, 310–311, 324
Branches of internal carotid artery to trigeminal ganglion **2**: 301
– – middle cerebral artery to angular gyrus **2**: 297, 302
– – oculomotor nerve to ciliary ganglion → Parasympathetic root of ciliary ganglion
– – portal triad **2**: 185
– – segmental artery of pulmonary artery **2**: 115
– – – bronchus **2**: 115
– to angular gyrus **2**: 297, 302
– – ciliary ganglion → Parasympathetic root of ciliary ganglion
– – trigeminal ganglion **2**: 301
Breast **1**: 70–74; **2**: 126
Broad face **2**: 2
– ligament of uterus **2**: 239–241, 246
– skull **2**: 2
Brodmann's areas of cerebral cortex **2**: 318
Bronchi → Bronchus(-i)
Bronchial branches of vagus nerve **1**: 25
– tree **1**: 114–115, 119–121
Broncho-aortic constriction of esophagus → Thoracic constriction of esophagus
Bronchography **2**: 120–121
Bronchomediastinal lymphatic trunk **1**: 15
– trunk → Bronchomediastinal lymphatic trunk
Bronchopulmonary lymph nodes **2**: 110–111, 113
– segments **2**: 115–117

Bronchus(-i) **2**: 105–106, 108–110, 119
Buccal artery **2**: 76, 86–87
– branches of facial nerve **2**: 84–85, 92, 98–99
– fat pad **2**: 28–29, 44
– nerve **2**: 82–87
– surface of tooth **2**: 39–40
– vein **2**: 80
Buccinator lymph node **2**: 81
– muscle **2**: 28, 30–32, 44, 48, 58, 80, 85–87
Bulb of occipital horn of lateral ventricle **2**: 320
– – penis **1**: 17, 259–260; **2**: 170, 250, 254, 267, 275, 277–278
– – rhombencephalon → Medulla oblongata
– – vestibule **2**: 250–251, 268–269, 280
Bulbar conjunctiva **2**: 364–365, 370–371, 374–375
Bulbospongiosus muscle **2**: 232, 234, 265–268, 274–276, 279–280
Bulbo-urethral gland **1**: 17; **2**: 250, 267, 277

C

Caecum → Cecum
Calcaneal anastomosis **1**: 266–268, 279–280
– branches of posterior tibial artery **1**: 267, 279–281
– fat body **1**: 279
– process of cuboid **1**: 186
– sulcus **1**: 187
– tendon **1**: 206–207, 210–213, 215, 217, 230, 232–234, 241, 267–268, 275–277, 279–280
– tubercle **1**: 186–187
– tuberosity **1**: 184–188, 212–213, 217, 232–234, 237–238
Calcaneocuboid joint **1**: 215
– ligament **1**: 206
Calcaneofibular ligament **1**: 206, 212, 214
Calcaneonavicular ligament **1**: 206
Calcaneus **1**: 184–188, 207–211, 214–215, 277
Calcarine branch of medial occipital artery **2**: 298–299, 302
– spur **2**: 322–323
– sulcus **2**: 304–305, 315, 317, 319, 322, 335, 346, 348, 355
Calf bone → Fibula
Callosomarginal artery **2**: 297, 299–300, 302, 347, 349, 354–355
Calvaria **1**: 87; **2**: 2–3, 17, 290, 336, 347, 349, 352, 354–362, 409
Canal for auditory tube → Canal for pharyngotympanic tube
– – pharyngotympanic tube **2**: 393, 396, 399
– – tensor tympani muscle **2**: 393, 396, 399
– – vertebral artery **1**: 31
Canaliculus for chorda tympani **2**: 393
Canine fossa of maxilla **2**: 24
– tooth/teeth **2**: 39–42
Caninus muscle **2**: 32, 37
Capillary lamina of choroid **2**: 373
Capitate **1**: 8, 92–94, 102–104, 123, 129
Capitulum of humerus **1**: 86, 90–91, 100–101, 149
Capsular branch of renal artery **2**: 162
Capsule of lens **2**: 375
– – prostate **2**: 237
Cardia **2**: 106–107, 113, 173, 198
Cardiac ganglia **2**: 167
– impression on mediastinal surface of left/right lung **2**: 111, 114
– nerve plexus **2**: 96, 149, 166–167
– notch of left lung **2**: 111–112

Cardial notch **2**: 173, 175
– orifice **2**: 174, 204
– part of stomach → Cardia
Cardinal ligament **2**: 239, 246, 251, 256
Cardiovascular system **1**: 12–14
Carina of trachea **2**: 155
Carotid canal **2**: 8–9, 11, 20, 393, 395–396, 398–400
– sheath **2**: 33
– sinus **2**: 76, 78–79, 292
– sulcus **2**: 10, 19
– tubercle **1**: 31; **2**: 37
Carpal articular surface of radius **1**: 88, 94, 99
– bones **1**: 8, 82–83, 92–94
– groove **1**: 94
– tendinous sheaths **1**: 130–131
– tunnel **1**: 103, 121–124, 166
Carpometacarpal joint(s) **1**: 82–83, 102, 104
– – of thumb **1**: 104
Carpus → Wrist
Cartilage(s) **1**: 9
– of acoustic meatus **2**: 390–392
– – auricle **2**: 390
– – larynx **2**: 64–65
Cartilaginous external acoustic meatus **2**: 391–392
– joint **1**: 9
– part of nasal septum **2**: 54
– – – pharyngotympanic tube **2**: 51, 395
Carunculae hymenales → Hymenal caruncles
Cauda equina **1**: 22, 39, 48, 55, 194; **2**: 225, 244, 284, 287
Caudal **1**: 5
Caudate lobe of liver **2**: 180–181, 183–184, 186, 191, 196, 204, 222, 248
– nucleus **2**: 300, 320, 322–323, 326, 329–334, 337–341, 344, 346–351, 354–357, 360–361
– process of caudate lobe of liver **2**: 181
Caval opening **1**: 69
Cave of septum pellucidum **2**: 322, 338, 350
Cavernous part of internal carotid artery **2**: 292–293, 301–302, 352, 359–360, 378
– sinus **2**: 62, 80, 293, 352–353, 359–360, 378, 380, 383
Cavity(-ies) of concha **2**: 390
– – heart **2**: 139
– – pharynx **1**: 16; **2**: 38, 50–53
Cecum **1**: 18–20, 194; **2**: 172, 177–178, 190, 192–196, 202–205, 225, 238
Celiac branches of posterior vagal trunk **2**: 167, 248
– ganglia **1**: 24–25; **2**: 167, 248–249
– lymph nodes **2**: 198, 203
– nerve plexus **1**: 25; **2**: 248–249
– trunk **1**: 12, 14; **2**: 105, 162, 196–200, 203, 211, 218–219
Celiacography **2**: 197
Cement **2**: 40
Central axillary lymph nodes **1**: 72–73
– canal of spinal cord **2**: 288, 304, 307, 310, 320–321, 324
– gray substance → Periaqueductal gray substance
– lobule of cerebellum **2**: 307–308
– nervous system **1**: 22; **2**: 303
– part of lateral ventricle **2**: 300, 320, 322–323, 326, 340–341, 346–347, 349, 354–356, 361, 408
– retinal artery **2**: 58, 372–374, 378, 384
– – vein **2**: 372–374, 378, 384
– sulcus of cerebrum **2**: 297–298, 304–305, 314, 316–317, 319, 323, 348, 362

Central sulcus of
– – – insula **2**: 323
– superior mesenteric lymph nodes **2**: 203
– tendon of diaphragm **1**: 69; **2**: 218
– thalamic radiation **2**: 333
– veins of suprarenal gland **2**: 216
Centromedian nucleus of thalamus **2**: 327, 340
Cephalic vein **1**: 72–73, 75, 105, 135–137, 140,
    145–147, 150–151, 156–157, 164; **2**: 98, 149
Ceratopharyngeal part of middle constrictor
    muscle **2**: 34, 46–47
Cerebellar cortex **2**: 309, 334
– fissures **2**: 308
– fossa of occipital bone **2**: 18
– hemisphere **2**: 295, 299, 303–304, 306, 308,
    342–343, 350, 352–353, 358–359, 361–362,
    400, 409
– peduncles **2**: 308
– tentorium → Tentorium cerebelli
Cerebellopontine angle **2**: 340
Cerebellorubral connections **2**: 334
– tract **2**: 309, 328, 334, 340
Cerebellum **1**: 22, 37; **2**: 13, 294, 299, 303,
    305–309, 321, 324, 334, 340, 342–343, 345,
    348, 350–353, 356–359, 361–362, 400, 409
Cerebral aqueduct → Aqueduct of midbrain
– arterial circle **2**: 292
– cortex **2**: 295, 299, 318–319, 322, 327, 338,
    346
– crus **2**: 309, 315, 328, 358, 385
– fossa of occipital bone **2**: 18
– gyri **2**: 316–317
– hemisphere **2**: 297, 299, 303–304, 313–319,
    324, 327, 329, 337–338
– lobes **2**: 312–313
– part of internal carotid artery **2**: 77, 301, 360,
    378
– peduncle **2**: 306, 309–311, 315, 328, 332–335,
    340–341, 344, 351, 358, 385
– sulci **2**: 316–317
– surface of greater wing of sphenoidal bone
    2: 19
– – – lesser wing of sphenoidal bone **2**: 19
– – – temporal bone **2**: 20
Cerebrospinal fluid **2**: 75, 294, 321
Cerebrum **1**: 22; **2**: 13, 289, 303–306, 312–319,
    323, 333, 336–343, 350–362, 384–387, 400,
    408–409
Ceruminous glands of external acoustic meatus
    2: 392
Cervical branch of facial nerve **2**: 84–85, 91–93,
    98–99
– canal of uterus **2**: 233, 240
– enlargement of spinal cord **1**: 22; **2**: 284
– fascia **1**: 64; **2**: 29, 33, 36, 44–45, 91–92
– lordosis **1**: 28
– lymph nodes **1**: 15; **2**: 81, 91, 163
– nerves [C 1–C 8] **1**: 22, 51, 60; **2**: 32, 37,
    82–83, 94–96, 166, 284, 286, 288–289, 291,
    294, 306, 311
– part of esophagus **2**: 53, 105–106
– – – internal carotid artery **2**: 77, 292,
    301–302
– – – sympathetic trunk **2**: 95–96, 100, 166
– – – thoracic duct **1**: 15
– – – vertebral artery **1**: 60; **2**: 72, 74, 79, 118,
    292, 302
– – – – column → Cervical spine
– pleura → Dome of pleura
– plexus **1**: 68; **2**: 34–35, 37, 94
– retinaculum **2**: 246

Cervical
– spine **1**: 28, 31, 36–37, 49–51; **2**: 285, 288
– vertebra(e) [C I–C VII] **1**: 28–31, 36–37, 40,
    50–51, 60, 82–83; **2**: 7, 33, 37, 53, 68, 71–75,
    79, 118, 284, 286, 289, 294, 302, 408
Cervicothoracic ganglion **1**: 25; **2**: 95–96,
    166–167
Cervix of tooth → Neck of tooth
– – uterus **1**: 17; **2**: 233, 239–240, 242, 246,
    251, 256–257, 260, 268
Check ligament of lateral rectus muscle
    2: 370–371, 379
Chest wall **1**: 68, 72–76, 79
Chiasmatic cistern **2**: 295, 321
Chin **2**: 44
Choana(e) **2**: 17, 23, 45, 50–51, 58, 63, 395
Cholecystocholangiography **2**: 186
Chondroglossus muscle **2**: 46
Chondropharyngeal part of middle constrictor
    muscle **2**: 34–35, 46–47
Chord of umbilical artery **2**: 246
Chorda tympani **2**: 84, 87–89, 391, 393, 398
Chordae tendineae of heart **2**: 132–134, 140
Chorionic lamina **2**: 243
– vessels **2**: 243
– villi **2**: 242
Choroid **2**: 373–376, 384
– enlargement of lateral ventricle **2**: 322–323
– line of fourth ventricle **2**: 308–311
– – – lateral ventricle **2**: 322, 326
– plexus(es) of forebrain **2**: 326
– – – fourth ventricle **2**: 306–309, 321, 340
– – – lateral ventricle **2**: 300, 322–323, 326,
    332, 340, 344, 346–349, 351, 354–356,
    361–362
– – – third ventricle **2**: 300, 307, 320–321, 326,
    340, 344
Choroidal fissure of lateral ventricle **2**: 322, 326
Chyle cistern → Cisterna chyli
Ciliary body **2**: 373, 376–377, 384–385
– folds → Ciliary plicae
– ganglion **2**: 381–382
– glands **2**: 366
– margin of iris **2**: 376
– muscle **2**: 374–375, 377
– part of retina **2**: 374–376, 384
– plicae **2**: 376
– processes **2**: 374–376
– zonule **2**: 373–377
Cingulate gyrus **2**: 304, 315, 317, 325–326,
    337–338, 346–348, 350, 354–355, 357,
    360–361
– sulcus **2**: 304–305, 317, 319, 337–338, 348
Circular folds of small intestine **2**: 174, 176,
    188, 194
– muscular layer of stomach **2**: 173
– sulcus of insula **2**: 323, 337, 344–345, 350
Circulation of cerebrospinal fluid **2**: 321
Circulatory system → Cardiovascular system
Circumflex branch of left coronary artery
    2: 107, 128–130, 135, 141–144, 147–148
– scapular artery **1**: 135, 139, 143
– vein **1**: 135
Cistern of lateral cerebral fossa **2**: 295
Cisterna ambiens **2**: 295, 357
– chyli **1**: 15; **2**: 163
– magna → Posterior cerebellomedullary
    cistern
Claustrum **2**: 323, 330–331, 337–338, 340,
    344, 346, 348, 350–351, 355–356, 360

Clavicle **1**: 18, 20–21, 43, 45, 62–63, 68, 73,
    75, 82, 84, 87, 95–97, 105–108, 110–112,
    136–137, 140, 142–143, 149; **2**: 33–36, 92,
    94, 96, 98, 126, 150, 172
Clavicular facet of scapula **1**: 85
– head of pectoralis major muscle **1**: 63–64
– notch **1**: 41, 45
– part of deltoid muscle **1**: 108
Clavipectoral fascia **1**: 64
– triangle **1**: 63, 136
Cleavage lines **1**: 11
Clinical crown of tooth **2**: 40
– root of tooth **2**: 40
Clitoris **1**: 17; **2**: 233, 240, 250–252, 260,
    268–269, 280–281
Clivus **2**: 10, 19, 290, 293–294
– branch(es) of cerebral part of internal carotid
    artery **2**: 301
Coccygeal cornu **1**: 34–35
– horn → Coccygeal cornu
– ligament → Dural part of filum terminale
– nerve **1**: 22; **2**: 226, 284
– plexus **2**: 227
Coccygeus muscle → Ischiococcygeus muscle
Coccyx [coccygeal vertebrae I–IV] **1**: 28, 34–35,
    38–40, 170–171, 173–175, 225; **2**: 232, 243,
    256–259, 265–266, 280, 284
Cochlea **2**: 361, 399–404, 406, 408–409
Cochlear aqueduct **2**: 405
– area **2**: 401–403
– canaliculus **2**: 20, 401, 405
– communicating branch of vestibular ganglion
    2: 405
– cupula **2**: 401, 403
– duct **2**: 391, 399, 404–405
– ganglion **2**: 404–405
– nerve **2**: 399, 405
– recess **2**: 402
Cockett's perforating veins **1**: 246
Coeliac → Celiac
Coeliacography → Celiacography
Colic impression on liver **2**: 181
– – – spleen **2**: 189
Collateral branch of posterior intercostal artery
    1: 76
– eminence of lateral ventricle **2**: 322–323, 348,
    350
– ligaments of interphalangeal joints of foot
    1: 206
– – – – – – hand **1**: 104
– – – knee joint → Fibular/tibial collateral
    ligament
– – – metatarsophalangeal joints **1**: 206
– sulcus **2**: 315, 317, 326, 340
– trigone **2**: 322–323, 354, 356, 362
Colliculus of arytenoid cartilage **2**: 64
Colon **2**: 171–172, 177–179, 182, 190, 192–196,
    200, 202–208, 220, 223–225, 230, 238,
    252–254, 257, 260–261
Column of fornix **2**: 307, 317, 320, 322,
    324–325, 328, 334, 338, 348–350, 355–356
Commissure of bulbs of vestibule **2**: 268
– – fornix **2**: 322, 324–325
Common anular tendon → Common tendinous
    ring of extra-ocular muscles
– bony limb of semicircular canals **2**: 401–402
– carotid artery **1**: 12, 14; **2**: 33, 36, 68, 71,
    74–75, 77–79, 93, 96–97, 99–100, 105–107,
    118, 122–125, 130–131, 139, 142–143, 149,
    156, 162–163, 165, 167, 292
– – nerve plexus **1**: 25; **2**: 100

Common
– fibular division of sciatic nerve **1**: 229, 235
– – nerve **1**: 229, 242–243, 245, 248, 254–256, 263–268, 271–272
– flexor sheath of hand **1**: 123, 130
– – tendon **1**: 115–116, 153
– hepatic artery **2**: 167, 196–200, 219
– – duct **2**: 183, 185–188
– iliac artery **1**: 12–14, 194; **2**: 162–163, 202, 218–219, 225, 228–230, 234, 238, 243–245, 252, 254, 260–261
– – lymph nodes **2**: 163
– – vein **1**: 12, 14, 194; **2**: 162–163, 218, 225, 228, 234, 243–245, 252, 254, 260–261
– interosseous artery **1**: 138–139, 153, 155
– membranous limb of semicircular ducts **2**: 405
– nasal meatus **2**: 23, 50, 58–59, 61–62
– palmar digital arteries **1**: 160–163, 165
– – – nerves of median nerve **1**: 132, 161–162
– – – – – ulnar nerve **1**: 132, 161
– peroneal nerve → Common fibular nerve
– plantar digital arteries **1**: 279–280
– – – nerves **1**: 279–280
– tendinous ring of extra-ocular muscles **2**: 370–371, 378–379, 381–382
– – sheath of fibulares muscles **1**: 214–215, 241
– – – – peronei muscles → Common tendinous sheath of fibulares muscles
Communicating branch of fibular artery **1**: 268, 279–280
– – – intermediate nerve with vagus nerve **2**: 398
– – – lacrimal nerve with zygomatic nerve **2**: 88, 379–380
– – – median nerve with ulnar nerve **1**: 161–162
– – – nasociliary nerve with ciliary ganglion → Sensory root of ciliary ganglion
– – – radial nerve with ulnar nerve **1**: 133, 164
– – with ciliary ganglion → Sensory root of ciliary ganglion
– – – recurrent laryngeal nerve **2**: 101
– – – ulnar nerve **1**: 133, 161–162, 164
– – – vagus nerve **2**: 398
– – – zygomatic nerve **2**: 88, 379–380
Compact bone **1**: 7, 10
– part of substantia nigra **2**: 328
Complete congenital inguinal hernia **2**: 273
Compressive stress trajectories **1**: 7
Compressor urethrae muscle **2**: 247
Concha of auricle **2**: 390
Conducting system of heart **2**: 132–134, 140
Condylar canal **1**: 50; **2**: 10, 18
– fossa **2**: 18
– process of mandible **2**: 6, 9, 25–26
Condyle of humerus **1**: 86
Confluence of sinuses **2**: 291, 294, 352–353, 359
Congenital inguinal hernia **2**: 273
Conjoint tendon → Inguinal falx
Conjunctiva **2**: 364–365, 370–371, 374–375
Conjunctival epithelium **2**: 375
– sac **2**: 385
Connective tissue of lesser pelvis **2**: 246–247
Conoid ligament **1**: 95–96
– tubercle of clavicle **1**: 84
Constrictions of esophagus **2**: 106
Conus arteriosus **2**: 132, 139, 142, 158
– branch of left coronary artery **2**: 135
– – – right coronary artery **2**: 135, 142
– elasticus **2**: 110
– medullaris **1**: 22; **2**: 284
Coraco-acromial ligament **1**: 9, 95–96

Coracobrachialis muscle **1**: 64, 106–107, 110, 112–113, 140–141, 144–145, 148–149; **2**: 93
Coracoclavicular ligament **1**: 9, 95–96, 106–107, 110
Coracohumeral ligament **1**: 95–96
Coracoid process **1**: 84–85, 87, 95–96, 106–107, 110, 140–141, 148–149
Corium → Dermis
Cornea **2**: 372–375, 384–385
Corneal epithelium **2**: 375
– limbus → Corneoscleral junction
– vertex **2**: 370
Corneoscleral junction **2**: 374–375
Corniculate cartilage **2**: 64–66
– tubercle **2**: 50–52, 68, 101
Corniculopharyngeal ligament **2**: 65
Corona ciliaris **2**: 374, 376
– of glans penis **2**: 275–277
– radiata **2**: 333
Coronal planes **1**: 5
– suture **2**: 3–4, 6, 10, 12, 17
Coronary angiography **2**: 146–147
– arteries of heart **2**: 135, 142–148
– – – –, variations **2**: 144–145
– ligament of liver **2**: 170, 180–181, 206–207
– sinus **2**: 125, 132, 135, 139–141, 143
– sulcus **2**: 124–125
Coronoid fossa of humerus **1**: 86
– process of mandible **2**: 6, 25–26, 41, 63, 73
– – – ulna **1**: 89–91, 99–100, 116
Corpus albicans **2**: 241
– callosum **2**: 13, 299–300, 304–305, 307, 315, 317, 319, 322, 324–326, 333–335, 337–350, 354–356, 360–361, 408
– cavernosum of clitoris **2**: 268
– – penis **1**: 17; **2**: 170, 232, 234, 258–259, 267, 274–275, 277–279
– luteum **2**: 241
– spongiosum penis **1**: 17; **2**: 170, 232, 234, 237, 266–267, 274–275, 277–278
– striatum **2**: 329, 332, 335, 338, 344, 348, 350
Corrugator supercilii muscle **2**: 32
Cortex of lens **2**: 375
– – suprarenal gland **2**: 216
Cortical labyrinth **2**: 212
Corticonuclear fibers **2**: 328, 332
Corticorubral fibers **2**: 334
Corticospinal fibers **2**: 328, 332
Corticotectal fibers **2**: 334
Costal arch **1**: 40–42, 62–63; **2**: 107, 150
– cartilage **1**: 41, 45
– facets of thoracic vertebra **1**: 32
– groove **1**: 44
– notches → Notches of sternum for ribs
– part of diaphragm **1**: 68–69; **2**: 222
– – – parietal pleura **2**: 150–151, 154–157
– process of lumbar vertebra **1**: 33, 38, 41, 48; **2**: 284
– surface of lung **2**: 112, 151
– – – scapula **1**: 85
– tubercular ligament(s) **1**: 47
Costocervical trunk **1**: 139; **2**: 79, 118
Costoclavicular ligament **1**: 45
Costodiaphragmatic recess **1**: 43; **2**: 126, 153–155, 182, 209, 222
Costomediastinal recess **2**: 157–159
Costotransverse foramen **1**: 46
– joint **1**: 47; **2**: 75
– ligament **1**: 47
Costovertebral joints **1**: 46–47
Costoxiphoid ligaments **1**: 45, 63
Cotyledones of placenta **2**: 243

Coverings of testis **2**: 270
Coxa valga **1**: 179
– vara **1**: 179
Coxal bone → Hip bone
Cranial **1**: 5
– arachnoid mater **2**: 295, 321, 326, 405
– base **2**: 8–11, 16, 37, 293, 394–395, 400
– cavity **1**: 22, 40; **2**: 294
– dura mater **1**: 51; **2**: 88, 289–293, 295, 297, 321, 352, 360, 362, 405
– nerves **1**: 22; **2**: 306
– pia mater **2**: 295, 326, 405
– root of accessory nerve **1**: 22; **2**: 289, 292, 294, 306, 311
Cranium **2**: 2–17, 32, 58–59, 61, 76–77, 290, 336, 394–395, 400
Cremaster muscle **1**: 63–67; **2**: 270–272, 274
Cremasteric fascia **1**: 67; **2**: 270–271, 274
Crest(s) of greater tubercle of humerus **1**: 86
– – head of rib **1**: 44
– – lesser tubercle of humerus **1**: 86
– – nail bed **1**: 11
– – neck of rib **1**: 44
Cribriform fascia **1**: 218, 249
– plate **2**: 7, 10, 12, 22–23, 55–56, 60, 88, 90, 291
Crico-arytenoid joint **2**: 65
– ligament **2**: 66
Cricoid cartilage **2**: 33, 36, 51–52, 64–68, 70, 101, 106, 108–110
Cricopharyngeal part of inferior constrictor muscle **2**: 33, 47
Cricothyroid branch of superior thyroid artery **2**: 98
– joint **2**: 65–68
– muscle **2**: 35, 47–48, 66, 68, 70, 97, 149
Cricotracheal ligament **2**: 65–66
Cricovocal membrane → Conus elasticus
Crista galli **2**: 5, 7, 10, 12–13, 22–23, 55–56, 58–60, 90, 294, 367, 369
– terminalis of right atrium of heart **2**: 132
Crown of tooth **2**: 40
Cruciate ligament(s) of atlas **1**: 50
– – – knee joint → Anterior/posterior cruciate ligament
Cruciform part of fibrous sheaths of digits of hand **1**: 121
– – – – – – toes **1**: 238
Crural chiasm **1**: 234
Crus/Crura of antihelix **2**: 390
– – clitoris **2**: 250–251, 260
– – diaphragm **2**: 196
– – fornix **2**: 322, 324–325
– – helix **2**: 390
– – penis **1**: 259–260; **2**: 234, 250, 254, 261, 267, 275–278
Cubital anastomosis **1**: 142–143, 154
– fossa **1**: 106
– lymph nodes **1**: 74
Cuboid **1**: 184–189, 209–211, 215
Cuboideonavicular joint **1**: 215
Culmen **2**: 307–308
Cuneate fasciculus **2**: 288, 310
– tubercle **2**: 310–311
Cuneiform bones **1**: 186, 189, 209
– tubercle **2**: 50–52, 68, 101
Cuneonavicular joint **1**: 215
Cuneus **2**: 317
Cupula(-ae) of diaphragm **2**: 150–151, 172
Cusps of mitral valve **2**: 133–135
– – tooth **2**: 39
– – tricuspid valve **2**: 132, 135

Cutaneous branch(es) of anterior branch of
    obturator nerve **1**: 228, 242–243, 248, 252,
    254–255, 266
– – – buccal nerve **2**: 85
– – – superficial cervical artery **2**: 91
– – – thoraco-acromial artery **2**: 91
– innervation of body wall **1**: 61, 78
– – – dorsal body wall **1**: 61
– – – head **2**: 82–83
– – – lower limb **1**: 242–243
– – – neck **2**: 82–83
– – – trunk **1**: 61, 78
– – – upper limb **1**: 132–133
– – – ventral body wall **1**: 78
– zone of anal canal **2**: 179
Cutis → Skin
Cymba conchae **2**: 390
Cystic artery **2**: 196–197, 200
– duct **2**: 181, 186–188, 198
– lymph node **2**: 198
– vein **2**: 196, 200
Cysts in spermatic cord **2**: 273

D

Dartos fascia **1**: 67; **2**: 271, 274
Deciduous canine tooth/teeth **2**: 42
– dentition **2**: 42–43
– incisor tooth/teeth **2**: 42
– premolar tooth/teeth **2**: 42
– tooth/teeth **2**: 42–43
Declive **2**: 307–308
Decussation of pyramids **2**: 306, 340
– – Stilling **2**: 334
– – superior cerebellar peduncles **2**: 309, 334
Deep artery of arm **1**: 138–143, 145–146
– – – penis **2**: 267, 277
– – – thigh **1**: 250–253, 256, 260, 262–263;
    2: 228
– auricular artery **2**: 77, 88–89, 392
– brachial artery → Deep artery of arm
– branch of lateral plantar nerve **1**: 279–280
– – – medial circumflex femoral artery **1**: 253
– – – – plantar artery **1**: 279–281
– – – radial nerve **1**: 113, 117, 140, 152–154,
    157
– – – transverse cervical artery **1**: 60
– – – ulnar nerve **1**: 152–153, 161–162
– cervical artery **1**: 60; **2**: 78–79, 118
– circumflex iliac artery **1**: 251–253; **2**: 228,
    234, 244–245
– – – vein **2**: 244
– dorsal vein of penis **2**: 267, 275–277
– external pudendal artery **1**: 252–253
– facial vein **2**: 80, 383
– fascia of leg **1**: 218, 230, 233–234, 241, 254,
    266–268, 270, 278–279
– – – penis **2**: 274–276
– femoral artery → Deep artery of thigh
– fibular nerve **1**: 235, 240, 242, 270–271,
    274–275, 278
– head of flexor pollicis brevis muscle
    1: 123–124, 167
– infrapatellar bursa **1**: 195
– inguinal lymph nodes **2**: 163
– – ring **1**: 67, 77; **2**: 272–273
– lateral cervical lymph nodes **2**: 81, 163
– – facial region **2**: 86–87
– layer of temporal fascia **2**: 30
– lingual artery **2**: 47
– medial facial region **2**: 88–90

Deep
– median cubital vein **1**: 136, 140, 151
– middle cerebral vein **2**: 300
– muscles of face **2**: 30
– – – neck **1**: 55
– palmar arch **1**: 138, 162–163
– – branch of ulnar artery **1**: 153, 161–163
– parotid lymph nodes **2**: 81
– part of masseter muscle **2**: 30, 98
– – – palpebral part of orbicularis oculi muscle
        → Lacrimal part of orbicularis oculi
        muscle
– perineal pouch **1**: 17; **2**: 233, 237, 243, 247,
    250–251, 267
– – space → Deep perineal pouch
– peroneal nerve → Deep fibular nerve
– petrosal nerve **2**: 88–89
– plantar arch **1**: 250, 279–281
– – artery **1**: 250, 271, 278, 280
– popliteal lymph nodes **1**: 245
– posterior sacrococcygeal ligament **1**: 190
– temporal arteries **2**: 87
– – nerves **2**: 87, 89
– transverse metacarpal ligament **1**: 102, 124,
    162
– – metatarsal ligament **1**: 213
– – perineal muscle **1**: 227; **2**: 232, 234, 250,
    261, 265–267, 276
– vein(s) of arm **1**: 145–146
– – – lower limb **1**: 246
– – – thigh **1**: 260, 262–263
Defloration **2**: 269
Deltoid branch of deep artery of arm **1**: 143
– – – profunda brachii artery → Deltoid
        branch of deep artery of arm
– – – thoraco-acromial artery **2**: 93
– fascia **1**: 53, 136
– ligament → Medial ligament of ankle joint
– muscle **1**: 52–53, 62–64, 96–97, 105–113,
    140–145, 148–149; **2**: 92
– region **1**: 4
– tuberosity of humerus **1**: 86
Deltopectoral lymph nodes **1**: 74
– triangle → Clavipectoral triangle
Dendritic renal pelvis **2**: 216
Dens axis **1**: 30–31, 36–37, 40, 50–51, 60; **2**: 5,
    52, 72–73, 294, 408
Dental alveoli of mandible **2**: 25
– – – maxilla **2**: 24
– arcade **2**: 5
– pulp **2**: 40
Dentate gyrus **2**: 317, 324–326
– nucleus **2**: 309, 334
Denticulate ligament **2**: 284–286, 289
Dentine **2**: 40
Depression of optic disc **2**: 374, 377
Depressor anguli oris muscle **2**: 28–29, 32, 44,
    48, 99
– labii inferioris muscle **2**: 28–29, 32, 99
– supercilii muscle **2**: 28, 366
Dermatomes of body wall **1**: 61, 78
– – head **2**: 82–83
– – lower limb **1**: 134, 242–244
– – neck **2**: 82–83
– – trunk **1**: 61, 78, 134, 244
– – upper limb **1**: 132–134, 244
Dermis **1**: 11
Descending aorta **1**: 12, 14; **2**: 78, 104–107,
    126, 157–163, 165
– branch of lateral circumflex femoral artery
    1: 251–253
– – – occipital artery **2**: 76

Descending
– colon **1**: 16, 18–19, 21, 194; **2**: 154, 171–172,
    182, 193, 196, 202, 204–208, 220, 223–225,
    238
– genicular artery **1**: 248, 250, 252, 269
– palatine artery **2**: 76–77, 87–89
– part of duodenum **2**: 155, 187–188, 191, 194,
    199–200, 223, 248
Detrusor muscle **2**: 235
Development of bones **1**: 8
– – hip bone **1**: 176–177
Dextrocardiogram **2**: 119
Diagonal band **2**: 315, 317, 335
– conjugate **1**: 178
Diaphragm **1**: 12–14, 16, 18–21, 25, 43, 68–69;
    2: 104–107, 113, 122, 126–131, 150–151,
    153–155, 160, 162, 164, 167, 172, 182, 185,
    189, 191, 196, 200, 208–209, 211, 218,
    220–223
Diaphragma sellae **2**: 55, 293–294, 378
Diaphragmatic constriction of esophagus
    2: 106–107
– part of parietal pleura **2**: 150
– surface of liver **2**: 180, 184–185, 191, 204
– – – lung **2**: 111–112, 114
– – – spleen **2**: 189
Diaphysis of metacarpal bone **1**: 8
– – phalanx of hand **1**: 8
– – radius **1**: 8
– – ulna **1**: 8
Diarthrosis → Synovial joint
Diastole **2**: 136–138
Diencephalon **2**: 303, 317, 334
Different positions of vermiform appendix
    2: 178
Digastric branch of facial nerve **2**: 84, 87
– fossa of mandible **2**: 25
– muscle **2**: 30, 32, 34, 36–37, 44–45, 47–51,
    87, 97–100
Digestive system → Alimentary system
Digits of foot **1**: 184–186, 188, 216–217
– – hand **1**: 92–94, 102, 121–122, 124, 130–131,
    161–165, 167
Diploic veins **2**: 295
Diploë **2**: 3, 295
Direct inguinal hernia **1**: 67; **2**: 273
Directions of motion **1**: 5
Distal **1**: 5
– carpal sulcus **1**: 105
– epiphysis of radius **1**: 8
– – – ulna **1**: 8
– interphalangeal joint of hand **1**: 104, 124–125
– phalanx of foot **1**: 184–186, 188
– – – hand **1**: 92–94, 104, 123, 167
– – – middle finger **1**: 167
– – – thumb **1**: 92–93, 123
– radio-ulnar joint **1**: 82–83, 99, 102, 104
– surface of tooth **2**: 39–40
Distobuccal cusp **2**: 39
Distopalatal cusp **2**: 39
Diverticulum in Laimer's triangle **2**: 49
Division of central nervous system **2**: 303
Dodd's perforating veins **1**: 246
Dolichocephalic skull **2**: 2
Dome of pleura **2**: 153
Dorsal **1**: 5
– arcuate ligament **1**: 102
– artery of clitoris **2**: 280
– – – foot → Dorsalis pedis artery
– – – penis **2**: 234, 267, 275–277, 279
– body wall **1**: 61

Dorsal
– branch(es) of posterior intercostal artery(-ies)
  1: 76; **2**: 285–286
– – – – vein(s) **2**: 285–286
– – – ulnar nerve **1**: 133, 150, 153–154, 162,
  164
– calcaneocuboid ligament **1**: 206–207
– carpal arch **1**: 138, 154, 165
– – branch of radial artery **1**: 155, 165
– – – – ulnar artery **1**: 138, 155, 161–163, 165
– – tendinous sheaths **1**: 130
– carpometacarpal ligaments **1**: 102
– cuboideonavicular ligament **1**: 206–207
– digital arteries of foot **1**: 271, 278, 281
– – – – hand **1**: 165, 167
– – branches of radial nerve → Dorsal digital
  nerves of radial nerve
– – expansion of foot **1**: 239
– – – – hand **1**: 124–126, 130, 165, 167
– – nerves of deep fibular nerve **1**: 271, 278
– – – – hand **1**: 164, 167
– – – – radial nerve **1**: 133, 161, 165
– – – – superficial fibular nerve **1**: 270, 278
– – – – thumb **1**: 161, 165
– – – – ulnar nerve **1**: 133, 165
– – veins of foot **1**: 278
– fascia of foot **1**: 230, 278
– – – hand **1**: 164
– funiculus of spinal cord → Posterior funiculus
  of spinal cord
– horn of spinal cord → Posterior horn
  of spinal cord
– intercarpal ligaments **1**: 102
– intermediate sulcus of spinal cord →
  Posterior intermediate sulcus of spinal cord
– interossei of foot → Dorsal interosseous
  muscles of foot
– – – hand → Dorsal interosseous muscles of
  hand
– interosseous muscles of foot **1**: 231, 236–240
– – – – hand **1**: 121–122, 124–130, 165–167
– median sulcus of medulla oblongata →
  Posterior median sulcus of medulla oblongata
– – – – spinal cord → Posterior median sulcus
  of spinal cord
– metacarpal arteries **1**: 165
– – ligaments **1**: 102
– – veins **1**: 164
– metatarsal arteries **1**: 271, 278, 281
– – ligaments **1**: 206–207
– – veins **1**: 278
– nasal artery **2**: 76
– nerve of clitoris **1**: 231, 280–281
– – – penis **1**: 78; **2**: 231, 267, 279
– nuclei of thalamus **2**: 326–327, 330, 340, 344
– pancreatic artery **2**: 188
– radiocarpal ligament **1**: 102
– ramus(-i) of cervical nerves → Posterior rami
  of cervical nerves
– – – lumbar nerves → Posterior rami of
  lumbar nerves
– – – sacral nerves → Posterior rami of
  sacral nerves
– – – spinal nerve → Posterior ramus of
  spinal nerve
– – – thoracic nerves → Posterior rami of
  thoracic nerves
– root ganglion → Spinal ganglion
– – of spinal nerve → Posterior root of spinal
  nerve
– rootlets of spinal nerve → Posterior rootlets
  of spinal nerve

Dorsal
– scapular nerve **1**: 60, 112, 134; **2**: 93–94, 98,
  149
– spinocerebellar tract → Posterior
  spinocerebellar tract
– surface of sacrum **1**: 35, 175
– tarsal ligaments **1**: 206–207, 212
– tarsometatarsal ligaments **1**: 206–207, 212
– tubercle of radius **1**: 88, 92, 102, 116, 125,
  130
– venous arch of foot **1**: 245, 270, 278
– – network of foot **1**: 278
– – – – hand **1**: 105, 164
Dorsalis pedis artery **1**: 250, 271, 278, 280–281
Dorsolateral nucleus of spinal cord →
  Posterolateral nucleus of spinal cord
– sulcus of medulla oblongata → Posterolateral
  sulcus of medulla oblongata
– – – spinal cord → Posterolateral sulcus of
  spinal cord
Dorsomedial nucleus of intermediate
  hypothalamus **2**: 328
Dorsum **1**: 2
– of foot **1**: 216, 230–232, 236, 278, 281
– – hand **1**: 125, 164–165
– – nose **2**: 44
– – penis **2**: 275–276
– – tongue **2**: 38, 46–47, 51, 101
– sellae **1**: 49; **2**: 7, 10, 19, 90, 293, 301,
  352–353, 359, 378, 385, 407
Duct of bulbo-urethral gland **2**: 277
Ductus arteriosus **1**: 13
– deferens **1**: 17, 67, 77; **2**: 234, 236–237, 244,
  255, 261, 270–272, 274, 276
– reuniens **2**: 405
– venosus **1**: 13
Duodenal cap → Ampulla of duodenum
– impression on liver **2**: 181
Duodenojejunal flexure **1**: 16; **2**: 154–155, 188,
  193–194, 199, 202, 204, 206
– fold → Superior duodenal fold
Duodenomesocolic fold → Inferior duodenal
  fold
Duodenum **1**: 16, 18–19; **2**: 155, 170–176,
  187–188, 191, 194, 199–200, 202–204,
  206–207, 223–224, 248
Dura mater **2**: 284–286, 289–293, 295, 297,
  321, 360, 362, 405
Dural part of filum terminale **2**: 284
– venous sinuses **2**: 291

E

Ear **2**: 391–392
Eardrum → Tympanic membrane
Echocardiography **2**: 136, 138
Efferent ductules of testis **2**: 270
– nerve fiber(s) **1**: 23
Effluent blood pathway of left ventricle of heart
  2: 133–134
– – – – right ventricle of heart **2**: 134
Ejaculatory duct **2**: 237, 277
Elbow joint **1**: 82–83, 90–91, 98–101, 116, 147,
  156
Elliptical recess of bony labyrinth **2**: 401–402
Emboliform nucleus → Anterior interpositus
  nucleus
Embryo **2**: 242
Enamel **2**: 40
Encephalon → Brain
Endocrine glands **1**: 15

Endolymphatic duct **2**: 399–400, 405
– sac **2**: 400, 405
– space of membranous labyrinth **2**: 405
Endometrium **2**: 233, 242
Endoscopic retrograde
  cholangiopancreatography **2**: 188
Endothelium of anterior chamber of eyeball
  2: 375
Enteric nerve plexus **2**: 248–249
Entrance into central canal of spinal cord **2**: 310
– to scala vestibuli **2**: 402
Ependyma **2**: 326
Epicardium → Visceral layer of serous
  pericardium
Epicranial aponeurosis **1**: 11, 53; **2**: 28–30, 85,
  290, 347, 349, 352–362, 409
Epicranius muscle **2**: 28–30
Epidermis **1**: 11
Epididymis **1**: 17, 67; **2**: 170, 232, 270–274, 278
Epidural space **1**: 39; **2**: 73, 232, 285–287
Epigastric fold → Lateral umbilical fold
– fossa → Epigastric region
– region **1**: 4; **2**: 182
Epiglottic cartilage **2**: 64–66, 68, 70
– tubercle **2**: 68
– vallecula **2**: 46, 53, 68
Epiglottis **2**: 46, 50–53, 64–65, 68–69, 101
Epimysium **1**: 10
Epiorchium → Visceral layer of tunica vaginalis
  testis
Epiphrenic dilatation of esophagus **2**: 107
Epiphysial cartilage **1**: 8–9
– line of radius **1**: 8, 93
– – – tibia **1**: 202, 208, 214
– plate of hip bone **1**: 176
Epiphysis of metacarpal bone **1**: 8
– – phalanx of hand **1**: 8
– – radius **1**: 8
– – ulna **1**: 8
Epiploic foramen → Omental foramen
Episcleral artery(-ies) **2**: 372–373
– layer **2**: 374–375
– space **2**: 384
– vein(s) **2**: 373
Epitympanic recess of tympanic cavity **2**: 391,
  398, 407
Eponychium **1**: 11
Epoöphoron **2**: 241
Equator of eyeball **2**: 373–374
– – lens **2**: 374–377
Erectile bodies of clitoris **2**: 268
– – – penis **2**: 275
Erector spinae muscle **1**: 52, 54–59, 194, 227;
  2: 213, 222–225, 287
Erigentes nerves → Pelvic splanchnic nerves
Eruption of deciduous teeth **2**: 42
– – permanent teeth **2**: 39
Esophageal branch(es) of inferior thyroid artery
  2: 100
– – – recurrent laryngeal nerve **2**: 101
– – – thoracic aorta **2**: 162
– hiatus **1**: 25, 69; **2**: 104, 155, 162, 199, 218
– impression on liver **2**: 181
– nerve plexus **1**: 25; **2**: 167
Esophagus **1**: 14, 16, 19; **2**: 47–50, 52–53, 75,
  100–101, 104–107, 113, 155–161, 164–165,
  173–175, 206–207
Ethmoid → Ethmoidal bone
Ethmoidal bone **2**: 10, 12–17, 22–23, 55–56,
  58–59, 62–63, 88, 90, 291, 367–369, 378, 385
– bulla **2**: 56–57

Ethmoidal
– cells **2**: 58, 60–62, 305, 336, 352–353,
  358–360, 365, 380, 385–387
– crest of maxilla **2**: 24, 57
– foveolae of frontal bone **2**: 21
– labyrinth **2**: 5, 7, 9, 11, 22, 58–59, 61, 367,
  369, 385, 395
– notch of frontal bone **2**: 21
– process of inferior concha **2**: 56–57
Euryprosopia **2**: 2
Eurysomatic person **1**: 6
Excretion urogram **2**: 217
Excretory ducts of lacrimal glands **2**: 365
– – – tarsal glands **2**: 366
Expiration **1**: 40–41; **2**: 153
Extension **1**: 5
Extensor carpi radialis brevis muscle **1**: 101,
  113–114, 118–119, 123, 125, 128, 130, 140,
  152–154, 156–157, 159, 165
– – – longus muscle **1**: 101, 105–109, 113–116,
    118–119, 123, 125, 128, 130, 140,
    142–143, 147–149, 152–154, 156–159,
    165
– – ulnaris muscle **1**: 105, 113, 117–119, 123,
    125, 128, 130, 154, 157–159, 165
– compartment of arm **1**: 148–149
– digiti minimi muscle **1**: 118–119, 123, 125,
  128, 130, 154, 157–159, 165
– digitorum brevis muscle **1**: 215, 231–232, 236,
  239–241, 278
– – longus muscle **1**: 216, 231–232, 235–236,
    239–241, 271, 273–278
– – muscle **1**: 103, 105, 109, 113, 118–119,
    123–125, 128, 130, 154, 157–159, 165
– hallucis brevis muscle **1**: 231–232, 236,
  240–241, 278
– – longus muscle **1**: 210–211, 231–232,
    235–236, 240–241, 271, 274–278
– indicis muscle **1**: 105, 117, 119, 125, 130, 154,
  157–159, 165
– pollicis brevis muscle **1**: 115, 117–119,
  125–126, 128, 130, 154, 157–159, 162, 165
– – longus muscle **1**: 105, 117–119, 123,
    125–126, 128, 130, 152, 154, 158, 165
– retinaculum of hand **1**: 118–119, 125, 130,
  150, 154, 164–165
External acoustic aperture → External acoustic
  pore
– – meatus **2**: 9, 11, 302, 361, 390–392,
    394–395, 400, 406, 408
– – opening **2**: 6–8, 20, 26, 47–48
– – pore **2**: 395
– anal sphincter muscle **2**: 179, 230–233, 243,
  251, 260–261, 265–266, 276, 279
– axis of eyeball **2**: 374
– branch of accessory nerve **2**: 100
– – – superior laryngeal nerve **2**: 96–98,
      100–101
– capsule **2**: 335, 337–338, 340, 344, 346, 348,
  350–351, 355–356, 360
– carotid artery **2**: 34, 73, 76–79, 81, 86–89,
  96–97, 99–100, 292, 301
– – nerve plexus **1**: 25; **2**: 87, 89, 96
– conjugate **1**: 178
– ear **2**: 390–391, 394
– iliac artery **1**: 12–14, 75, 77, 250–253;
  2: 162–163, 220–221, 228–230, 233–234, 238,
  244–245, 250, 252, 256, 258–259
– – lymph nodes **2**: 163
– – vein **1**: 14, 75, 77, 247, 252; **2**: 163,
    220–221, 228, 230, 233–234, 238, 244–245,
    250, 252, 256, 258–259

External
– intercostal muscle **1**: 54–55, 57–59, 64–65;
  2: 37, 93, 164
– jugular vein **2**: 33, 80, 85, 91–93, 97–99, 122,
  149, 162, 164
– medullary lamina of corpus striatum →
  Lateral medullary lamina of corpus striatum
– – – – thalamus **2**: 327, 340, 344
– nasal artery → Dorsal nasal artery
– – nerve **2**: 82–83, 85–86, 90, 383
– – veins **2**: 80
– nose → Nose
– oblique muscle **1**: 53–55, 57, 63–68, 194,
  226–228; **2**: 196, 220–221, 225, 228, 274
– occipital crest **2**: 18
– – protuberance **1**: 53, 55, 57–58; **2**: 8, 12,
    17–18
– opening of carotid canal **2**: 8, 20
– – – cochlear canaliculus **2**: 405
– – – tympanic canaliculus **2**: 20
– os of uterus **2**: 233, 239–240, 243, 268
– pudendal veins **1**: 248
– spermatic fascia **1**: 67; **2**: 270–271, 274
– surface of cochlear duct **2**: 404
– – – cranial base **2**: 8, 16–17, 37, 395
– – – cranium **2**: 394
– – – frontal bone **2**: 21
– table of calvaria **2**: 3
– urethral orifice **1**: 17; **2**: 232–233, 240, 265,
  268–269, 276–277, 280
– – sphincter muscle **2**: 235, 256, 267
Extrahepatic bile ducts **2**: 186–187
Extra-ocular muscles **2**: 59, 370–371, 378–379,
  381–382
Extraperitoneal organ(s) **2**: 171
– position **2**: 171
– space **2**: 171
Extreme capsule **2**: 337–338, 340, 344, 346,
  348, 350–351, 355–356, 360
Extrinsic muscles of eyeball → Extra-ocular
  muscles
Eye **2**: 364–366
Eyeball **2**: 9, 11, 59, 61–62, 352–353, 358–359,
  362, 370–375, 378, 381–382, 384–386
Eyebrow(s) **2**: 364
Eyelash(es) **2**: 364, 366
Eyelid(s) **2**: 364–366

F

Facet on atlas for dens axis **1**: 30
– – talus for plantar calcaneonavicular ligament
    1: 187, 207
Facial area of internal acoustic meatus **2**: 403
– artery **2**: 44, 76–77, 79, 81, 85–87, 92,
  98–100, 383
– canal **2**: 89, 393, 396, 399, 402
– colliculus **2**: 310–311, 320
– lymph nodes **2**: 81
– muscles → Muscles of face
– nerve [VII] **1**: 22, 25, 51; **2**: 32, 34, 37, 84–85,
  87–89, 91–93, 98–100, 284, 289, 291–292,
  294–295, 306, 308–309, 311, 340, 383, 391,
  398–399, 408–409
– region **2**: 84–85
– vein **2**: 80–81, 85, 92, 98–99, 383
Falciform ligament of liver **2**: 171, 180, 190–191,
  204, 206, 222
– margin of saphenous opening **1**: 65, 218, 248
– process of sacrotuberous ligament **1**: 190
False chordae tendineae of heart **2**: 132–134
Falx cerebelli **2**: 294

Falx
– cerebri **2**: 58, 289, 291, 294–295, 300, 336,
  339, 343, 347, 354–358, 360–361
Fascia glutea **1**: 53–54, 218, 226
– lata **1**: 53–54, 65, 218, 222–223, 226, 230,
  246, 248, 254, 256, 266
– of arm **1**: 135–137
– – dorsum of foot → Dorsal fascia of foot
– – – – hand → Dorsal fascia of hand
– – forearm → Antebrachial fascia
– – leg → Deep fascia of leg
– – lower limb **1**: 218, 230, 254, 266
– – neck → Cervical fascia
– – penis **2**: 274–276
– – thigh **1**: 218, 254
– – upper limb **1**: 135–137, 150–151, 164
Fascial sheath of eyeball **2**: 384
Fasciculi proprii of spinal cord **2**: 288
Fasciolar gyrus **2**: 317, 325
Fastigial nucleus **2**: 309
Fastigium **2**: 307, 320
Fatty appendices of colon → Omental
  appendices
Female endocrine glands **1**: 15
– external genitalia **2**: 269
– genital system **1**: 17; **2**: 233
– internal genitalia **2**: 239–243, 245
– larynx **2**: 64
– lesser pelvis **2**: 238–243, 245–247, 250–253,
  256–257, 260
– pelvic organs **2**: 233, 238–243, 245–247
– – viscera **2**: 233, 238–243, 245–247
– pelvis **1**: 172, 174–175, 178; **2**: 233, 243
– perineum **2**: 265, 269, 280–281
– urethra **1**: 17; **2**: 233, 243, 250, 256–257, 260
– urogenital system **2**: 233
Femoral artery **1**: 14, 64–65, 75, 219, 248–253,
  259–260, 262–263, 269; **2**: 163, 228, 256–259
– branch of genitofemoral nerve **1**: 78, 242, 248;
  2: 227
– hernia **1**: 249
– nerve **1**: 227–229, 235, 242, 244, 248–249,
  252, 270; **2**: 226–228, 245, 248, 256–258
– septum **1**: 249
– triangle **1**: 4, 249
– vein **1**: 14, 64–65, 75, 218–219, 246–249,
  259–260, 262–263; **2**: 163, 228, 256–259
Femur **1**: 7, 9–10, 170–171, 173, 177, 179–181,
  193–194, 196–200, 202–204, 220–226, 229,
  233–234, 247, 251, 258–265, 269, 277; **2**: 205,
  209, 254–259
Fetal kidney **2**: 210
– lobulation of kidney **2**: 210
– peritoneal cavity **2**: 170
– suprarenal gland **2**: 210
Fetus **2**: 243
Fibrocartilaginous ring of tympanic membrane
  2: 392, 398
Fibrous appendix of liver **2**: 154, 180–181, 191
– capsule of kidney **2**: 212
– joint **1**: 9
– layer of articular capsule **1**: 10–11
– – – eyeball **2**: 372
– membrane of articular capsule → Fibrous
  layer of articular capsule
– pericardium **2**: 107, 122–123, 149, 151,
  164–165
– rings of heart **2**: 135
– sheath(s) **1**: 10
– – of digits of hand **1**: 102, 121–122, 124, 130,
    162
– – – toes **1**: 237–238

Fibrous
− tissue **1**: 9
− trigones of heart **2**: 135
Fibula **1**: 170–171, 182–183, 195–197, 199, 202–203, 205, 208–210, 214, 216, 220–222, 226, 230–233, 235, 247, 255–256, 266–269, 271–277
Fibular artery **1**: 250, 266–268, 271, 273–274, 278–279
− articular facet on tibia **1**: 183
− collateral ligament **1**: 195–196, 199–200, 220, 272
− notch of tibia **1**: 183
− nutrient artery **1**: 268
− trochlea of calcaneus **1**: 187–188
− veins **1**: 247, 273–274
Fibularis brevis muscle **1**: 206–208, 213–215, 231–236, 240–241, 267–268, 271, 273–277
− longus muscle **1**: 206, 208, 213–215, 231–235, 238, 240–241, 267–268, 271, 273–277
− tertius muscle **1**: 231–232, 236, 240–241, 278
Filiform papillae **2**: 39
Filum terminale **1**: 22; **2**: 284
− − externum → Dural part of filum terminale
− − internum → Pial part of filum terminale
Fimbria(e) of hippocampus **2**: 324–326, 340, 351
− − uterine tube **1**: 17; **2**: 233, 239–240
Fimbriated fold of tongue **2**: 38
Fingernail → Nail
Fingers including thumb → Digits of hand
First cervical vertebra → Atlas [C I]
− functional areas of cerebral cortex **2**: 319
Fissura antitragohelicina **2**: 390
Fissure for ligamentum teres **2**: 181
− − − venosum **2**: 181
− − round ligament → Fissure for ligamentum teres
Flank → Lateral region of abdomen
Flexion **1**: 5
Flexor carpi radialis muscle **1**: 101, 105–106, 113–116, 121–124, 128, 130, 151–153, 156–159, 161–162
− − ulnaris muscle **1**: 101–102, 105, 113–117, 121–124, 128, 130, 152–153, 156–158, 161–162
− compartment of arm **1**: 148–149
− digiti minimi brevis muscle of foot **1**: 237–238, 240
− − − − − hand **1**: 121–124, 128, 130, 162, 166
− digitorum brevis muscle **1**: 208, 211, 214, 237–238, 240, 279–280
− − longus muscle **1**: 208, 214–215, 231, 233–235, 238, 240–241, 267–268, 273–277, 280
− − profundus muscle **1**: 101, 116–117, 121–124, 128, 153, 156–159, 162, 166–167
− − superficialis muscle **1**: 101, 113–117, 121–124, 128, 130, 152–153, 156–159, 162, 166–167
− hallucis brevis muscle **1**: 237–238, 240, 279
− − longus muscle **1**: 208, 211, 213–215, 233–235, 237–238, 240–241, 267–268, 273–277, 280
− pollicis brevis muscle **1**: 103, 121, 123–124, 128, 130, 162, 166–167
− − longus muscle **1**: 114–117, 121–124, 128, 130–131, 152–153, 157–159, 162, 166–167
− retinaculum of foot **1**: 233–234, 238, 241, 267–268, 279–280
− − − hand **1**: 102–103, 121–124, 130, 152–153, 161–162, 166

Flocculus **2**: 308–309, 340
Floor of fourth ventricle → Rhomboid fossa
− − oral cavity **2**: 36, 39
− − orbit **2**: 58–59
Flumina pilorum → Hair streams
Fold(s) of chorda tympani **2**: 398
− − iris **2**: 376
− − superior laryngeal nerve **2**: 50
− − uterine tube **2**: 241
Foliate papillae **2**: 39, 46
Folium(-ia) of cerebellum **2**: 308
− − vermis **2**: 307–308
Foot **1**: 2, 184–189, 206–217, 230–232, 236–241, 270–271, 278–281
Footplate of stapes → Base of stapes
Foramen cecum of frontal bone **2**: 10, 21
− − − medulla oblongata **2**: 306, 340
− − − tongue **2**: 46, 50, 101
− for basivertebral vein **1**: 39, 47–48
− lacerum **2**: 8–10, 17, 399–400
− magnum **1**: 22, 40, 50; **2**: 8–10, 12, 18, 72, 290–291, 394–395
− ovale **1**: 13; **2**: 8–10, 19, 133, 301, 395, 399–400
− rotundum **2**: 10, 19, 301, 368, 400
− singulare **2**: 401, 403
− spinosum **2**: 8–10, 19, 395, 399–400
− transversarium of atlas **1**: 30, 49–50
− − − axis **1**: 30
− − − cervical vertebra **1**: 30–31, 49–50; **2**: 289
Forearm **1**: 2, 99, 105, 114–119, 137, 150–159
Forebrain **2**: 303, 306
Foreskin → Prepuce of penis
Fornix cerebri **2**: 299–300, 304–305, 307, 317, 320, 322, 324–326, 328, 334, 338, 340, 344, 346, 348–350, 355–356, 361
− of lacrimal sac **2**: 365
− − stomach **2**: 173–176, 191
Fossa for gallbladder **2**: 181
− − lacrimal gland **2**: 21, 367–368
− − − sac **2**: 4, 367–369
− of oval window **2**: 396
− − round window **2**: 396, 398
− ovalis **1**: 12; **2**: 132, 140
Fourth ventricle **2**: 304–311, 320–321, 324, 340, 342–343, 359, 409
Fovea centralis **2**: 374, 377
− for ligament of head of femur **1**: 179–180
Foveola of retina **2**: 377
Free border of nail **1**: 11
− − − ovary **2**: 239–240
− part of column of fornix **2**: 324, 328
− tenia **2**: 177, 179, 192–193, 202, 204
Frenulum of clitoris **2**: 269
− − ileal orifice **2**: 177–178
− − labia minora **2**: 269
− − lower lip **2**: 38
− − prepuce **2**: 274–276
− − superior medullary velum **2**: 310–311
− − tongue **2**: 38–39
Frill of iris **2**: 376
Frontal angle of parietal bone **2**: 22
− belly of occipitofrontalis muscle **2**: 28–30, 85, 366
− bone **1**: 87; **2**: 3–4, 6–7, 10, 12–17, 21, 23, 55–56, 58, 336, 347, 349, 356–357, 360, 367–369, 384, 387
− border of parietal bone **2**: 22
− branch(es) of callosomarginal artery **2**: 297
− − − middle meningeal artery **2**: 77, 290, 380
− − − superficial temporal artery **2**: 76, 85–86

Frontal
− connective tissue strands of lesser pelvis **2**: 246
− crest **2**: 3, 10, 21
− eminence → Frontal tuber
− forceps of radiation of corpus callosum → Minor forceps of radiation of corpus callosum
− horn of lateral ventricle **2**: 300, 302, 320, 322–323, 332, 337–339, 344, 346–350, 354–355, 360
− lobe **2**: 305, 312–313, 323, 329, 336, 339, 345, 347, 349, 354–358, 360, 362, 384, 386–387
− margin of greater wing of sphenoidal bone **2**: 19
− − − lesser wing of sphenoidal bone **2**: 19
− nerve **2**: 58, 84, 379–382, 384
− notch **2**: 4, 21, 367
− operculum of frontal lobe **2**: 323
− planes **1**: 5
− pole **2**: 296, 306, 314–316, 348
− process of maxilla **2**: 4, 12, 24, 54, 57, 367–369
− − − zygomatic bone **2**: 367
− sinus **2**: 5, 7, 12–13, 23, 52, 55–62, 88, 90, 291, 294, 305, 347, 357, 362, 367, 369–370, 380–382, 386
− suture **2**: 3, 17
− tuber **2**: 17, 21
− veins **2**: 297
Fronto-ethmoidal suture **2**: 10, 12
Frontolacrimal suture **2**: 4
Frontomaxillary suture **2**: 4, 365, 367
Frontonasal suture **2**: 4
Frontopontine fibers **2**: 328, 332
Frontozygomatic suture **2**: 4, 6, 368
Fundiform ligament of penis **1**: 66
Fundus of bladder **2**: 235, 258
− − gallbladder **2**: 186, 190–191
− − internal acoustic meatus **2**: 403
− − stomach **1**: 43; **2**: 128, 130, 155, 173–176, 182, 191
− − uterus **1**: 17; **2**: 172, 233, 238–240, 242, 245, 250–251, 260
Fungiform papillae **2**: 46
Funiculus separans **2**: 310
Furrow of nail matrix **1**: 11

G

Gallbladder **1**: 16, 18, 20; **2**: 154, 172, 180–181, 183, 186–187, 190–191, 196, 198, 200, 204, 208, 223, 248
Ganglion impar **1**: 25
− of sympathetic trunk **1**: 23, 79; **2**: 285
Gastric areas **2**: 174
− folds **2**: 174–175
− impression on liver **2**: 181
− − − spleen **2**: 189
− lymph nodes **2**: 198
− nerve plexus(es) **1**: 25
− pits **2**: 174
− rugae → Gastric folds
Gastrocnemius muscle **1**: 195, 200, 203–204, 217, 221–222, 224, 226, 229, 231–234, 252, 255–256, 265, 267–268, 272–274, 276–277
Gastrocolic ligament **2**: 190–191, 196, 204
Gastroduodenal artery **2**: 196–198, 200, 203
Gastro-omental lymph nodes **2**: 198
Gastrophrenic ligament **2**: 206
Gastrosplenic ligament **2**: 171, 191
Gemellus inferior muscle **1**: 223–224, 226–227, 229, 256; **2**: 253, 279

Gemellus
– superior muscle **1**: 223–224, 226–227, 229, 256; **2**: 253, 279
Genial spines of mandible → Mental spines of mandible
Genicular anastomosis **1**: 250, 252
Geniculate ganglion **2**: 84, 87–89, 399
Geniculocalcarine fibers → Optic radiation
Geniculotemporal fibers → Acoustic radiation
Geniculum of facial nerve **2**: 84, 89
Genioglossus muscle **2**: 30, 32, 35–36, 38, 45–48, 97, 99
Geniohyoid muscle **2**: 30, 32, 34–36, 45–48, 87, 97–99
Genital branch of genitofemoral nerve **1**: 78, 242; **2**: 227, 274
– systems **1**: 17
Genitofemoral nerve **1**: 242, 244, 248; **2**: 226–228, 274
Genu of corpus callosum **2**: 307, 317, 322, 334, 345–350, 354–355
– – internal capsule **2**: 332–333, 348, 355–356
Gingiva **2**: 40
Gingival margin **2**: 40
– papilla(e) **2**: 38
Glabella **2**: 21
Glands of tongue **2**: 38
Glandular branches of facial artery **2**: 76
Glans of clitoris **2**: 268–269, 281
– penis **1**: 17; **2**: 170, 232, 274–278
Glenohumeral joint **1**: 9, 82–83, 95–97, 109–110
– ligaments **1**: 95–96
Glenoid cavity of scapula **1**: 84–85, 87, 96–97
– labrum of scapula **1**: 96–97
Globose nucleus → Posterior interpositus nucleus
Globus pallidus **2**: 334–335, 338–339, 344, 348, 350, 356
– – external segment → Globus pallidus lateral segment
– – internal segment → Globus pallidus medial segment
– – lateral segment **2**: 329–330, 332, 335, 338–339, 344, 348, 350, 356
– – medial segment **2**: 329–330, 332, 335, 338–339, 344, 348, 350, 356
Glossopharyngeal nerve [IX] **1**: 22, 25, 51; **2**: 34–35, 37, 89, 96–97, 100, 284, 289, 291–292, 294–295, 306, 311, 340
– part of superior constrictor muscle **2**: 46–47
Glottis **2**: 68
Gluteal fascia → Fascia glutea
– fold **1**: 218
– region **1**: 4, 254–257
– surface of ilium **1**: 175–176, 191, 221, 225
– tuberosity of femur **1**: 180
Gluteus maximus muscle **1**: 52–54, 194, 217–218, 222–224, 226–227, 229, 255–258, 261–262; **2**: 225, 230, 253, 255–259, 265–266, 278, 280
– medius muscle **1**: 52–54, 194, 217, 219, 223–224, 226–227, 229, 256–258; **2**: 225, 230, 252–259
– minimus muscle **1**: 194, 224, 227, 229, 257–258; **2**: 225, 252–259
Gracile fasciculus **2**: 288, 310
– lobule of cerebellum **2**: 308–309
– tubercle **2**: 310–311
Gracilis muscle **1**: 200, 219–224, 227–228, 231, 233, 235, 252–253, 255–256, 259–265, 267, 272
Granular foveolae of calvaria **2**: 3

Gray commissure of spinal cord **2**: 288
– matter/substance of cerebrum **2**: 289, 338
– – – spinal cord **2**: 285
– ramus communicans of spinal nerve **1**: 23, 79; **2**: 95–96, 166–167, 285
Great arteries of abdomen **2**: 218–219, 229
– auricular nerve **1**: 60–61, 78; **2**: 82–83, 85, 91–94, 96, 98
– cardiac vein **2**: 107, 129–130, 133, 135, 142–143
– cerebral vein **2**: 291, 299–300, 307, 342–343, 346
– saphenous vein **1**: 75, 245–249, 252, 254, 262–267, 270, 272, 274, 278; **2**: 163, 228, 256–259
– toe [I] **1**: 184–186, 188, 216–217
– veins of abdomen **2**: 218
Greater curvature of stomach **2**: 173–176, 198
– horn of hyoid bone **2**: 27, 35–36, 46–49, 65–68, 70, 100–101
– occipital nerve **1**: 60; **2**: 82–83, 85, 91–93
– omentum **1**: 63; **2**: 170, 173, 190–193, 196, 202, 204
– palatine artery **2**: 88–89
– – canal **2**: 368
– – foramen **2**: 24
– – groove of maxilla **2**: 24
– – nerve **2**: 84, 88–89
– pancreatic artery **2**: 188
– petrosal nerve **2**: 84, 88–89, 398–399
– sciatic foramen **1**: 190–191, 193, 257
– – notch **1**: 172, 175–176
– splanchnic nerve **1**: 25; **2**: 167, 248–249
– supraclavicular fossa **1**: 63; **2**: 36
– trochanter **1**: 173, 177, 179–180, 192, 194, 216–217, 220–221, 223–225, 254–255, 257–258; **2**: 209, 253–254, 257, 259
– tubercle of humerus **1**: 86–87, 95, 97, 109, 111
– vestibular gland **2**: 251, 269, 280
– wing of sphenoidal bone **2**: 4, 6, 8, 10, 12, 17, 19, 31, 58, 60, 63, 367–368
Grey → Gray
Groin → Inguinal region
Groove(s) for aorta **2**: 111
– – azygos vein **2**: 111
– – greater petrosal nerve **2**: 10, 396, 400, 402
– – inferior petrosal sinus **2**: 10, 18, 20
– – lesser petrosal nerve **2**: 396, 400
– – meningeal arteries **2**: 3, 12, 290
– – middle meningeal artery **2**: 19, 22, 400
– – – temporal artery **2**: 20
– – occipital artery **2**: 20
– – popliteus muscle **1**: 180–181
– – radial nerve **1**: 86
– – sigmoid sinus **2**: 10–11, 18, 20, 22, 400, 402, 406–407
– – spinal nerve **1**: 30–31
– – subclavian artery **1**: 44; **2**: 111–112
– – subclavius muscle **1**: 84
– – superior petrosal sinus **2**: 10
– – – sagittal sinus **2**: 3, 10, 18, 20–22, 295
– – – vena cava **2**: 111
– – tendon of fibularis longus muscle **1**: 186–187
– – – – flexor digitorum longus muscle **1**: 213
– – – – – hallucis longus muscle **1**: 187, 212–213
– – transverse sinus **2**: 10, 12, 18
– – ulnar nerve **1**: 86
– – vena cava → Groove on liver for inferior vena cava
– – vertebral artery **1**: 30–31, 49, 59; **2**: 289

Groove(s)
– of promontory of tympanic cavity **2**: 396
– on first rib for subclavian artery **1**: 44
– – liver for inferior vena cava **2**: 181
– – lung for aorta **2**: 111
– – – – azygos vein **2**: 111
– – – – subclavian artery **2**: 111–112
– – – – superior vena cava **2**: 111
Gubernaculum of testis **2**: 272
Gum → Gingiva
Gyrus(-i) of cerebrum → Cerebral gyri
– – insula → Insular gyri

H

Habenula **2**: 307, 325
Habenular commissure **2**: 307, 310, 320, 324, 340, 348
– nuclei **2**: 331, 348
– trigone **2**: 310–311, 348
Hair(s) **1**: 11
– cells of spiral organ **2**: 404
– streams **1**: 11
Hamate **1**: 8, 92–94, 102–104, 123–124, 129
Hamstrings of thigh → Posterior muscles of thigh
Hamulus of spiral lamina **2**: 402–403
Hand **1**: 2, 92–94, 102, 104–105, 121–131, 160–167
Handle of malleus **2**: 391–392, 397–400
Hard palate **1**: 51; **2**: 13, 38–39, 41, 45, 52, 55, 57, 62, 73, 336, 365, 386–387, 395
Haustrum(-a) of colon **2**: 177–179
Head **1**: 2; **2**: 13
– of caudate nucleus **2**: 320, 322–323, 329–334, 337–339, 346–351, 354–357, 360
– – epididymis **2**: 170, 270–272, 278
– – femur **1**: 173, 177, 179–180, 193–194, 251, 258; **2**: 195, 205, 220–221, 250, 252, 254, 256–259
– – fibula **1**: 181–183, 195–197, 199, 202–203, 205, 216, 220–222, 226, 231–233, 247, 255–256, 266–268, 271–272, 276–277
– – humerus **1**: 73, 85–87, 96–97, 137, 148–149
– – malleus **2**: 391, 397–400
– – mandible **2**: 6, 11, 25–26, 63, 395
– – metacarpal bone **1**: 94, 123, 125, 129
– – metatarsal bone **1**: 186
– – muscle **1**: 10
– – pancreas **2**: 188, 198–200, 202–203, 223–224, 248
– – phalanx of foot **1**: 186
– – – – hand **1**: 94
– – posterior horn of spinal cord **2**: 288
– – radius **1**: 88, 90–91, 99–101
– – rib **1**: 41, 44, 46–47
– – stapes **2**: 391, 397–398
– – talus **1**: 186–188, 210, 215
– – ulna **1**: 89, 92, 94, 116
Head's zone(s) **1**: 79
– – of diaphragm **1**: 79
– – – esophagus **1**: 79
– – – gallbladder **1**: 79
– – – heart **1**: 79
– – – inner organs **1**: 79
– – – kidney **1**: 79
– – – large intestine **1**: 79
– – – liver **1**: 79
– – – small intestine **1**: 79
– – – stomach **1**: 79
– – – testis **1**: 79
– – – urinary bladder **1**: 79

Heart **1**: 18, 43; **2**: 104, 107, 119, 122, 124–148, 153–155, 158–161, 166–167, 172
Heel bone → Calcaneus
Helicine arteries of penis **2**: 277
Helicotrema **2**: 403
Helix **2**: 390
Hemi-azygos vein **1**: 14; **2**: 162–163, 167
Hemisphere of cerebellum → Cerebellar hemisphere
– – cerebrum → Cerebral hemisphere
Hemorrhoidal zone of anal canal → Anal pecten
Hepatic artery proper **2**: 181, 183–185, 196–199, 203
– blood vessels **2**: 183
– branches of anterior vagal trunk **2**: 248–249
– lymph nodes **2**: 183, 198
– nerve plexus **1**: 25; **2**: 248–249
– portal vein **1**: 12–13; **2**: 181, 183, 185, 188, 196, 198–199, 201, 203, 213, 248
– segmentation → Segmentation of liver
– veins **1**: 12–14; **2**: 131, 160, 162, 180, 182, 185, 199, 206–207, 218, 221–222
Hepatoduodenal ligament **2**: 171, 183, 191, 204, 206
Hepatogastric ligament **2**: 170, 183, 191
Hepatorenal ligament **2**: 170, 207
– recess of subhepatic space **2**: 171
Hernial contents **1**: 63, 67; **2**: 273
– orifices of femoral hernia **1**: 249
– ring **1**: 63; **2**: 273
– sac **1**: 63, 67, 249; **2**: 273
Hiatus for greater petrosal nerve **2**: 396, 398, 400
– – lesser petrosal nerve **2**: 393, 396, 398–400
Highest nasal concha **2**: 52
– nuchal line **2**: 18
Hilum of dentate nucleus **2**: 309
– – kidney **2**: 208, 210, 220–221
– – lung **2**: 126
– – ovary **2**: 239, 241
Hindbrain **2**: 303
Hip **1**: 222–226
– bone **1**: 40, 170, 172, 176–177, 227–228; **2**: 194–195, 205, 217, 252, 254
– joint **1**: 170–171, 173, 177, 192–194, 220, 225; **2**: 220–221, 256
Hippocampal sulcus **2**: 315, 317, 326, 334
Hippocampus **2**: 324–326, 333, 340–341, 344, 348, 350–351, 356–358, 361–362, 408
Histological internal os of uterus → Internal os of uterus
Homologous parts of vertebrae **1**: 29
Hook of hamate **1**: 93–94, 102–103, 123–124
Horizontal fissure of cerebellum **2**: 307–308, 340
– – – right lung **2**: 111–112, 150, 154–155
– part of duodenum → Inferior part of duodenum
– – – middle cerebral artery → Sphenoidal part of middle cerebral artery
– planes **1**: 5
– plate of palatine bone **2**: 8, 12, 17, 24, 57–58
Horseshoe kidney **2**: 211
Humeral axillary lymph nodes **1**: 72
– head of flexor carpi ulnaris muscle **1**: 113
– – – pronator teres muscle **1**: 113, 115–116
– lymph nodes → Humeral axillary lymph nodes
Humeroradial joint **1**: 82–83, 90–91, 100
Humero-ulnar head of flexor digitorum superficialis muscle **1**: 113, 115, 117
– joint **1**: 82–83, 90–91, 100–101

Humerus **1**: 73, 82–83, 86–87, 90–91, 95–98, 100–101, 105, 107–109, 111, 113–116, 118–119, 135–137, 139–150, 152–154
Hymen **2**: 269
Hymenal caruncles **2**: 240, 269
Hyo-epiglottic ligament **2**: 66
Hyoglossus muscle **2**: 34–35, 45–48, 97–99
Hyoid bone **1**: 18, 20–21; **2**: 27, 34–36, 44–49, 52–53, 65–68, 70, 78–79, 93, 98–101
Hypertonic stomach **2**: 174
Hypochondrium **1**: 4
Hypogastric nerve **1**: 25; **2**: 231, 248–249
Hypoglossal canal **1**: 49–50; **2**: 9–10, 12, 18, 27, 400
– nerve [XII] **1**: 22, 51; **2**: 32, 34, 37, 47, 81, 87, 94, 96–100, 284, 291–292, 294–295, 306, 311
– trigone **2**: 310–311
Hyponychium **1**: 11
Hypopharynx → Laryngopharynx
Hypophysial arteries **2**: 301
– fossa **2**: 7, 10, 12, 19, 52, 55, 90, 290, 294, 302
Hypophysis → Pituitary gland
Hypothalamic nuclei **2**: 328
– sulcus **2**: 307, 324, 328
Hypothalamus **1**: 15; **2**: 307, 325, 328, 350–351
Hypothenar eminence **1**: 105, 114–115, 120, 160
Hypotonic stomach **2**: 174
Hypotympanic recess **2**: 391
Hysterosalpingography **2**: 240

I

Ileal arteries **2**: 188, 200–204, 219
– orifice **2**: 177–178, 194–195, 205
– papilla **2**: 177, 195
– veins **2**: 188, 200–201, 204
Ileocecal fold **2**: 177
Ileocolic artery **2**: 200–203, 219
– lymph nodes **2**: 203
– vein **2**: 201–202
Ileum **1**: 16, 18, 20–21; **2**: 170, 172, 177–178, 190, 192–196, 200, 202, 204–205, 220–221, 225, 232, 238, 243, 252, 256–261
Iliac branch of iliolumbar artery **2**: 228
– crest **1**: 53, 69, 172–176, 191, 194, 217–219, 223, 226, 255–257; **2**: 211, 218, 227, 287
– fossa **1**: 172, 176, 191, 220
– nerve plexus **1**: 25; **2**: 248
– tuberosity **1**: 174, 176
Iliacus muscle **1**: 69, 77, 194, 219–220, 227–228, 252–253, 258; **2**: 211, 218, 225, 228, 230, 252, 254
Iliococcygeus muscle **2**: 264–266
Iliocostalis cervicis muscle **1**: 56–58; **2**: 74
– lumborum muscle **1**: 54, 56–58
Iliofemoral ligament **1**: 192–193, 225
Iliohypogastric nerve **1**: 61, 78, 242–244, 248, 254–255; **2**: 209, 226–228, 248
Ilio-inguinal nerve **1**: 78, 244, 248; **2**: 209, 226–228, 248, 274, 280
Iliolumbar artery **2**: 228, 230, 234, 245
– ligament **1**: 58–59, 190
Iliopectineal arch **1**: 190, 219, 249
Iliopsoas muscle **1**: 194, 219–220, 224, 229, 249, 258; **2**: 256–259
Iliopubic eminence **1**: 174, 176, 178
– nerve → Iliohypogastric nerve
Iliotibial tract **1**: 195, 218–219, 222–224, 226, 230–232, 255–256, 259–260, 271; **2**: 228
Ilium **1**: 172–177, 191, 194, 220–221, 225, 258; **2**: 205, 220–221, 225, 230, 251–257, 264

Impression(s) for costoclavicular ligament **1**: 84
– of cerebral gyri **2**: 10
Inca bone **2**: 3
Incisive bone **2**: 17, 23–24
– canal **2**: 12, 24, 45, 55–57, 90
– foramina **2**: 24
– fossa **2**: 8, 24
– papilla **2**: 38–39
Incisor tooth/teeth **1**: 36; **2**: 39–42, 59
Incisura of tentorium → Tentorial notch
Inclination of pelvis **1**: 178
Incudomallear joint **2**: 397
Incudostapedial joint **2**: 397
Incus **2**: 391, 397–400, 405–406
Index finger **1**: 92–93, 105
Indirect inguinal hernia **1**: 67; **2**: 273
Indusium griseum **2**: 317, 324–326, 334–335, 338, 340, 345
Infantile hip bone **1**: 176–177
– pelvic girdle **1**: 177
– thymus **2**: 104
Inferior **1**: 5
– aberrant ductule of epididymis **2**: 270
– alveolar artery **2**: 76–77, 85–89
– – nerve **2**: 84, 86–89
– – vein(s) **2**: 80
– anal nerves **1**: 254–255; **2**: 231, 279–281
– angle of scapula **1**: 84–85, 108, 111
– articular facet of vertebra → Articular facet of inferior articular process of vertebra
– – process of axis **1**: 30
– – – vertebra **1**: 30–33, 36, 38, 46, 55; **2**: 286
– – surface of atlas **1**: 30
– – – – tibia **1**: 183
– belly of omohyoid muscle **1**: 106–107, 110, 140, 143; **2**: 34–36, 92, 98
– border of liver **2**: 180
– – – lung **2**: 111–112, 153–154
– – – spleen **2**: 189
– branch(es) of oculomotor nerve **2**: 379, 381–382
– – – transverse cervical nerve **2**: 91–92
– cerebellar peduncle **2**: 308, 310–311
– cerebral veins **2**: 291, 295, 300
– cervical cardiac branches of vagus nerve **1**: 25; **2**: 96, 149
– – – nerve **2**: 95–96, 166–167
– clunial nerves **1**: 61, 243, 254–255; **2**: 279–280
– colliculus **2**: 310–311
– conjunctival fornix **2**: 364–365, 384
– constrictor muscle **2**: 33, 35, 46–49, 68, 74, 99–101
– costal facet of thoracic vertebra **1**: 32
– deep lateral cervical lymph nodes **2**: 163
– dental nerve plexus **2**: 84, 86
– diaphragmatic lymph nodes **2**: 113
– duodenal flexure **2**: 188
– – fold **2**: 206
– – fossa **2**: 193, 206
– epigastric artery **1**: 17, 67, 75, 77, 252–253; **2**: 196, 200, 228, 234, 244–246, 272–273
– – vein **1**: 67, 75, 77, 252; **2**: 196, 200, 244, 246, 272–273
– extensor retinaculum of foot **1**: 230–232, 236, 241, 271
– extremity of kidney **2**: 208, 215, 217–218
– – – thyroid gland → Inferior pole of thyroid gland
– eyelid **2**: 362, 364, 379, 384
– fascia of pelvic diaphragm **2**: 250–251
– fibular retinaculum **1**: 206, 232, 241

Inferior
– fovea of fourth ventricle **2**: 310
– frontal gyrus **2**: 314–316, 337–338, 348
– – sulcus **2**: 314, 316
– ganglion of vagus nerve **2**: 100
– gemellus muscle → Gemellus inferior muscle
– genial spine of mandible → Inferior mental
  spine of mandible
– glenohumeral ligament **1**: 95–96
– gluteal artery **1**: 256–257; **2**: 230, 234,
  244–245
– – line of ilium **1**: 176
– – nerve **1**: 227, 229, 244, 256–257; **2**: 226,
  279
– – vein(s) **1**: 257
– horn of falciform margin of saphenous
  opening **1**: 218
– – – lateral ventricle → Temporal horn of
  lateral ventricle
– – – thyroid cartilage **2**: 64–65, 68
– hypogastric nerve plexus **1**: 24–25; **2**: 231,
  248–249
– hypophysial artery **2**: 301
– ileocecal recess **2**: 177
– labial branch of facial artery **2**: 76, 85–86
– – vein(s) **2**: 80, 383
– lacrimal canaliculus **2**: 365, 383
– – papilla **2**: 364–365
– laryngeal nerve **2**: 101
– lateral brachial cutaneous nerve **1**: 132–133,
  135–136, 142–143, 150
– – cutaneous nerve of arm → Inferior lateral
  brachial cutaneous nerve
– – genicular artery **1**: 250, 267, 269, 271
– ligament of epididymis **2**: 270
– lingular bronchus of left lung [B V]
  2: 108–109, 114
– – segment of left lung [S V] **2**: 117
– lobar arteries of left lung **2**: 119
– – – – right lung **2**: 113, 119
– lobe of left lung **2**: 111–112, 114, 117,
  149–150, 154–156, 160
– – – right lung **2**: 111–114, 116, 149–150, 155,
  160, 165
– longitudinal fasciculus **2**: 333
– – muscle of tongue **2**: 38, 46–47
– – lumbar triangle **1**: 53–55, 57, 226
– macular arteriole **2**: 377
– – venule **2**: 377
– medial genicular artery **1**: 250, 267–269, 271
– mediastinum **2**: 104
– medullary velum **2**: 307, 309
– mental spine of mandible **2**: 25
– mesenteric artery **1**: 12, 14; **2**: 162, 199, 202,
  211, 218–219, 230–231, 234
– – ganglion **1**: 24–25; **2**: 248
– – nerve plexus **1**: 25; **2**: 248–249
– – vein **2**: 188, 200, 202–203
– nasal concha **2**: 4–5, 8, 12, 14, 23, 50, 52,
  55–59, 62, 88–89, 305, 336, 360, 365, 369,
  386–387
– – meatus **2**: 23, 52, 55–58, 365, 367
– – retinal arteriole **2**: 377
– – venule **2**: 377
– nuchal line **1**: 55; **2**: 8, 18
– oblique muscle **2**: 370–371, 384, 386
– olivary complex **2**: 309
– olive **2**: 311, 340
– ophthalmic vein **2**: 58, 80, 379, 383–384
– orbital fissure **2**: 4, 8, 23, 58, 367–369, 379
– palpebral branches of infra-orbital nerve **2**: 85,
  87

Inferior
– pancreatic lymph nodes **2**: 203
– pancreaticoduodenal artery **2**: 188, 198, 200,
  219
– – lymph nodes **2**: 203
– parathyroid gland **1**: 15; **2**: 49–50, 101
– parietal lobule **2**: 314, 316, 323
– part of duodenum **2**: 170, 175, 188, 194, 199,
  202, 206, 224
– – – vestibular nerve **2**: 405
– peroneal retinaculum → Inferior fibular
  retinaculum
– petrosal sinus **2**: 291, 294
– phrenic artery **1**: 14; **2**: 162, 196, 200, 203
– pole of kidney → Inferior extremity of kidney
– – – testis → Lower pole of testis
– – – thyroid gland **2**: 71
– pubic ligament **1**: 190, 193
– – ramus **1**: 172–173, 175–176, 221; **2**: 250,
  268, 281
– recess of omental bursa **2**: 170
– rectal artery **2**: 230–231, 276, 279–280
– – nerve plexus **2**: 231
– – nerves → Inferior anal nerves
– – vein(s) **2**: 276
– rectus muscle **2**: 58, 63, 360, 362, 370–371,
  379, 382, 384–387
– root of ansa cervicalis **2**: 93–94, 97–98
– sagittal sinus **2**: 291, 294, 300, 321, 326
– segmental artery of kidney **2**: 212, 214
– semilunar lobule of cerebellum **2**: 307–309
– superficial inguinal lymph nodes **1**: 245
– suprarenal artery **2**: 162, 215
– surface of tongue **2**: 38, 47
– tarsus **2**: 365, 383–384
– temporal gyrus **2**: 315–316, 338
– – line of parietal bone **2**: 6, 22
– – retinal arteriole **2**: 377
– – – venule **2**: 377
– – sulcus **2**: 316
– thoracic aperture **1**: 41
– thyroid artery **2**: 79, 97, 100–101, 118, 149
– – notch **2**: 64, 70
– – tubercle **2**: 64
– – vein **2**: 97, 122, 149, 151, 162, 164
– tibiofibular joint → Tibiofibular syndesmosis
– tracheobronchial lymph nodes **2**: 104, 110,
  113
– transverse scapular ligament **1**: 95, 143
– trunk of brachial plexus **1**: 134; **2**: 94–95, 166
– ulnar collateral artery **1**: 138, 140–141,
  152–153
– veins of cerebellar hemisphere **2**: 295
– vena cava **1**: 12–15; **2**: 123, 125–127, 131–132,
  134, 139–141, 143, 154–155, 159–160, 162,
  164, 167, 171, 180–183, 185–186, 196,
  198–199, 203, 206–208, 211, 213–214, 218,
  220, 222–224, 228, 248
– vertebral notch **1**: 32–33
– vesical artery **2**: 230, 234, 244–247, 276
– – vein(s) **2**: 276
– vestibular area of internal acoustic meatus
  2: 401, 403
Inferolateral margin of cerebral hemisphere
  2: 337
Inferomedial margin of cerebral hemisphere
  2: 337
Infra-auricular lymph nodes **2**: 91
Infraclavicular fossa **1**: 4
– lymph nodes → Deltopectoral lymph nodes
– part of brachial plexus **1**: 134, 140–141
Infraglenoid tubercle **1**: 84–85, 95–96

Infraglottic cavity **2**: 68
Infrahyoid branch of superior thyroid artery
  2: 98
– lymph nodes **2**: 81
– muscles **2**: 74
Infra-orbital artery **2**: 58, 76, 85–87, 379, 383
– canal **2**: 59, 61, 367–369
– foramen **2**: 4, 6, 24, 367–368
– groove **2**: 4, 24, 58, 367–368
– margin **2**: 4–5, 367, 371
– – of maxilla **2**: 24, 367–368
– nerve **2**: 58, 82–87, 379, 383–384
– suture of maxilla **2**: 367
– vein **2**: 80
Infrapatellar branch of saphenous nerve **1**: 242,
  248, 252, 270
– fat pad **1**: 10, 195, 198, 200, 202–204
– synovial fold **1**: 198, 200
Infrapiriform foramen **1**: 223–225, 257; **2**: 264,
  281
Infrascapular region **1**: 4
Infraspinatus muscle **1**: 95, 97, 109, 111–113,
  142–144, 148
Infraspinous fascia **1**: 53–54, 108
– fossa **1**: 84–85, 87, 95
Infrasternal angle **1**: 41
Infratemporal crest of greater wing of
  sphenoidal bone **2**: 19, 31
– fossa **2**: 88–89
– surface of greater wing of sphenoidal bone
  2: 19
– – – maxilla **2**: 24
Infratrochlear nerve **2**: 82–83, 85–87, 381–383
Infundibular nucleus of hypothalamus →
  Arcuate nucleus of hypothalamus
– recess **2**: 293, 307, 320, 338
Infundibulopelvic ligament → Suspensory
  ligament of ovary
Infundibulum of pituitary gland **2**: 291–293, 304,
  307, 315, 330–331, 334–335, 358, 378, 385
– – right ventricle of heart → Conus arteriosus
– – uterine tube **2**: 239–240
Inguinal canal **1**: 17, 66–67; **2**: 234, 272–273
– falx **1**: 66, 77
– hernia(e) **1**: 67; **2**: 273
– ligament **1**: 14, 64–66, 75, 77, 190, 218–219,
  248–249, 252; **2**: 209, 227–228
– lymph nodes **1**: 15
– region **1**: 4, 63–67, 77, 216, 249; **2**: 272–273
Inion **2**: 8, 18
Inner border of iris **2**: 376
– hernial orifice of femoral hernia **1**: 249
– lip of iliac crest **1**: 174, 176
– muscles of larynx **2**: 67
– sheath of optic nerve **2**: 372–374, 378, 384
– spiral sulcus **2**: 404
Innervation of lacrimal gland **2**: 88
– – mucous membrane of nasal cavity **2**: 88–90
– – – – – palate **2**: 88
– – parotid gland **2**: 89
– – sublingual gland **2**: 87
– – submandibular gland **2**: 87
– – teeth **2**: 86
Innominate line of cranium **2**: 59, 367
Insertion of muscle **1**: 10
Inspiration **1**: 40–41; **2**: 153
Insula **2**: 323, 337–340, 344–346, 348, 350–351,
  355, 361
Insular arteries **2**: 300, 339
– gyri **2**: 337, 348, 360
– lobe → Insula
– part of middle cerebral artery **2**: 298, 300

Insular
– threshold → Limen insulae
Interalveolar septa of mandible 2: 25
– – – maxilla 2: 24
Interarytenoid fold of rima glottidis 2: 69
– notch 2: 46, 50, 67, 101
Interatrial septum 2: 131–132, 140
Intercapitular arteries of hand 1: 161–162, 165
– veins of foot 1: 278
– – – hand 1: 164
Intercartilaginous part of rima glottidis 2: 69
Intercavernous sinus(es) 2: 293–294
Interclavicular ligament 1: 45
Intercondylar eminence 1: 182–183, 197–198
– fossa 1: 180–181, 199
– line 1: 180
Intercostal lymph nodes 2: 163
– nerves 1: 25, 61, 68, 78, 132–133, 136,
  227–228; 2: 93, 96, 166–167
– space 1: 41
Intercostobrachial nerve(s) 1: 72, 132, 136;
  2: 93, 149
Intercrural fibers of superficial inguinal ring 1: 66
– fissure of cerebellum → Horizontal fissure of
  cerebellum
Interdental papilla(e) → Gingival papilla(e)
Interfascicular fasciculus 2: 288
Interfoveolar ligament 1: 66, 77
Interganglionic branch(es) of sympathetic trunk
  1: 23, 25; 2: 166–167
Intergluteal cleft 2: 256–259
Intermaxillary suture 2: 4
Intermediate cuneiform 1: 184–186, 188–189,
  210–211, 215
– dorsal cutaneous nerve 1: 270, 278
– hepatic vein 2: 185
– hypothalamus 2: 328
– lumbar lymph nodes 2: 198
– nerve 1: 22; 2: 84, 87–88, 284, 289, 291–292,
  294–295, 306, 308–309, 311, 340, 398–399,
  408–409
– part of urethra 2: 235–237, 266–267, 277
– sacral crest 1: 34–35
– supraclavicular nerves 1: 136; 2: 82–83, 91–92
– tendon of digastric muscle 2: 97
– tract of dorsal digital expansion of hand
  1: 125
– zone of iliac crest 1: 174, 176
Intermediomedial frontal branch of
  callosomarginal artery 2: 299
Intermembranous part of rima glottidis 2: 69
Intermesenteric nerve plexus 2: 248
Internal acoustic meatus 2: 20, 395, 399,
  401–403, 406–407, 409
– – opening 2: 10, 12, 20, 27, 400, 403
– anal sphincter muscle 2: 179, 243, 251
– axis of eyeball 2: 374
– branch of accessory nerve 2: 100
– – – superior laryngeal nerve 2: 96–101
– capsule 2: 300, 330–335, 337–341, 344,
  346–351, 354–357, 360–361
– carotid artery 2: 61–63, 72–73, 76–79, 86–89,
  95–97, 100, 166, 291–295, 298–299, 301–302,
  339, 351–353, 358–360, 378–380, 382, 385,
  391, 395, 409
– – nerve 2: 100
– – – plexus 1: 25; 2: 87–88, 95–96, 166, 382
– cerebral veins 2: 299–300, 326, 341, 344, 355,
  361
– ear 2: 391, 401, 403
– iliac artery 1: 12–14, 251; 2: 162–163,
  220–221, 228–231, 234, 244–247, 253, 255

Internal iliac
– – vein 1: 14; 2: 163, 220–221, 228, 234,
  244–245, 253, 255
– intercostal membrane 1: 47
– – muscle 1: 64–65, 68; 2: 164
– jugular vein 1: 12, 14; 2: 33, 36, 49, 68, 71,
  73–75, 80–81, 92–93, 96–100, 122, 149,
  162–164, 383, 395
– medullary lamina of corpus striatum →
  Medial medullary lamina of corpus striatum
– – – thalamus 2: 327, 340, 344
– oblique muscle 1: 53–55, 57, 64–67, 194,
  226–228; 2: 196, 220–221, 225, 228
– occipital crest 2: 10, 18
– – protuberance 2: 10–11, 18, 409
– opening of carotid canal 2: 20, 399–400
– os of uterus 2: 243
– pudendal artery 1: 256–257; 2: 230–231, 234,
  244–245, 251, 255–256, 267, 276, 279–280
– – vein 1: 257; 2: 251, 255–256, 276, 279–280
– spermatic fascia 1: 67; 2: 270–271, 274
– surface of cranial base 2: 10, 16, 293, 394,
  400
– – – frontal bone 2: 21
– – table of calvaria 2: 3
– thoracic artery 1: 75–76, 139; 2: 78–79, 97,
  118, 122, 149, 154, 162
– – vein(s) 1: 75–76; 2: 97, 122, 149, 151, 154,
  162
– urethral orifice 1: 17; 2: 232–233, 235, 246,
  258, 277
– – sphincter muscle 2: 235
– vertebral venous plexuses 2: 285–287
Internasal suture 2: 4
Interneuron 1: 23, 79
Interossei → Interosseous muscles
Interosseous border of fibula 1: 182–183
– – – radius 1: 88
– – – tibia 1: 182–183
– – – ulna 1: 89
– intercarpal ligaments 1: 104
– membrane of forearm 1: 98–99, 102,
  116–117, 122, 153–154, 157–158
– – – leg 1: 195–196, 205–206, 214, 235, 271,
  278
– metacarpal ligaments 1: 104
– muscles of foot 1: 239
– – – hand 1: 126–127, 129
– sacro-iliac ligament 1: 190
Interparietal bone 2: 3
Interpectoral lymph nodes 1: 73–74
Interpeduncular cistern 2: 295, 321, 358
– fossa 2: 306–307, 309, 344, 351
– nucleus 2: 325
Interphalangeal joints of foot 1: 206, 213
– – – hand 1: 82–83, 104, 124–125, 165
Interpubic disc 1: 172, 174, 190, 193
Interradicular septum(-a) of mandible 2: 25
– – – maxilla 2: 24
– – – vertebral canal 2: 285–286
Intersegmental part(s) of pulmonary vein
  2: 113, 115
Intersigmoid recess 2: 204
Interspinales cervicis muscles 1: 55
Interspinous ligament(s) 1: 39, 48
Intertendinous connections of extensor
  digitorum muscle 1: 125, 130
Interthalamic adhesion 2: 307, 320, 324,
  326–328, 348, 356
Intertragic incisure 2: 390
– notch → Intertragic incisure

Intertransversarii laterales lumborum muscles
  → Lateral lumbar intertransversarii muscles
Intertransverse ligament(s) 1: 46–47, 59
Intertrochanteric crest 1: 180, 192
– line 1: 179, 192
Intertubercular sulcus of humerus 1: 86
– tendon sheath 1: 95–96, 106
Interureteric crest 2: 235
Interventricular foramen 2: 300, 307, 320–322,
  324, 326, 355
– septal branches of left coronary artery 2: 144
– – – – right coronary artery 2: 144
– septum 2: 132–134, 137, 139, 145, 159
Intervertebral disc 1: 31, 36–39, 43, 47–49, 51;
  2: 72, 156, 158–159, 182, 221, 294
– foramen 1: 28, 36, 38, 48, 51, 55
– surface of vertebral body 1: 30–32
– vein(s) 2: 287
Intestinal border of mesentery 2: 176
– loops 1: 67; 2: 242, 273
– lymphatic trunk(s) 1: 15; 2: 163
– surface of uterus 2: 242
– trunk(s) → Intestinal lymphatic trunk(s)
Intra-articular sternocostal ligament 1: 45
Intrabiventral fissure of cerebellum 2: 308–309
Intracanalicular part of optic nerve → Part of
  optic nerve in canal
Intracranial part of optic nerve 2: 358, 370, 378
– – – vertebral artery 2: 79, 292, 302
Intragluteal injection 1: 257
Intrahepatic bile ducts 2: 183
Intrajugular process of occipital bone 2: 18
– – – temporal bone 2: 20
Intralaminar nuclei of thalamus 2: 327
Intralimbic gyrus 2: 317, 325, 334
Intramural part of ureter 2: 235
– – – uterine tube → Uterine part of tube
Intraparietal sulcus 2: 314, 316
Intraperitoneal organ 2: 171
– position 2: 171
– viscera of abdomen 2: 192–193
Intrapulmonary lymph nodes 2: 110
Intravenous excretion urogram 2: 217
Investing layer of cervical fascia 2: 29, 33,
  44–45, 91–92
– structures of spinal cord 2: 286
Iridial part of retina 2: 374–375, 384
– vein(s) 2: 373
Iridocorneal angle 2: 373–375, 384
Iris 2: 364, 370–376, 384
Ischial spine 1: 172, 174–176, 190–191, 220–221,
  224–226; 2: 244, 264, 281
– tuberosity 1: 175–176, 190–191, 193, 221,
  223–226, 249, 256, 258; 2: 230, 251, 253,
  255–259, 265–267, 278–279, 281
Ischio-anal fossa 1: 194, 261; 2: 251, 253,
  255–259, 261, 265–266, 278
Ischiocavernosus muscle 1: 227; 2: 234, 261,
  265–268, 275, 279–280
Ischiococcygeus muscle 1: 219, 227–228; 2: 230,
  234, 244–245, 264–266, 279
Ischiofemoral ligament 1: 192–193
Ischiorectal fossa → Ischio-anal fossa
Ischium 1: 172–173, 175–177, 194, 220–221,
  261; 2: 253, 255, 257, 268
Isthmus of cartilaginous auricle 2: 390
– – cingulate gyrus 2: 304, 315, 317
– – prostate 2: 237
– – thyroid gland 2: 36, 52, 70–71
– – uterine tube 2: 239–240
– – uterus 2: 233, 240, 256–257, 260

J

Jejunal arteries **2**: 188, 200–204, 219
– veins **2**: 188, 200–201, 204
Jejunum **1**: 16, 18, 20–21; **2**: 154–155, 170, 172, 175–176, 192–194, 199, 208, 223–224
Joint capsule → Articular capsule
Joints **1**: 9–10
– of auditory ossicles → Articulations of auditory ossicles
– – foot **1**: 170–171, 206–215
– – hand **1**: 102, 104
– – head of rib **1**: 47
– – larynx **2**: 65
– – pelvic girdle **1**: 190–191
Jugular foramen **2**: 10, 27, 399–400
– fossa **2**: 8–9, 11–12, 20, 393, 395, 400, 402
– lymphatic trunk **1**: 15, 72, 76; **2**: 81, 149, 163
– nerve **2**: 96, 100
– notch of occipital bone **2**: 18
– – – petrous part of temporal bone **2**: 20
– – – sternum **1**: 45
– process of occipital bone **2**: 18
– trunk → Jugular lymphatic trunk
– tubercle of occipital bone **2**: 18
– venous arch **2**: 33, 97
Jugulodigastric lymph node **2**: 81
Jugulo-omohyoid lymph node **2**: 81
Jugum sphenoidale **2**: 10, 19, 291
Juxta-esophageal lymph nodes **2**: 113
Juxta-intestinal mesenteric lymph nodes **2**: 203

K

Kidney **1**: 14, 17, 19–20; **2**: 171, 182, 186, 199, 208–215, 217–218, 220–224, 248
– lobes **2**: 210
Knee **1**: 252
– cap → Patella
– joint **1**: 10, 170–171, 195–204, 265

L

Labial commissure of mouth **2**: 38, 44
– part of orbicularis oris muscle **2**: 28–30
– surface of tooth **2**: 40
Labium majus **1**: 17, 259; **2**: 233, 250, 252, 269, 281
– minus **1**: 17; **2**: 233, 240, 243, 250, 252, 269, 281
Labyrinthine artery(-ies) **2**: 77, 289, 292, 298–299
– wall of tympanic cavity **2**: 396, 398
Lacrimal apparatus **2**: 365
– artery **2**: 77, 378–382
– bone **2**: 6, 14–15, 17, 55–57, 367–368
– canaliculus **2**: 365, 383
– caruncle **2**: 364–365
– fold **2**: 365
– fossa → Fossa for lacrimal gland
– gland **2**: 80, 365, 379–383, 385–386
– groove in maxilla **2**: 24
– margin of maxilla **2**: 24
– nerve **2**: 58, 82–86, 88, 379–382
– notch of maxilla **2**: 24, 367
– papilla **2**: 364–365
– part of orbicularis oculi muscle **2**: 32
– punctum **2**: 364–365
– sac **2**: 365, 383
Lacrimomaxillary suture **2**: 6, 368
Lactiferous duct(s) **1**: 70–71
– sinus(es) **1**: 70–71

Lacunar inguinal ligament **1**: 77, 190, 219, 249
Laimer's triangle **2**: 49
Lambdoid border of occipital bone **2**: 18
– suture **2**: 3, 5–8, 10, 12
Lamellated corpuscles **1**: 161–162
Lamina affixa **2**: 300, 322, 326
– cribrosa of sclera **2**: 374
– of cricoid cartilage **2**: 51–52, 64–68, 101, 109
– – modiolus cochleae **2**: 402
– – septum pellucidum **2**: 322
– – thyroid cartilage **2**: 64–66, 68, 70, 149
– – vertebral arch **1**: 33
– terminalis **2**: 307
Large intestine **2**: 202–205
Laryngeal cartilages **2**: 64–65
– fat body **2**: 65
– inlet **2**: 46, 50–51, 101
– prominence of thyroid cartilage **2**: 33–34, 36, 44, 64–65, 70, 97, 99, 149, 164
– ventricle **2**: 52, 68
– vestibule **2**: 68, 74
Laryngopharyngeal branches of superior cervical ganglion **2**: 96, 100
Laryngopharynx **1**: 16; **2**: 50, 52–53, 68, 106, 165
Laryngoscopy **2**: 69
Larynx **1**: 16; **2**: 47, 64–70, 101, 106
Lateral **1**: 5
– ampullary nerve **2**: 405
– angle of eye **2**: 364
– antebrachial cutaneous nerve **1**: 132–133, 136, 140–143, 151–153
– aperture of fourth ventricle **2**: 308, 310–311, 321
– arch of foot **1**: 189
– arcuate ligament of diaphragm **1**: 69; **2**: 105
– atlanto-axial joint **1**: 36, 49–51; **2**: 72
– axillary lymph nodes → Humeral axillary lymph nodes
– basal segment of left lung [S IX] **2**: 117
– – – – right lung [S IX] **2**: 116
– – segmental bronchus of left lung [B IX] **2**: 108–109, 114
– – – – right lung [B IX] **2**: 108–109, 114, 120–121
– bony ampulla **2**: 401–402
– border of foot **1**: 216–217
– – – humerus **1**: 86, 98
– – – kidney **2**: 208
– – – scapula **1**: 84–85
– branch(es) of accessory saphenous vein **1**: 248
– – – left coronary artery **2**: 144, 147–148
– – – posterior rami of spinal nerves **1**: 23, 61
– – – supra-orbital nerve **2**: 82–83, 85–87, 380–381, 383
– calcaneal branches of sural nerve **1**: 266–267
– cerebral fossa **2**: 295, 316, 323, 331, 337, 345
– – sulcus **2**: 306, 315–317, 319, 338, 344, 348, 351, 355, 361–362
– cervical lymph nodes **2**: 81, 91, 163
– – region **1**: 4, 62; **2**: 36
– circumflex femoral artery **1**: 250–253; **2**: 228
– – – vein **1**: 247
– condyle of femur **1**: 10, 179–181, 196–199, 202–204, 259–261, 265, 277
– – – tibia **1**: 10, 182–183, 197–200, 202–203, 226, 232, 276–277
– condylopatellar line **1**: 181, 198
– cord of brachial plexus **1**: 134, 140–141; **2**: 94–95, 166
– corticospinal tract **2**: 288
– costotransverse ligament **1**: 47

Lateral
– crico-arytenoid muscle **2**: 67
– crus of major alar cartilage of nose **2**: 54
– – – superficial inguinal ring **1**: 66
– cuneiform **1**: 184–186, 188–189, 211, 215
– cutaneous branch(es) of dorsal branch of posterior intercostal artery **1**: 76
– – – – iliohypogastric nerve **1**: 242–243, 248, 254–255
– – – – intercostal nerves **1**: 61, 78, 132–133, 136; **2**: 93
– – – – posterior intercostal artery **1**: 76
– – – – – rami of spinal nerves **1**: 61
– – – – – – thoracic nerves **1**: 61, 133
– – nerve of forearm → Lateral antebrachial cutaneous nerve
– – – – thigh → Lateral femoral cutaneous nerve
– direct veins of lateral ventricle **2**: 300
– division of lumbar erector spinae → Lumbar part of iliocostalis lumborum muscle
– dorsal cutaneous nerve **1**: 242, 266–267, 278
– epicondyle of femur **1**: 179–181
– – – humerus **1**: 86, 90, 98, 105, 108–109, 116, 118–119, 135, 142–143, 148, 150, 154
– femoral cutaneous nerve **1**: 61, 78, 242–244, 248–249, 252, 254–255, 266; **2**: 209, 226–228, 248
– frontobasal artery **2**: 298
– funiculus of medulla oblongata **2**: 310, 340
– – – spinal cord **2**: 288
– geniculate body **2**: 310–311, 326, 330, 332, 334–335, 340, 350, 357
– – nuclei **2**: 327
– glosso-epiglottic fold **2**: 46
– head of flexor hallucis brevis muscle **1**: 240
– – – gastrocnemius muscle **1**: 195, 200, 203–204, 222, 224, 226, 229, 232–234, 256, 265, 267–268, 272, 276–277
– – – triceps brachii muscle **1**: 105, 108–109, 111, 113, 118–119, 142–143, 145–146, 148–149
– horn of spinal cord **1**: 79; **2**: 288
– hypothalamic area **2**: 328
– inguinal fossa **1**: 67, 77; **2**: 238, 244, 272
– – hernia **1**: 67; **2**: 273
– intercondylar tubercle **1**: 182, 197, 204–205
– intermuscular septum of arm **1**: 108–109, 118–119, 135, 142–143, 150, 154
– lacunae of superior sagittal sinus **2**: 295, 297
– lemniscus **2**: 311
– ligament of temporomandibular joint **2**: 26, 31
– lip of bicipital groove → Crest of greater tubercle of humerus
– – – linea aspera **1**: 180
– longitudinal stria **2**: 322, 324, 334–335, 338, 345
– malleolar arterial network **1**: 271, 278
– – branches of fibular artery **1**: 250, 266–268
– – facet of talus **1**: 187–188
– malleolus **1**: 182–183, 205, 208, 212, 214, 216–217, 230–233, 236, 241, 276–278
– mammary branches of lateral cutaneous branch of posterior intercostal artery **1**: 76
– – – – – thoracic artery **1**: 72
– margin of humerus **1**: 86
– marginal vein of foot **1**: 278
– mass of atlas **1**: 30–31, 36, 51; **2**: 72–73, 408
– medullary lamina of corpus striatum **2**: 335, 338, 344, 348, 350
– membranous ampulla **2**: 405
– meniscus **1**: 10, 196, 198–203

Lateral
- nasal branches of anterior ethmoidal nerve
  2: 88
- – cartilage **2**: 54
- occipital artery **2**: 298, 302
- occipitotemporal gyrus **2**: 304, 315, 317
- olfactory region of nasal mucosa **2**: 90
- – stria **2**: 306, 335
- orbitofrontal artery → Lateral frontobasal
  artery
- palpebral commissure **2**: 364
- – ligament **2**: 365, 383
- – raphe **2**: 364
- part of occipital bone **1**: 49; **2**: 17–18
- – – sacrum **1**: 34–35
- – – vaginal fornix **2**: 240
- patellar retinaculum **1**: 195, 200, 265
- pectoral cutaneous branch of intercostal
  nerve **1**: 23
- – nerve **1**: 68, 112–113, 134; **2**: 93–94, 149
- plantar artery **1**: 214, 250, 279–281
- – nerve **1**: 214, 240, 243, 268, 279–280
- – veins **1**: 214
- plate of pterygoid process of sphenoidal bone
  2: 19, 23–24, 48, 368, 395
- posterior nucleus of thalamus **2**: 327
- process of calcaneal tuberosity **1**: 186–187
- – – malleus **2**: 392, 397
- – – talus **1**: 187
- prolapse of intervertebral disc **1**: 48
- pterygoid muscle **2**: 26, 30–32, 37, 49–50, 63,
  73, 80, 86–87
- recess of fourth ventricle **2**: 308–311, 320
- rectus muscle **2**: 58, 352–353, 360, 370–371,
  374, 379–382, 385, 387
- region of abdomen **1**: 4
- root of median nerve **1**: 140–141; **2**: 93
- – – optic tract **2**: 335
- rotation **1**: 5
- sacral arteries **2**: 230, 234, 244–245
- – crest **1**: 34–35
- – veins **2**: 244, 287
- segment of right lung [S IV] **2**: 116
- segmental bronchus of right lung [B IV]
  2: 108–109, 114, 120–121
- semicircular canal **2**: 396, 398–402, 406–407
- – duct **2**: 399, 405–407
- spinothalamic tract **2**: 288
- supraclavicular nerves **1**: 135–136, 142;
  2: 82–83, 91–93
- supracondylar line of femur **1**: 180
- – ridge of humerus → Lateral
  supra-epicondylar ridge of humerus
- supra-epicondylar ridge of humerus **1**: 86, 98
- sural cutaneous nerve **1**: 242–243, 248,
  254–256, 266–268
- surface of fibula **1**: 182–183, 205
- – – tibia **1**: 182–183, 205
- – – radius **1**: 88
- – – testis **2**: 270
- – – zygomatic bone **2**: 26, 58, 367
- talocalcaneal ligament **2**: 206–207
- tarsal artery **1**: 250, 271, 278, 281
- thoracic artery **1**: 72, 139; **2**: 93, 149
- – vein **2**: 93
- thyrohyoid ligament **2**: 65–67, 101
- tracts of dorsal digital expansion of hand
  1: 125
- tuberal nuclei of hypothalamus → Tuberal
  nuclei of hypothalamus
- tubercle of posterior process of talus **1**: 187

Lateral tubercle of
- – – talus → Lateral tubercle of posterior
  process of talus
- umbilical fold **1**: 77; **2**: 196, 200, 238, 246
- ventricle **2**: 289, 300, 302, 320, 322–323, 326,
  332–335, 337–344, 346–351, 354–358,
  360–362, 385, 408
- wall of nasal cavity **2**: 55–57, 88–90
- – – orbit **2**: 11, 58, 371
- – – tympanic cavity → Membranous wall of
  tympanic cavity
Latissimus dorsi muscle **1**: 52–55, 63–65, 72,
  105–107, 110, 113, 140–141, 148–149,
  226–227; **2**: 93
Least splanchnic nerve **2**: 167
Left anterior lateral segment of liver [III] **2**: 184
- – medial segment of liver [IVb] **2**: 184
- atrioventricular orifice **2**: 133, 135, 139, 141
- – valve → Mitral valve
- atrium of heart **1**: 12–13; **2**: 104, 107, 122,
  125, 127, 131, 133, 136–137, 139–141, 143,
  155, 158, 161
- auricle of heart **2**: 122, 124–126, 129–130,
  132–133, 139–143, 154, 158, 166
- branch of hepatic artery proper **2**: 183–184,
  196–197
- – – – portal vein **1**: 12–13; **2**: 183
- bundle of atrioventricular bundle **2**: 140
- colic artery **2**: 202, 219
- – flexure **2**: 154–155, 172, 200, 205, 248
- – vein **2**: 202
- coronary artery **2**: 107, 124, 128–130,
  132–135, 141–144, 147–148, 162
- – cusp of aortic valve → Left semilunar cusp
  of aortic valve
- – vein → Great cardiac vein
- crus of lumbar part of diaphragm **1**: 69;
  2: 105–106, 182, 189, 196, 200
- cupula of diaphragm **2**: 150–151
- fibrous ring of heart **2**: 133, 135
- – trigone of heart **2**: 135, 141
- gastric artery **2**: 167, 196–200, 203–204, 219
- – lymph nodes **2**: 198
- – vein **2**: 196, 200
- gastro-epiploic artery → Left gastro-omental
  artery
- – vein → Left gastro-omental vein
- gastro-omental artery **2**: 196–198
- – lymph nodes **2**: 198
- – vein **2**: 196
- hepatic duct **2**: 183
- – vein **2**: 185
- inferior lobar bronchus **2**: 108–109, 114, 127,
  164
- – pulmonary vein **2**: 123, 125, 133, 139, 141,
  143, 158, 164
- infracolic space **2**: 171
- lamina of thyroid cartilage → Lamina of
  thyroid cartilage
- lobe of liver **2**: 154, 172, 180–183, 190–191,
  196, 200, 204, 222, 248
- – – prostate **2**: 237
- – – thyroid gland **2**: 35, 49–50, 68, 71, 75, 97,
  100–101, 150–151, 164–165, 167
- lumbar lymph nodes → Lumbar lymph nodes
- lung **1**: 16, 21; **2**: 108–109, 111–114, 116–117,
  119, 126, 128–131, 149–152, 154–161, 172,
  191, 209, 220, 222
- main bronchus **1**: 16; **2**: 96, 105–111, 114,
  119–121, 127, 155, 157
- marginal branch of left coronary artery
  2: 135, 143, 147

Left marginal
- – vein of great cardiac vein **2**: 143
- medial segment of liver [IV] **2**: 184
- parietocolic space **2**: 171
- posterior lateral segment of liver [II] **2**: 184
- – medial segment of liver [IVa] **2**: 184
- pulmonary artery **1**: 13; **2**: 96, 107, 111, 119,
  122–125, 131, 139, 142–143, 155, 157, 165
- – veins **2**: 96, 111, 140, 157
- semilunar cusp of aortic valve **2**: 133–135, 137
- – – – pulmonary valve **2**: 132, 135, 141
- superior lobar bronchus **2**: 108–109, 114, 165
- – pulmonary vein **2**: 107, 123–125, 131, 133,
  139, 141, 143, 164
- triangular ligament of liver **2**: 180, 206–207
- venous angle **1**: 15
- ventricle of heart **1**: 12–13; **2**: 107, 122,
  124–126, 128–135, 137–143, 145, 154,
  159–160, 166–167
Leg **1**: 2, 182–183, 205, 216–217, 230–235,
  266–268, 270–277
Lens **2**: 61–62, 353, 359, 373–377, 384–385
- epithelium **2**: 375
- fibers **2**: 377
- star **2**: 377
Lenticular fasciculus **2**: 340
- nucleus → Lentiform nucleus
- process of incus **2**: 397–398
Lenticulostriate arteries → Anterolateral central
  arteries
Lentiform nucleus **2**: 300, 329, 332
Leptomeningeal septum **2**: 285–286
- space → Subarachnoid space
- – of optic nerve → Subarachnoid space of
  optic nerve
Leptomeninx **2**: 295–296
Leptoprosopia **2**: 2
Leptosomatic person **1**: 6; **2**: 153
Lesser curvature of stomach **2**: 173–176, 198
- horn of hyoid bone **2**: 27, 36, 46, 65–66, 70
- occipital nerve **1**: 60–61; **2**: 82–83, 85, 91–94,
  96, 98
- omentum **2**: 170–171, 173, 191
- palatine arteries **2**: 89
- – foramina **2**: 24, 27
- – nerves **2**: 84, 89
- pelvis **1**: 77; **2**: 232–247, 250–261
- petrosal nerve **2**: 89, 393, 398
- sciatic foramen **1**: 190–193, 225, 257
- – notch **1**: 175–176
- splanchnic nerve **1**: 25; **2**: 167
- supraclavicular fossa **1**: 63
- trochanter **1**: 173, 177, 179–180, 192–193,
  220–221, 224–225, 258; **2**: 209, 256–257
- tubercle of humerus **1**: 86–87, 97
- wing of sphenoidal bone **2**: 5, 10, 12, 19, 58,
  60, 367–368, 380
Levator anguli oris muscle **2**: 28
- ani muscle **1**: 194, 227–228; **2**: 179, 231, 234,
  236, 244, 250–251, 253–259, 261, 264–266,
  276, 279–281
- labii superioris alaeque nasi muscle **2**: 28–30,
  32, 85, 366
- – – muscle **2**: 28–29, 32, 48, 366
- palpebrae superioris muscle **2**: 58, 360,
  365–366, 370–371, 379–384, 386–387
- scapulae muscle **1**: 54, 60, 110–112, 142;
  2: 30, 33–36, 74–75, 81, 92–93, 98, 149
- veli palatini muscle **2**: 37, 48, 51, 73, 395
Levatores costarum breves muscles **1**: 56,
  58–59
- – longi muscles **1**: 56, 58–59

Ligament(s) of foot **1**: 206–208, 212–215
– – head of femur **1**: 193; **2**: 256
– – inferior vena cava **2**: 181
– – larynx **2**: 66
– – ovary **1**: 17; **2**: 238–241
– – pelvic girdle **1**: 190–191
– – temporomandibular joint **2**: 26–27
Ligamenta flava → Ligamentum flavum
Ligamentum arteriosum (Ductus arteriosus)
    1: 12; **2**: 107, 122–124, 142–143
– flavum **1**: 37, 39, 47, 49; **2**: 75, 285–286
– nuchae **1**: 60; **2**: 33, 73–74
– teres of liver → Round ligament of liver
– – – uterus → Round ligament of uterus
– venosum **1**: 12; **2**: 181
Limbic lobe **2**: 312–313, 319
– system **2**: 325
Limbus fossae ovalis **2**: 132
– of Giacomini **2**: 317, 325, 334
– – osseous spiral lamina **2**: 404
Limen insulae **2**: 323
– nasi **2**: 52, 55, 57
Linea alba **1**: 63–66, 68, 77; **2**: 232
– aspera **1**: 180, 223–224
– semilunaris **1**: 62, 65
– terminalis of pelvis **1**: 34, 172–174; **2**: 195, 217
Lines of human body **1**: 4
Lingual aponeurosis **2**: 46–47
– artery **2**: 76–77, 79, 86–87, 96–100
– glands **2**: 38, 47
– gyrus **2**: 315, 317
– nerve **2**: 45, 47, 84, 86–88, 97, 99
– septum **2**: 46–47
– surface of tooth **2**: 39–40
– tonsil **2**: 45–46, 50, 101
Lingula of cerebellum **2**: 307–309, 351
– – left lung **2**: 111–112, 150, 160
– – mandible **2**: 25, 27
Little finger **1**: 105
– toe **1**: 186
Liver **1**: 12–13, 16, 18–21, 148; **2**: 128–131,
    154–155, 160, 164, 170–172, 180–186,
    190–191, 196, 199–200, 204, 206–208, 213,
    218, 220–224, 248
– of newborn child **2**: 181
Lobe(s) of ear → Lobule of auricle
– – mammary gland **1**: 70–71
– – thymus **2**: 104
Lobulated kidney **2**: 210
Lobule(s) of auricle **2**: 390
– – mammary gland **1**: 70
– – testis **2**: 270–271
– – thymus **2**: 104
Locus caeruleus **2**: 310
Long ciliary nerves **2**: 372, 382
– gyrus of insula **2**: 323, 344
– head of biceps brachii muscle **1**: 64, 95–97,
    106–107, 109–112, 141, 144
– – – femoris muscle **1**: 199, 221–224,
        226–227, 232–234, 255–256, 258,
        261–263, 267–268
– – – triceps brachii muscle **1**: 95, 105–112,
        141–146, 148–149
– limb of incus **2**: 391, 397–398
– plantar ligament **1**: 212–214, 238
– posterior ciliary arteries **2**: 372–373
– saphenous vein → Great saphenous vein
– skull **2**: 2
– thoracic nerve **1**: 68, 72, 112, 134; **2**: 93–94,
    98, 149
Longissimus capitis muscle **1**: 56–58, 60; **2**: 32,
    37, 73–74

Longissimus
– cervicis muscle **1**: 56–58; **2**: 74
– thoracis muscle **1**: 54, 56–58
Longitudinal arch of foot **1**: 189
– axes **1**: 5
– bands of cruciate ligament of atlas **1**: 50
– canals of modiolus cochleae **2**: 403
– cerebral fissure **2**: 58, 296, 306, 314–315,
    336–343, 347–350, 354–358, 360–361
– duct of epoöphoron **2**: 241
– fascicles of palmar aponeurosis **1**: 120
– – – plantar aponeurosis **1**: 237
– muscular layer of stomach **2**: 173
– pontine fibers **2**: 340, 361
Longus capitis muscle **2**: 35, 37, 63, 73, 294
– colli muscle **2**: 33, 35, 37, 71, 74–75
Lower abdomen **2**: 171, 192–193, 202, 225
– accessory renal artery **2**: 214–215
– dental arcade → Mandibular dental arcade
– eyelid → Inferior eyelid
– jaw **2**: 5, 61
– leg → Leg
– limb **2**: 134, 170–171, 216–217, 242–247,
    250–251, 269
– lip **2**: 38, 44–45, 47, 52
– lobe of left/right lung → Inferior lobe of
    left/right lung
– pleura-free triangle **2**: 150
– pole of testis **2**: 270
– trunk of brachial plexus → Inferior trunk of
    brachial plexus
Lowest splanchnic nerve → Least splanchnic
    nerve
Lumbar artery(-ies) **1**: 14; **2**: 162, 228–229, 234
– ganglia **1**: 25; **2**: 248–249
– intertransversarii muscles **1**: 58–59
– lordosis **1**: 28
– lymph nodes **2**: 163
– lymphatic trunk(s) **1**: 15; **2**: 163
– nerves [L 1–L 5] **1**: 22; **2**: 226, 284
– part of diaphragm **1**: 69; **2**: 105–106, 155, 182,
    189, 208, 220–223
– – – iliocostalis lumborum muscle **1**: 56–58
– – – longissimus thoracis muscle **1**: 56
– – – vertebral column → Lumbar spine
– plexus **1**: 227–229, 244; **2**: 209, 226–227
– region **1**: 4, 54–55
– spine **1**: 28, 38–39, 48, 228; **2**: 287–288
– splanchnic nerves **1**: 25; **2**: 248–249
– triangle → Inferior lumbar triangle
– trunk(s) → Lumbar lymphatic trunk(s)
– veins **1**: 14; **2**: 162
– vertebra(e) [L I–L V] **1**: 28–29, 33, 38–41,
    48, 55, 82–83, 170–171, 173, 190–191, 219;
    2: 105, 182, 194, 203, 205, 208, 213–214,
    217, 220–221, 223–224, 243–245, 253, 264,
    284, 287
Lumbocostal triangle **1**: 69
Lumbosacral enlargement of spinal cord **1**: 22;
    2: 284
– plexus **1**: 244; **2**: 226–227
– trunk **2**: 226, 231, 234, 248
Lumbrical muscles of foot **1**: 237–238
– – – hand **1**: 120–124, 127, 130, 160, 162, 165,
    167
Lunate **1**: 8, 92–94, 102, 104, 129, 159
– sulcus **2**: 316
– surface of acetabulum **1**: 172, 176, 190–191, 193
Lung(s) **1**: 12–13, 16, 18–21; **2**: 72, 108–109,
    111–114, 116–117, 119–121, 126, 128–131,
    149, 151–161, 164–165, 172, 191, 209, 220,
    222

Lunule of nail **1**: 11
– – radius **1**: 86, 88
Lymph node(s) around cardia **2**: 198
– – of abdomen **2**: 163, 198, 203
– – – anterior border of omental foramen →
        Lymph node of omental foramen
– – – axilla **1**: 72–74
– – – bronchi **2**: 110
– – – chest wall **1**: 72–74
– – – head **2**: 81
– – – inguinal region **2**: 163
– – – lower limb **1**: 245, 248
– – – lung **2**: 113
– – – mesentery **2**: 203
– – – neck **2**: 81
– – – omental foramen **2**: 198
– – – pelvis **2**: 163
– – – retroperitoneal organs of upper abdomen
        2: 203
– – – thigh **1**: 248
– – – thorax **2**: 163
– – – trachea **2**: 110
– – – upper abdomen **2**: 198
– – – – limb **1**: 74
Lymphatic drainage of lung **2**: 113
– ducts **1**: 15
– trunks **1**: 15
– vessels of abdomen **2**: 163, 198, 203
– – – axilla **1**: 72–74
– – – breast **1**: 72–74
– – – bronchi **2**: 110
– – – chest wall **1**: 72–74
– – – head **2**: 81
– – – inguinal region **2**: 163
– – – lower limb **1**: 245
– – – lung **2**: 113
– – – mesentery **2**: 203
– – – neck **2**: 81
– – – pelvis **2**: 163
– – – retroperitoneal organs of upper abdomen
        2: 203
– – – thorax **2**: 76; **2**: 163
– – – trachea **2**: 110
– – – upper abdomen **2**: 198
– – – – limb **1**: 74
Lymphoid nodules of lingual tonsil **2**: 45–46, 101
– organs **1**: 15
– system **1**: 15

M

M1 segment of middle cerebral artery →
    Sphenoidal part of middle cerebral artery
M2 segment of middle cerebral artery →
    Insular part of middle cerebral artery
Macula cribrosa superior **2**: 402
– of retina **2**: 374, 377
Main first functional areas of cerebral cortex
    2: 319
Major alar cartilage of nose **2**: 54
– calyx/calices **1**: 17; **2**: 212, 216–217
– circulus arteriosus of iris **2**: 372–373
– duodenal papilla **2**: 187–188
– fontanelle → Anterior fontanelle
– forceps of radiation of corpus callosum
    2: 345–346
– renal calyx/calices → Major calyx/calices
– sublingual duct **2**: 45
Male endocrine glands **1**: 15
– external genitalia **2**: 270–271, 274, 276
– genital system **1**: 17; **2**: 232
– internal genitalia **2**: 244

Male
– larynx 2: 64
– lesser pelvis 2: 236–237, 244, 246–247, 250–251, 254–255, 258–259, 261
– pelvic organs 2: 232, 234, 236–237, 244, 246–247
– – viscera 2: 232, 234, 236–237, 244, 246–247
– pelvis 1: 172, 174; 2: 232, 234, 244
– perineum 2: 266–267, 279
– urethra 1: 17; 2: 170, 232, 235–237, 250, 258–259, 266–267, 275, 277–278
Malleolar fossa of lateral malleolus 1: 182
– groove of lateral malleolus 1: 182–183
– – – medial malleolus 1: 182, 212
– prominence 2: 392
– stria 2: 392
Malleus 2: 391–392, 397–400, 405–406
Mammary gland 1: 70–75
Mammillary body 2: 300, 306, 315, 324–325, 328, 330–331, 334–335, 344, 351
– process of lumbar vertebra 1: 33
Mammillotegmental fasciculus 2: 328
Mammillothalamic fasciculus 2: 324, 328, 334, 344, 350
Mandible 1: 36, 51; 2: 4–7, 9, 11, 14–15, 17, 25–27, 31–32, 40–41, 44–48, 51, 58, 63, 73, 85–87, 99–100, 395
Mandibular canal 2: 41, 86
– dental arcade 2: 5
– division of trigeminal nerve → Mandibular nerve [V₃]
– foramen 2: 25, 27
– fossa of temporal bone 2: 8, 11, 20, 26, 395
– lymph node 2: 44, 81
– nerve [V₃] 1: 22; 2: 82–84, 86–87, 89, 293, 295, 306, 380, 395
– notch 2: 25
Manubriosternal joint 1: 40–41, 45
Manubrium of sternum 1: 40–41, 45; 2: 118, 154
Margin of tongue 2: 46
Marginal loops at sclerocorneal boundary 2: 372–373
– mandibular branch of facial nerve 2: 84–85, 92, 98–99
Massa intermedia → Interthalamic adhesion
Masseter muscle 2: 28, 30, 32, 34–37, 44, 49, 51, 58, 63, 73, 81, 85–86, 92, 98–99
Masseteric artery 2: 76
– fascia 2: 29, 33, 91
– tuberosity of mandible 2: 25, 31
Mastoid angle of parietal bone 2: 22
– antrum 2: 393–396, 400
– border of occipital bone 2: 18
– branch of occipital artery 2: 76–77
– cells 2: 7, 9, 11, 302, 361, 393–396, 399–400, 406–407
– fontanelle 2: 17
– foramen 2: 8, 20
– lymph nodes 2: 81
– notch of temporal bone 2: 20, 27
– process 1: 55, 59–60; 2: 4, 6, 8, 12, 20, 26–27, 35, 49–50, 73, 92, 100, 393, 395, 399
Maxilla 2: 4, 6, 8, 12, 14–17, 23–24, 48, 54–59, 62, 88, 90, 367–369
Maxillary artery 2: 76–77, 86–89, 99
– division of trigeminal nerve → Maxillary nerve [V₂]
– hiatus 2: 24, 55–57, 369
– nerve [V₂] 1: 22; 2: 82–84, 86–90, 293, 295, 306, 380
– process of zygomatic bone 2: 58

Maxillary
– sinus 2: 5, 7, 24, 41, 58–63, 73, 80, 336, 360, 362, 365, 367–370, 379, 383–384, 386–387
– surface of greater wing of sphenoidal bone 2: 19
– tuberosity 2: 24, 368
– veins 2: 80, 99, 383
Medial 1: 5
– angle of eye 2: 364
– antebrachial cutaneous nerve 1: 132–134, 136, 140–141, 150–151, 160; 2: 93–94, 149
– arch of foot 1: 189
– arcuate ligament of diaphragm 1: 69; 2: 105
– basal segment of right lung [S VII] 2: 116
– – segmental bronchus of right lung [B VII] 2: 108–109, 114, 120–121
– border of foot 1: 216–217
– – – humerus 1: 86, 98
– – – kidney 2: 208
– – – scapula 1: 84–85, 111, 142
– – – tibia 1: 182
– brachial cutaneous nerve 1: 61, 78, 132–136, 140–142, 150–151; 2: 94, 149
– branch(es) of accessory saphenous vein 1: 245, 248
– – – posterior rami of cervical nerves 1: 60–61
– – – – – spinal nerves 1: 23, 61
– – – supra-orbital nerve 2: 82–83, 85–87, 380–381, 383
– calcaneal branches of tibial nerve 1: 242, 267–268, 270, 279
– canthic fold → Palpebronasal fold
– circumflex femoral artery 1: 250–253, 256
– clunial nerves 1: 61, 243, 254–255
– collateral artery of deep artery of arm 1: 138, 143
– condyle of femur 1: 179–181, 196–199, 202–204, 220, 259–261, 265, 277
– – – tibia 1: 182–183, 197–200, 202–203, 276–277
– condylopatellar line 1: 181, 198
– cord of brachial plexus 1: 134, 140–141; 2: 94–95, 166
– crest of fibula 1: 182–183
– crural cutaneous nerve 1: 242–243, 266, 270, 278
– crus of major alar cartilage of nose 2: 54
– – – superficial inguinal ring 1: 66
– cuneiform 1: 184–186, 188–189, 210, 215
– cutaneous branch(es) of dorsal branch of posterior intercostal artery 1: 76
– – – – posterior rami of spinal nerves 1: 61
– – nerve of arm → Medial brachial cutaneous nerve
– – – – forearm → Medial antebrachial cutaneous nerve
– – – – leg → Medial crural cutaneous nerve
– division of lumbar erector spinae muscle → Lumbar part of longissimus thoracis muscle
– dorsal cutaneous nerve 1: 270, 278
– eminence of rhomboid fossa 2: 309–311
– epicondyle of femur 1: 179–181
– – – humerus 1: 86, 90–91, 98, 105–107, 114–116, 136, 140–141, 148, 152–153
– femoral intermuscular septum 1: 220
– frontal gyrus 2: 337, 348
– frontobasal artery 2: 299
– geniculate body 2: 310–311, 330–332, 334–335, 350, 357
– – nuclei 2: 327
– head of flexor hallucis brevis muscle 1: 240

Medial head of
– – – gastrocnemius muscle 1: 195, 200, 203–204, 221–222, 224, 229, 231, 233–234, 252, 256, 265, 267–268, 272, 276–277
– – – triceps brachii muscle 1: 105–107, 109–110, 113–116, 118–119, 141–143, 145–146, 148–149, 152
– inguinal fossa 1: 67, 77; 2: 238, 272–273
– – hernia 1: 67; 2: 273
– intercondylar tubercle 1: 182, 197, 204–205
– intermuscular septum of arm 1: 106–107, 114–116, 140–141, 152–153
– internal nasal branch(es) of anterior ethmoidal nerve 2: 90
– lacunar external iliac lymph node 1: 249
– lemniscus 2: 328
– ligament of ankle joint 1: 212
– lip of bicipital groove → Crest of lesser tubercle of humerus
– – – linea aspera 1: 180, 223
– longitudinal stria 2: 322, 324, 334–335, 338, 345
– malleolar arterial network 1: 278
– – branches of posterior tibial artery 1: 250, 266–268
– – facet of talus 1: 187
– malleolus 1: 182–183, 205, 208–209, 212, 214, 216–217, 230–231, 233–234, 236–238, 241, 270, 276, 278–279
– mammary branches of perforating branches of internal thoracic artery 1: 76
– medullary lamina of corpus striatum 2: 335, 338, 344, 348, 350
– meniscus 1: 196, 198–203
– muscles of thigh 1: 216–217, 220–221; 2: 234, 252, 254, 258, 278
– nuclei of thalamus 2: 326–327, 331, 340, 344
– occipital artery 2: 297–299, 302
– occipitotemporal gyrus 2: 315, 317, 333, 338
– olfactory stria 2: 306, 335
– orbitofrontal artery → Medial frontobasal artery
– palpebral commissure 2: 364
– – ligament 2: 28, 365–366, 383
– patellar retinaculum 1: 195, 200, 265
– pectoral nerve 1: 68, 112–113, 134; 2: 93–94, 149
– plantar artery 1: 214, 250, 279–281
– – nerve 1: 214, 240, 243, 268, 279–280
– – veins 1: 214
– plate of pterygoid process of sphenoidal bone 2: 19, 23–24, 30, 89, 395
– process of calcaneal tuberosity 1: 186–187
– prolapse of intervertebral disc 1: 48
– pterygoid muscle 2: 30–32, 36–37, 49–51, 63, 73, 80, 86–87, 89, 100
– rectus muscle 2: 58, 352–353, 360, 370–373, 379, 382, 385–387
– root of median nerve 1: 140–141; 2: 93
– – – optic tract 2: 335
– rotation 1: 5
– segment of right lung [S V] 2: 116
– segmental bronchus of right lung [B V] 2: 108–109, 114, 120–121
– subtendinous bursa of gastrocnemius muscle 1: 233
– supraclavicular nerves 2: 82–83, 91–92
– supracondylar line of femur 1: 180
– – ridge of humerus → Medial supra-epicondylar ridge of humerus

Medial
- supra-epicondylar ridge of humerus **1**: 86, 98
- sural cutaneous nerve **1**: 255–256, 266–268
- surface of arytenoid cartilage **2**: 64
- – – fibula **1**: 182–183
- – – ovary **2**: 239–240
- – – testis **2**: 270
- – – tibia **1**: 230–231, 241, 270
- – – ulna **1**: 89
- talocalcaneal ligament **1**: 207, 212
- tarsal arteries **1**: 271, 278
- tubercle of posterior process of talus **1**: 187–188
- – – talus → Medial tubercle of posterior process of talus
- umbilical fold **1**: 77; **2**: 196, 200, 238, 246
- – – ligament **1**: 12, 67, 77; **2**: 234, 245
- vein of lateral ventricle **2**: 300
- wall of orbit **2**: 11, 58–59, 367, 371
- – – tympanic cavity → Labyrinthine wall of tympanic cavity
Median antebrachial vein **1**: 105, 136, 151
- aperture of fourth ventricle **2**: 304, 307–308, 321
- arcuate ligament of diaphragm **1**: 69; **2**: 105
- artery **1**: 153
- atlanto-axial joint **1**: 49–51; **2**: 294
- conjugate(s) of pelvic contraction **1**: 178
- – – – expansion **1**: 178
- – – – inlet **1**: 178
- – – – outlet **1**: 178
- – – – pelvis **1**: 178
- cricothyroid ligament **2**: 48, 65–68, 70
- cubital vein **1**: 105, 136–137, 140, 151
- glosso-epiglottic fold **2**: 46
- nerve **1**: 113, 117, 123, 128, 132–134, 140–141, 145–147, 151–153, 156–162; **2**: 93–94, 149
- nuclei of thalamus **2**: 327
- palatine suture **2**: 8, 24
- plane **1**: 5
- sacral artery **1**: 14; **2**: 162, 202, 218, 228–230, 234, 244, 255
- – crest **1**: 34–35, 194; **2**: 265
- – vein **1**: 14; **2**: 162, 218, 234, 244, 255
- sulcus of fourth ventricle → Median sulcus of rhomboid fossa
- – – rhomboid fossa **2**: 284, 310–311, 320
- – – tongue → Midline groove of tongue
- thyrohyoid ligament **2**: 47–48, 65–66, 68, 70
- umbilical fold **1**: 77; **2**: 196, 200, 238, 246
- – – ligament **1**: 67; **2**: 235, 245
- vein of forearm → Median antebrachial vein
Mediastinal part of parietal pleura **2**: 150–151
- surface of lung **2**: 111, 151
- veins **2**: 122
Mediastinum **2**: 104, 107, 149, 164–165, 191
- of testis **2**: 270–271
Medulla oblongata **1**: 22, 25, 37; **2**: 13, 95, 166, 294, 303–306, 309–310, 321, 340, 342–343, 361, 408
- of suprarenal gland **2**: 216
Medullary cavity **1**: 7
- cone → Conus medullaris
- rays of kidney **2**: 212
- striae of fourth ventricle **2**: 310–311, 320
Membranous labyrinth **2**: 405
- lamina of pharyngotympanic tube **2**: 395
- part of interventricular septum **2**: 133
- urethra → Intermediate part of urethra
- wall of trachea **2**: 49–50, 65–66, 109
- – – tympanic cavity **2**: 398

Mendosa suture **2**: 17
Meningeal arteries **2**: 290
- branch(es) of cerebral part of internal carotid artery **2**: 301
- – – mandibular nerve **2**: 380
- – – maxillary nerve **2**: 380
- – – spinal nerve → Meningeal ramus of spinal nerve
- – – vagus nerve **2**: 100
- – – vertebral artery **2**: 77
- ramus(-i) of cervical nerves **2**: 286
- – – – spinal nerve **1**: 23; **2**: 285–286
- veins **2**: 290
Meninges **2**: 285–286, 294–296
Menisci of knee joint → Lateral/medial meniscus
Mental branch of inferior alveolar artery **2**: 76, 85–86
- foramen **2**: 4, 6, 25, 41
- nerve **2**: 82–86
- protuberance of mandible **2**: 4, 25
- spines of mandible **2**: 25
- tubercle of mandible **2**: 25
Mentalis muscle **2**: 28–30, 32
Mentolabial sulcus **2**: 44
Mesencephalic arteries **2**: 289, 298–299
Mesencephalon → Midbrain
Mesenteric lymph nodes **2**: 203
Mesentery **2**: 170–171, 176, 193, 199, 202–204, 206–207, 224–225, 252, 260
Mesial surface of tooth **2**: 39
Mesiobuccal cusp **2**: 39
Mesiopalatal cusp **2**: 39
Meso-appendix **2**: 177, 204
Mesocolic tenia **2**: 177
Mesocolon **2**: 230
Mesometrium **2**: 239–240
Mesosalpinx **2**: 239–241
Mesotendon **1**: 10
Mesovarian border of ovary **2**: 239–240
Mesovarium **2**: 239–241
Metacarpal bone(s) → Metacarpals [I–V]
Metacarpals [I–V] **1**: 8, 82–83, 92–94, 102–104, 123–127, 129, 165–167
Metacarpophalangeal joints **1**: 82–83, 102, 104, 124
Metacarpus **1**: 129, 166–167
Metatarsal bone(s) → Metatarsals [I–V]
- interosseous ligaments **1**: 215
Metatarsals [I–V] **1**: 170–171, 184–186, 188, 209–211, 215
Metatarsophalangeal joints **1**: 206, 213
Metencephalon **2**: 303
Midbrain **2**: 289, 303–305, 309–310, 315, 320–321, 324, 328, 334–335, 340, 350–353, 357–359, 361
Midcarpal joint **1**: 104
Midclavicular line **1**: 4
Middle cardiac vein **2**: 135, 143
- carpal sulcus **1**: 105
- cerebellar peduncle **2**: 306, 308–311, 340, 343, 361
- cerebral artery **2**: 292, 297–302, 339, 351, 358, 362
- cervical cardiac nerve **2**: 95, 100, 166–167
- – ganglion **1**: 25; **2**: 95–96, 100, 149, 166–167
- clinoid process **2**: 10
- colic artery **2**: 200–203
- – lymph nodes **2**: 203
- – vein **2**: 200, 202
- constrictor muscle **2**: 34–35, 46–49, 100
- cranial fossa **2**: 10–11, 60, 291, 369, 380, 382, 394, 399, 406–407

Middle
- cuneiform → Intermediate cuneiform
- ear **2**: 391, 393–394, 399
- ethmoidal cells **2**: 57, 60, 62, 359, 369, 385
- facet on talus for calcaneus **1**: 187, 207
- finger **1**: 104–105, 124–125, 165, 167
- frontal gyrus **2**: 314, 316, 337–338, 348
- – sulcus **2**: 316
- genicular artery **1**: 267
- glenohumeral ligament **1**: 95–96
- lobar artery of right lung **2**: 119
- – bronchus **2**: 108–110, 114, 120–121
- lobe of prostate **2**: 237
- – – right lung **2**: 111–114, 116, 149–150, 155, 160, 165
- mediastinum **2**: 104
- meningeal artery **2**: 76–77, 86–89, 290–291, 294, 380, 395
- – branch of maxillary nerve **2**: 380
- – veins **2**: 80, 290
- nasal concha **2**: 5, 22–23, 50, 52, 55–59, 62–63, 88, 305, 336, 360, 365, 369, 386–387
- – – meatus **2**: 23, 52, 55–58, 365
- phalanx of foot **1**: 184–186, 188
- – – hand **1**: 11, 92–94, 104, 167
- – – middle finger **1**: 167
- rectal artery **2**: 230–231, 234, 244–247, 276
- – nerve plexus **2**: 231, 248–249
- – veins **2**: 276
- retinal arteriole **2**:377
- – venule **2**:377
- scalene muscle **1**: 68; **2**: 33–37, 72, 75, 81, 92–93, 96, 165
- suprarenal artery **1**: 14; **2**: 162
- talar articular surface of calcaneus **1**: 187, 207
- temporal artery **2**: 76
- – branch of middle cerebral artery **2**: 302
- – gyrus **2**: 316, 338
- – vein **2**: 85
- thyroid vein(s) **2**: 97, 149
- trunk of brachial plexus **1**: 134; **2**: 94–95, 166
Midline groove of tongue **2**: 39, 46
- sulcus of tongue → Midline groove of tongue
Minor calyx/calices **2**: 212, 216–217
- circulus arteriosus of iris **2**: 372–373
- duodenal papilla **2**: 188
- fontanelle → Posterior fontanelle
- forceps of radiation of corpus callosum **2**: 345–346, 348
- renal calyx/calices → Minor calyx/calices
- sublingual ducts **2**: 45
Mitral valve **2**: 104, 133–138, 140
Modiolus cochleae **2**: 402–404
Molar tooth/teeth **2**: 39–41, 58, 369, 387
Mons pubis **2**: 269, 281
Motor areas of cerebral cortex **2**: 319
- decussation → Decussation of pyramids
- root of cervical/sacral/spinal/thoracic nerve → Anterior root of cervical/sacral/spinal/thoracic nerve
- – – trigeminal nerve **2**: 89, 295, 306, 380
- speech area of cerebral cortex **2**: 319
Mouth **2**: 38–39, 44
Mucosa → Mucous membrane
Mucosal folds of gallbladder **2**: 186
- – – male urethra **2**: 277
Mucous membrane of bladder **2**: 235, 277
- – – cheek **2**: 45
- – – dorsum of tongue **2**: 46
- – – esophagus **2**: 51
- – – hard palate **2**: 39, 45
- – – mouth **2**: 39

Mucous membrane of
– – – nasal cavity **2**: 55–57, 90
– – – oral cavity proper **2**: 45
– – – palate **2**: 39, 45, 58
– – – pharynx **2**: 50–51
– – – stomach **2**: 173
– – – tongue **2**: 38, 46
– – – trachea **2**: 68
– – – urinary bladder **2**: 235, 277
– – – uterus → Endometrium
– – – vagina **2**: 233
Multifidus cervicis muscle **1**: 58–59; **2**: 33, 74–75
– lumborum muscle **1**: 54–56, 59
– thoracis muscle **1**: 58
Multiparous woman **2**: 268
Multiple renal arteries **2**: 214
Muscle(s) **1**: 10
– attachments to base of skull **2**: 37
– – – bones of foot **1**: 240
– – – – – hand **1**: 128
– – – femur **1**: 229
– – – fibula **1**: 235
– – – hip bone **1**: 227–228
– – – humerus **1**: 113
– – – hyoid bone **2**: 34–35
– – – interosseous membrane of forearm **1**: 117
– – – – – – leg **1**: 235
– – – lumbar spine **1**: 228
– – – pectoral girdle **1**: 112
– – – pelvic girdle **1**: 228
– – – radius **1**: 117
– – – skull **2**: 32
– – – thorax **1**: 68
– – – tibia **1**: 235
– – – ulna **1**: 117
– of abdomen **1**: 62–66
– – anal triangle **2**: 265–266
– – arm **1**: 106–111
– – back **1**: 52–55, 60; **2**: 37
– – – proper **1**: 56–59
– – dorsum of foot **1**: 231–232, 236
– – – – hand **1**: 125
– – face **2**: 28–30, 37, 366
– – floor of oral cavity **2**: 36
– – foot **1**: 231–232, 236–238
– – forearm **1**: 114–116, 118–119
– – gluteal region **1**: 257
– – hand **1**: 121–125
– – hip **1**: 222–226
– – larynx **2**: 47, 66–67
– – leg **1**: 10, 231–234
– – lower limb **1**: 219–224, 226, 231–234, 236–238
– – lumbar region **1**: 55
– – neck **1**: 53–55, 60; **2**: 34–37
– – pelvic diaphragm **2**: 264–266
– – pharynx **2**: 47–49
– – scalp **2**: 28–30
– – shoulder **1**: 106–111
– – soft palate **2**: 395
– – sole of foot **1**: 237–238
– – thigh **1**: 219–222, 224, 226
– – thorax **1**: 68
– – tongue **2**: 38, 46
– – upper limb **1**: 106–111, 114–116, 118–119, 121–125
– – urogenital triangle **2**: 265–267
Muscular branch(es) of femoral nerve **1**: 252
– – – lateral circumflex femoral artery **2**: 228
– – – median nerve **1**: 152–153, 161–162
– – – musculocutaneous nerve **1**: 141
– – – radial nerve **1**: 140

Muscular branch(es) of
– – – sciatic nerve **1**: 256
– – – superior gluteal nerve **2**: 228
– coat → Muscular layer
– layer of bladder **2**: 235
– – – esophagus **2**: 47, 49, 106
– – – pharynx → Muscles of pharynx
– – – stomach **2**: 173
– – – urinary bladder **2**: 235
– – – uterine tube **2**: 241
– – – uterus → Myometrium
– – – vagina **2**: 233
– part of interventricular septum **2**: 134, 145
– process of arytenoid cartilage **2**: 64–65
Musculocutaneous nerve **1**: 112–113, 117, 132–134, 140–141, 145–146; **2**: 93–94, 149
Musculotubal canal **2**: 11, 20, 393, 396, 398
Musculus(-i) pectinati → Pectinate muscles
– uvulae **2**: 51, 395
Myelencephalon → Medulla oblongata
Mylohyoid branch of inferior alveolar artery **2**: 76–77, 87, 89
– groove of mandible **2**: 25, 27
– line of mandible **2**: 25
– muscle **2**: 30, 32, 34–36, 44–48, 86–87, 97–99
Myocardium **2**: 131, 133–135, 138, 141, 145
Myometrium **2**: 233, 242–243

N

Nail **1**: 11, 167
– bed **1**: 11
– matrix **1**: 11
– wall **1**: 11
Naris/Nares **2**: 44, 54
Narrow face **2**: 2
Nasal bone **1**: 87; **2**: 4, 6, 12, 14–15, 17, 23, 54–56, 62, 90, 368–369
– cavity **1**: 16, 51; **2**: 5, 9, 11, 41, 55–63, 73, 88–89, 336, 352–353, 359–360, 365, 369, 385–387
– crest of maxilla **2**: 24
– margin of frontal bone **2**: 21
– notch of maxilla **2**: 24
– opening of nasolacrimal canal **2**: 57
– septum **1**: 51; **2**: 5, 9, 11, 23, 41, 50–51, 54, 58–63, 90, 336, 352, 359–360, 365, 367, 369, 385–387
– spine of frontal bone **2**: 21
– surface of maxilla **2**: 24
– – – palatine bone **2**: 58
– vestibule **2**: 52, 55–57
Nasalis muscle **2**: 28–30, 32, 366
Nasociliary nerve **2**: 84, 379–382
– root of ciliary ganglion → Sensory root of ciliary ganglion
Nasofrontal vein **2**: 80
Nasolabial sulcus **2**: 44
Nasolacrimal canal **2**: 57, 365, 368
– duct **2**: 56, 365, 369, 385
Nasomaxillary suture **2**: 4, 6
Nasopalatine nerve **2**: 88, 90
Nasopharyngeal meatus **2**: 55, 57
Nasopharynx **1**: 16; **2**: 45, 50, 52–53, 55, 63, 73
Natal cleft → Intergluteal cleft
Navicular **1**: 184–186, 188, 207, 209–211, 215, 279
– articular surface of talus **1**: 187, 207
– fossa **1**: 17; **2**: 232, 275, 277–278
Neck **1**: 2, 55, 60; **2**: 33, 47, 72–75, 91–101, 118, 149, 164–166

Neck
– of bladder **2**: 235, 258
– – femur **1**: 173, 179–180, 194; **2**: 254, 257, 259
– – fibula **1**: 183
– – gallbladder **2**: 186
– – glans penis **2**: 275–277
– – malleus **2**: 397
– – mandible **2**: 25–26
– – posterior horn of spinal cord **2**: 288
– – radius **1**: 88, 90–91, 98, 100
– – rib **1**: 44
– – scapula **1**: 84–85, 95, 97
– – talus **1**: 187–188, 210, 215
– – tooth **2**: 40
Neck-shaft angle of thigh bone **1**: 179
Neostriatum → Striatum
Nerve(s) fascicles of cerebrum **2**: 333
– fiber(s) bundles of optic nerve **2**: 378
– – to spiral ganglion **2**: 404
– of anterior region of elbow **1**: 140–141
– – arm **1**: 140–143
– – axilla **2**: 93, 149
– – dorsum of foot **1**: 278
– – – – hand **1**: 165
– – face **2**: 85–90
– – female pelvis **2**: 245
– – fingers **1**: 165
– – foot **1**: 271, 278–280
– – forearm **1**: 152–154
– – gluteal region **1**: 255–257
– – hand **1**: 160–162, 165
– – head **2**: 84–90
– – knee **1**: 252
– – larynx **2**: 101
– – leg **1**: 267–268, 271
– – lesser pelvis **2**: 234, 244–245
– – male pelvis **2**: 234, 244
– – mediastinum **2**: 149
– – neck **2**: 92–93, 97–99, 149
– – palm of hand **1**: 160–162
– – perineum **2**: 279–281
– – peripharyngeal space **2**: 100
– – popliteal fossa **1**: 255–256, 267–268
– – posterior abdominal wall **2**: 228
– – – region of elbow **1**: 142–143
– – pterygoid canal **2**: 88–89
– – rectum **2**: 231
– – shoulder **1**: 140, 142–143
– – sole of foot **1**: 279–280
– – thigh **1**: 252, 255–256; **2**: 228
– – thorax **2**: 93, 97
– – thyroid gland **2**: 101
– – tongue **2**: 97
– – upper limb **1**: 132
– – – thorax **2**: 97
– to mylohyoid muscle **2**: 84, 87, 89
Nervous system **1**: 22
Nervus(-i) erigentes → Pelvic splanchnic nerves
– spinosus → Meningeal branch of mandibular nerve
Neural layer of retina **2**: 374
Neurohypophysis **2**: 293, 307, 328
Nipple **1**: 70–71, 73–74
Nodal point of axes of eyeball **2**: 374
Node(s) → Lymph node(s)
Nodule(s) of semilunar cusps of aortic valve **2**: 133, 135
– – – – – pulmonary valve **2**: 132, 135
– – vermis **2**: 307–309
Noncartilaginous external acoustic meatus → Bony external acoustic meatus

Noncoronary cusp of aortic valve → Posterior
  semilunar cusp of aortic valve
Nose 2: 23, 44, 54, 63, 90, 358–359
Nostril → Naris
Notch(es) of cardiac apex 2: 125, 132, 141
– – liver for ligamentum teres 2: 181, 190
– – sternum for ribs 1: 45
Nuchal fascia 2: 33, 75
– ligament → Ligamentum nuchae
– lines 2: 18
– plane 2: 8, 18
Nucleus(-i) lateralis cerebelli → Dentate
  nucleus
– medialis cerebelli → Fastigial nucleus
– of forebrain 2: 329–332
– – hypothalamus 2: 328
– – lens 2: 375
– – mammillary body 2: 328
– – midbrain 2: 330–331
– – thalamus 2: 327, 340
– pulposus of intervertebral disc 1: 39, 48
Nulliparous woman 2: 268
Nutrient artery of humerus 1: 143

O

Obex 2: 310–311
Oblique arytenoid muscle 2: 51–52, 67, 101
– cord of interosseous membrane of forearm
  1: 98–99
– diameter of pelvis 1: 178
– fissure of left lung 2: 111–112, 150, 155
– – – right lung 2: 111–112, 150, 154–155
– head of adductor hallucis muscle 1: 238, 240
– – – – pollicis muscle 1: 122, 124
– line of mandible 2: 25
– – – thyroid cartilage 2: 64, 66
– muscle fibers of stomach 2: 173
– part of cricothyroid muscle 2: 66, 70
– pericardial sinus 2: 123, 143
– popliteal ligament 1: 195, 221, 233–234
– vein of left atrium of heart 2: 143
Obliquus capitis inferior muscle 1: 55, 58–60
– – superior muscle 1: 55, 58–60; 2: 32, 37, 73
Oblong fovea of arytenoid cartilage 2: 64
Obturator artery 1: 193, 252; 2: 230, 234,
  244–245, 252, 254, 256
– branch of inferior epigastric artery 2: 244
– – – – – vein 2: 244
– canal 1: 190–191, 193, 225, 249; 2: 264
– crest 1: 176
– externus muscle 1: 220, 224, 227–229,
  258–260; 2: 250–252, 254, 256–257, 259
– fascia 2: 250–251, 264–266, 279–280
– foramen 1: 172–173, 175–176, 190, 192–193,
  220
– groove 1: 176
– internus muscle 1: 194, 223–227, 229, 256;
  2: 230, 244, 250–259, 264–266, 279–281
– membrane 1: 77, 190–191, 193, 249;
  2: 250–251, 256–257
– nerve 1: 227–229, 235, 242–244, 248, 252,
  254–255, 266; 2: 226–228, 234, 244–245, 248,
  256
– vein(s) 2: 244, 252, 254, 256
Occipital angle of parietal bone 2: 22
– artery 1: 60; 2: 76–77, 85–86, 91–93,
  98–100
– belly of occipitofrontalis muscle 1: 53–54, 60;
  2: 29–30, 32–33, 85, 91–92

Occipital
– bone 1: 37, 49–51, 60, 87; 2: 3, 6–8, 10,
  12–13, 15–18, 49, 51, 72, 290, 294, 321, 347,
  349, 352–359, 362, 409
– border of parietal bone 2: 22
– branch of posterior auricular artery 2: 91–92
– – – – – nerve 2: 84
– condyle 1: 40, 60; 2: 8, 18, 72, 395
– emissary vein 2: 49
– forceps of radiation of corpus callosum →
  Major forceps of radiation of corpus callosum
– genu of optic radiation 2: 335
– gyri 2: 314
– horn of lateral ventricle 2: 300, 320, 322–323,
  332, 335, 342–343, 346–349, 354–356, 362
– lobe 2: 305, 312–313, 329, 345, 347, 349,
  354–359, 362
– lymph nodes 2: 81
– margin of temporal bone 2: 20
– plane 2: 18
– pole 2: 296, 306, 314–316, 334, 348
– region 1: 4
– sinus 2: 291, 294
– sulci 2: 316
– vein(s) 1: 60; 2: 80, 85, 297
Occipitofrontalis muscle 1: 53–54, 60; 2: 28–30,
  32–33, 85, 91–92, 366
Occipitomastoid suture 2: 6, 8, 10, 12
Occipitotemporal sulcus 2: 315, 317
Occlusal surface of first molar 2: 39
– – – tooth 2: 39
Ocular movements 2: 371
Oculomotor nerve [III] 1: 22, 25; 2: 88,
  291–295, 298, 306, 315, 344, 358, 379–382
– root of ciliary ganglion → Parasympathetic
  root of ciliary ganglion
Odontoblast layer 2: 40
Oesophageal → Esophageal
Oesophagus → Esophagus
Olecranon 1: 89–91, 98–101, 105, 108–109,
  118–119, 135, 142, 149–150
– fossa 1: 86, 91, 98, 148
Olfactory bulb 1: 22; 2: 295, 298, 304, 306, 315,
  324–325, 335
– nerve(s) [I] 1: 22; 2: 88, 90, 298, 306, 315
– region of nasal mucosa 2: 90
– striae 2: 306, 335
– sulcus 2: 315, 317, 335
– tract 1: 22; 2: 298, 306, 315, 324–325, 333,
  335, 337, 387
– trigone 2: 306, 315, 325, 333, 338
Olive → Inferior olive
Omental appendices 2: 177, 179
– branches of left gastro-omental artery 2: 196
– – – right gastro-omental artery 2: 196, 202
– bursa 2: 170–171, 191, 204, 206–207
– eminence of pancreas 2: 188
– foramen 2: 170–171, 191
– tenia 2: 177
– tuberosity of liver 2: 181
Omoclavicular triangle 1: 63; 2: 36
Omohyoid muscle 1: 106–107, 110, 112, 140,
  143; 2: 33–36, 44, 81, 92–93, 97–99
Opening(s) of cochlear canaliculus 2: 20, 405
– – diaphragm for inferior vena cava → Caval
  opening
– – duct of bulbo-urethral gland 2: 277
– – ethmoidal labyrinth 2: 22
– – frontal sinus 2: 21, 59, 62
– – greater vestibular gland 2: 269
– – inferior vena cava 2: 132, 134
– – left coronary artery 2: 133–134

Opening(s) of
– – nasolacrimal duct 2: 365
– – prostatic ducts 2: 235
– – pulmonary trunk 2: 141
– – – veins 2: 155
– – right coronary artery 2: 133–134, 140
– – sphenoidal sinus 2: 11, 19, 55–56
– – superior vena cava 2: 132
– – vestibular canaliculus 2: 20
Opercular part of inferior frontal gyrus 2: 316,
  338
Ophthalmic artery 2: 58, 76–77, 86, 88–89,
  291–293, 301, 378–383, 385
– division of trigeminal nerve → Ophthalmic
  nerve [V₁]
– nerve [V₁] 1: 22; 2: 82–84, 86, 89, 293, 295,
  306, 379–382
Opponens digiti minimi muscle of foot 1: 232,
  238, 240
– – – – – hand 1: 103, 121–124, 128, 130, 162,
  166
– pollicis muscle 1: 103, 121–124, 128, 130, 166
Optic axis 2: 374
– canal 2: 4, 10, 19, 58, 301, 367–368, 371, 378
– chiasm 1: 22; 2: 13, 60, 293, 301, 304–305,
  307, 328, 335, 358, 360, 378
– disc 2: 373–374, 377, 384
– nerve [II] 1: 22; 2: 58, 88–89, 291–295, 298,
  301, 304, 306, 315, 324, 335–336, 338,
  352–353, 358–360, 362, 370–374, 378–382,
  384–385, 387
– part of retina 2: 374, 376, 384
– radiation 2: 332, 335, 348, 350, 355–357
– tract 1: 22; 2: 293, 315, 333–335, 338–339,
  344, 351
Ora serrata retinae 2: 373–374, 376
Oral cavity 2: 38–39
– – proper 1: 16; 2: 38–39, 45, 52, 55, 58, 61,
  336, 386–387
– fissure 2: 44
– opening → Oral fissure
– vestibule 1: 16; 2: 45, 52
Orbicularis oculi muscle 2: 28–30, 32, 48, 85,
  366, 384–385
– oris muscle 2: 28–30, 32
Orbiculus ciliaris 2: 374, 376
Orbit(s) 2: 5, 11, 58–63, 336, 360, 362, 365,
  367–371, 378–379, 383–387
Orbital branch of middle meningeal artery 2: 77,
  380
– cavity 2: 58, 336, 367–369, 379–382, 384–387
– fat body → Retrobulbar fat
– gyri 2: 315, 335, 337
– opening 2: 368
– part of frontal bone 2: 4, 7, 12, 21, 336, 357,
  360, 384, 387
– – – inferior frontal gyrus 2: 315–316
– – – lacrimal gland 2: 365
– – – optic nerve 2: 336, 352–353, 359–360,
  362, 370, 378, 384–385, 387
– – – orbicularis oculi muscle 2: 28–30, 32, 366
– plate of ethmoidal bone 2: 22, 59, 62–63,
  368–369, 378, 385
– process of palatine bone 2: 57, 368
– region 2: 366, 383
– septum 2: 365, 383–384
– sulci 2: 315, 335
– surface of frontal bone 2: 21, 58, 367–369
– – – greater wing of sphenoidal bone 2: 19,
  58, 368
– – – lesser wing of sphenoidal bone 2: 19, 58
– – – maxilla 2: 24, 58, 62, 367, 369

Orbital surface of
– – – sphenoidal bone **2**: 19, 58, 368
– – – zygomatic bone **2**: 58, 367–368
– veins **2**: 383
Organ of Corti → Spiral organ
– – hearing **2**: 391
Orifice of bile duct **2**: 187
– – ileal papilla → Ileal orifice
– – pancreatic duct **2**: 187
– – vermiform appendix **2**: 177–178
Origin(s) of coronary arteries **2**: 135
– – extra-ocular muscles **2**: 379
– – muscle **2**: 10
Oropharynx **1**: 16; **2**: 13, 38, 45, 52–53
Orthotonic stomach **2**: 174
Osseous joint → Bony union
– spiral lamina **2**: 402–404
Ossification center of head of femur **1**: 177
Osteogenesis **1**: 8
Otic ganglion **2**: 89
Otoscopy **2**: 392
Outer border of iris **2**: 376
– hernial orifice of femoral hernia **1**: 249
– lip of iliac crest **1**: 174, 176
– sheath of optic nerve **2**: 371–372, 374, 378, 384
– spiral sulcus **2**: 404
Oval fossa → Fossa ovalis
– window **2**: 393, 396, 401–402
Ovarian artery **1**: 14; **2**: 162–163, 215, 238–239, 241, 245
– branch(es) of uterine artery **2**: 241, 245
– cortex **2**: 241
– fimbria **2**: 239
– medulla **2**: 241
– nerve plexus **1**: 25; **2**: 248–249
– stroma **2**: 241
– vein(s) **1**: 14; **2**: 162–163, 238–239
Ovary **1**: 15, 17; **2**: 163, 233, 238–241, 245, 251–252

P

P1 segment of posterior cerebral artery →
Precommunicating part of posterior cerebral artery
P2 segment of posterior cerebral artery →
Postcommunicating part of posterior cerebral artery
P3 segment of posterior cerebral artery →
Lateral occipital artery
P4 segment of posterior cerebral artery →
Medial occipital artery
Palatal surface of tooth **2**: 39–40
Palate **2**: 7–8, 13, 38–39, 41, 45, 50–52, 55–56, 58, 62, 88, 336, 365, 395
Palatine aponeurosis **2**: 395
– bone **2**: 8, 12, 15–17, 23–24, 55–58, 368
– grooves in maxilla **2**: 24
– process of maxilla **2**: 8, 12, 17, 23–24, 55–56, 59, 88, 90, 369
– raphe **2**: 38–39
– rugae → Transverse palatine folds
– spines of maxilla **2**: 24
– tonsil **2**: 38–39, 45–46, 50–52, 101
Palatoglossal arch **2**: 38–39, 50, 52
Palatoglossus muscle **2**: 46–47
Palatopharyngeal arch **2**: 38–39, 45, 50, 52
Palatopharyngeus muscle **2**: 45, 51
Palatovaginal groove of sphenoidal bone **2**: 19
Palm of hand **1**: 105, 160–162
Palmar aponeurosis **1**: 114–116, 120, 160, 166

Palmar
– branch of anterior interosseous nerve →
Palmar branch of median nerve
– – – median nerve **1**: 132, 151–153, 160–161
– – – ulnar nerve **1**: 132, 151–153, 160
– carpal anastomosis **1**: 162
– – branch of radial artery **1**: 152–153, 161–162
– – – – ulnar artery **1**: 162
– – tendinous sheaths **1**: 130–131
– carpometacarpal ligaments **1**: 102
– interossei → Palmar interosseous muscles
– interosseous muscles **1**: 124, 126–127, 162, 167
– metacarpal arteries **1**: 162–163
– – ligaments **1**: 102
– radiocarpal ligament **1**: 102
– region of hand → Palm of hand
– ulnocarpal ligament **1**: 102
Palmaris brevis muscle **1**: 116, 120, 152, 160, 166
– longus muscle **1**: 101, 105, 114–116, 120, 123, 151–152, 160, 162
Palmate folds of cervical canal **2**: 233
Palpebral branch of lacrimal nerve **2**: 82–83, 85–86
– conjunctiva **2**: 364–365
– fissure **2**: 364, 384
– part of lacrimal gland **2**: 365
– – – orbicularis oculi muscle **2**: 28–30, 366
Palpebronasal fold **2**: 364
Pampiniform venous plexus **1**: 67; **2**: 270–272, 274, 278
Pancreas **1**: 16, 18–19; **2**: 154–155, 170–172, 186, 188, 191, 196, 198–200, 202–204, 206–208, 223–224, 248
Pancreatic branches of splenic artery **2**: 197
– duct **2**: 187–188
– islets **1**: 15
– notch **2**: 188
– veins **2**: 188
Pancreaticocolic ligament **2**: 154
Pancreaticoduodenal lymph nodes **2**: 198
– veins **2**: 188
Papilla of parotid duct **2**: 45
Papillary muscles of left ventricle of heart **2**: 140
– – – right ventricle of heart **2**: 140
Paracentral branch(es) of pericallosal artery **2**: 297, 299
– lobule **2**: 314, 317
Parafascicular nucleus of thalamus **2**: 327
Paraflocculus **2**: 309
Parahippocampal gyrus **2**: 304, 315, 317, 325–326, 331, 333–334, 338, 340, 348, 351, 361
Paramammary lymph nodes **1**: 73–74
Paramedian planes **1**: 5
Paranasal sinuses **2**: 59–63, 336, 369, 386–387
Para-olfactory sulci **2**: 304, 317
Parasternal line **1**: 4
– lymph nodes **1**: 73, 76
Parasympathetic ganglion(-ia) **1**: 25
– innervation of eyeball **2**: 382
– nervous system **1**: 24–25; **2**: 249
– – – in lesser pelvis **2**: 231
– – – – retroperitoneal space **2**: 248–249
– part of autonomic division of peripheral nervous system → Parasympathetic nervous system
– pathways **1**: 24
– root of ciliary ganglion **2**: 381–382
– – – otic ganglion → Lesser petrosal nerve
– – – pelvic ganglia → Pelvic splanchnic nerves

Parasympathetic root of
– – – pterygopalatine ganglion → Greater petrosal nerve
– – – sublingual ganglion → Chorda tympani
– – – submandibular ganglion → Chorda tympani
Paraterminal gyrus **2**: 304, 317, 334, 337
Parathyroid gland **2**: 50, 100–101
Paratracheal lymph nodes **2**: 110, 113
Para-umbilical veins **1**: 75
Paraventricular nucleus of hypothalamus **2**: 328
Paravertebral line **1**: 4
Paravesical fossa **2**: 238
Parenchyma of testis **2**: 271
Parietal bone **1**: 87; **2**: 3–4, 6–7, 12–17, 22, 290, 295, 368
– border of temporal bone **2**: 20
– branch of medial occipital artery **2**: 299
– – – middle meningeal artery **2**: 77, 290, 380
– – – superficial temporal artery **2**: 76, 85–86
– eminence → Parietal tuber
– emissary vein **2**: 295
– foramen **2**: 3, 12, 22
– layer of serous pericardium **2**: 104, 123, 132, 142–143, 154–155
– – – synovial sheath **1**: 10
– – – tunica vaginalis testis **2**: 270–271, 274
– lobe **2**: 305, 312–313, 329, 341–343, 347, 354, 361–362, 408
– margin of frontal bone **2**: 21
– – – greater wing of sphenoidal bone **2**: 19
– – notch of temporal bone **2**: 20
– operculum of inferior parietal lobule **2**: 323
– peritoneum **1**: 63, 67, 77, 249; **2**: 171, 196, 200, 204, 218, 222, 230, 232–233, 247, 273, 276
– pleura **1**: 74; **2**: 150–151, 153–157, 209
– region **1**: 4
– tuber **2**: 17, 22
– veins **2**: 297, 300
Parietomastoid suture **2**: 6, 10
Parieto-occipital branch of medial occipital artery **2**: 297, 302
– notch of cerebrum **2**: 316
– sulcus **2**: 304–305, 314–317
Parietopontine fibers **2**: 328
Parotid duct **2**: 28, 30, 44–45, 48, 86–87, 98
– fascia **2**: 29, 33, 36, 44, 91
– gland **2**: 28, 36, 44–45, 49–50, 58, 63, 72–73, 85, 89, 92–93, 98, 100, 408
– lymph nodes **2**: 81
– nerve plexus **2**: 84–85, 98–99
Pars flaccida of tympanic membrane **2**: 392
– tensa of tympanic membrane **2**: 392
Part(s) of human body **1**: 2
– – optic nerve in canal **2**: 378
Patella **1**: 10, 170, 181, 195–198, 200, 202–204, 216, 219–221, 226, 230–231, 247, 259, 265, 270–271
Patellar anastomosis **1**: 248, 252, 271
– ligament **1**: 10, 195–196, 198, 202–205, 218–220, 230–232, 235, 265, 272
– surface of femur **1**: 179, 181, 196, 198
Patent part of umbilical artery **2**: 230
Pecten pubis → Pectineal line of pubis
Pectinate line of anal canal **2**: 179
– muscles of left atrium of heart **2**: 133
– – – right atrium of heart **2**: 132
Pectineal inguinal ligament **1**: 192–193, 219
– line of femur **1**: 180
– – – pubis **1**: 172, 174, 176

Pectineus muscle **1**: 219–220, 227–229, 249, 252–253, 258–260; **2**: 227–228, 252, 257–259
Pectoral axillary lymph nodes **1**: 72–73
– branches of thoraco-acromial artery **2**: 93
– fascia **1**: 70, 74
– girdle **1**: 43, 84, 87, 112
– lymph nodes → Pectoral axillary lymph nodes
– region **1**: 4
Pectoralis major muscle **1**: 62–65, 68, 70–74, 97, 105–107, 110–113, 140–141, 144; **2**: 92–93
– minor muscle **1**: 64, 68, 72, 97, 106–107, 110, 112, 140–141, 144; **2**: 93, 149
Pedicle of vertebral arch **1**: 32–33, 47
Peduncle of flocculus **2**: 309
– – tonsil of cerebellum **2**: 309
Peduncular branches of posterior cerebral artery **2**: 299
Pelvic bone → Hip bone
– contraction **1**: 178
– diaphragm **2**: 250–251, 264–266
– expansion **1**: 178
– floor → Pelvic diaphragm
– ganglia **2**: 249
– girdle **1**: 2, 172–175, 177, 190–191
– inclination **1**: 178
– inlet **1**: 172, 178
– lymph nodes **1**: 15
– measurements **1**: 178
– nerve plexus → Inferior hypogastric nerve plexus
– organs **2**: 232–234, 236–247
– outlet **1**: 178
– splanchnic nerves **1**: 25; **2**: 226, 231, 248–249
– surface of sacrum **1**: 35, 172
– viscera **2**: 232–234, 236–247
Pelvis **1**: 172–174, 178, 228; **2**: 232–233, 250–261
Pendulous position of vermiform appendix **2**: 178
Penis **1**: 17, 260; **2**: 170, 232, 234, 250, 254, 258–259, 261, 266–267, 274–279
Perforating arteries of deep artery of thigh **1**: 250–251, 253, 256, 262–263
– branch(es) of deep palmar arch **1**: 162
– – – fibular artery **1**: 250, 271, 278
– – – internal thoracic artery **1**: 76
– veins of deep vein of thigh **1**: 262–263
– – – lower limb **1**: 246, 270
Periaqueductal gray substance **2**: 315, 328, 335, 340
Peribronchial lymphatic vessels **2**: 113
Pericallosal artery **2**: 297, 299–300, 302
Pericardial branch(es) of phrenic nerve **2**: 149
– – – thoracic aorta **2**: 162
– cavity **2**: 104, 123, 129, 155, 159
– sac **2**: 122–123
Pericardium **2**: 107, 122–125, 142, 172
Perichondrium **1**: 9
Perilymphatic space **2**: 405
Perimetrium **2**: 233, 243
Perineal artery **2**: 267, 276, 279–280
– body **1**: 17; **2**: 237, 243, 265–266
– branches of posterior femoral cutaneous nerve **2**: 279–280
– fascia **2**: 250–251, 265–266, 279
– flexure of anal canal → Anorectal flexure of anal canal
– membrane **2**: 250–251, 267, 276, 279–280
– muscles **2**: 265–267
– nerves **1**: 255; **2**: 267, 279–281
– raphe **2**: 269

Perineal
– region **2**: 279–280
– veins **2**: 276, 279
Perinephric fat → Perirenal fat capsule
Perineum **2**: 265–267, 269, 279–281
Periodontium **2**: 40
Periorbita **2**: 58, 379, 381, 384
Periorchium → Parietal layer of tunica vaginalis testis
Periosteum **1**: 9–10, 200; **2**: 285–286
Peripharyngeal space **2**: 100
Peripheral nervous system **1**: 22, 25
Perirenal fat capsule **2**: 208, 210, 213, 220–222, 224
Peritendon **1**: 10
Peritoneal cavity **2**: 154, 170–171, 252–255, 272
– serosa **2**: 171
– subserosa **2**: 171
Peritoneum **1**: 67,77; **2**: 171, 176, 193, 200, 204, 218, 222, 230, 232–233, 241, 247, 250–251, 272–273, 276
Permanent dentition **2**: 39
– teeth **2**: 5, 39–41, 43
Peroneal → Fibular
Peroneus brevis/longus/tertius muscle → Fibularis brevis/longus/tertius muscle
Perpendicular plate of ethmoidal bone **2**: 12–13, 22–23, 58
– – – palatine bone **2**: 55–57
Persisting frontal suture **2**: 3
Pes anserinus **1**: 219, 221, 231, 272
– hippocampi **2**: 320, 323–325, 344
Petro-occipital fissure **2**: 10, 12
Petrosal branch of middle meningeal artery **2**: 380
– fossula **2**: 20
Petrosquamous fissure **2**: 20
Petrotympanic fissure **2**: 20
Petrous bone → Petrous part of temporal bone
– part of internal carotid artery **2**: 292, 301–302, 378
– – – temporal bone **2**: 5, 10, 17, 20, 302, 352–353, 359, 362, 393, 395–396, 399–400, 402, 405–409
Phalanx/Phalanges of foot **1**: 170–171, 184–185, 188
– – hand **1**: 8, 82–83, 92–94
Pharyngeal branch of descending palatine artery **2**: 88
– – – vagus nerve **2**: 100
– cavity → Cavity of pharynx
– diverticulum in Laimer's triangle **2**: 49
– glands **2**: 49
– lymphoid ring **2**: 45
– muscles → Muscles of pharynx
– nerve plexus **2**: 96, 100
– opening of auditory tube → Pharyngeal opening of pharyngotympanic tube
– – – pharyngotympanic tube **2**: 45, 52, 55, 57, 88, 90
– raphe **2**: 49, 100
– recess **2**: 50–51, 57
– tonsil **2**: 13, 45, 50–51, 57, 63
– tubercle of occipital bone **2**: 18, 47, 395
– venous plexus **2**: 100
Pharyngobasilar fascia **2**: 47, 49, 100
Pharyngo-epiglottic fold **2**: 50–51
Pharyngo-esophageal constriction **2**: 53, 106
– diverticulum **2**: 49
Pharyngotympanic tube **2**: 45, 51–52, 55, 57, 88, 90, 393–396, 398, 405–406
Pharynx **2**: 45–53, 73, 100

Phase of expiration **1**: 40–41
– – inspiration **1**: 40–41
Philtrum **2**: 38,44
Phrenic nerve **2**: 33, 93–94, 96, 149
Phrenicocolic ligament **2**: 191, 207
Physiological cup → Depression of optic disc
Pia mater **2**: 285–286, 295, 326, 405
Pial part of filum terminale **2**: 284
Pigmented epithelium of iris **2**: 375
– layer of retina **2**: 374
Pineal body → Pineal gland
– gland **1**: 15; **2**: 299, 310–311, 315, 324, 332, 335, 346, 348, 356, 361
– recess **2**: 307, 320, 324
Pinna → Auricle
Piriform fossa **2**: 46, 50, 53, 68, 74, 101
– recess → Piriform fossa
Piriformis muscle **1**: 219, 223–226, 228–229, 256–258; **2**: 230, 234, 264–265, 281
Pisiform **1**: 8, 92–94, 102–104, 121–124, 130, 152–153, 161–162
– joint **1**: 104
Pisohamate ligament **1**: 102, 124
Pisometacarpal ligament **1**: 102
Pituitary gland **1**: 15; **2**: 13, 291–293, 295, 298, 301, 304–307, 315, 321, 330–331, 334–335, 358, 360, 378, 385
Placenta **1**: 13; **2**: 243
Plane(s) **1**: 5
– of right/left symmetry **1**: 5
Plantar aponeurosis **1**: 188, 210–211, 213, 237–238, 279
– calcaneocuboid ligament **1**: 211–213
– calcaneonavicular ligament **1**: 207, 212–213
– chiasm **1**: 238
– cuneonavicular ligaments **1**: 213
– interossei → Plantar interosseous muscles
– interosseous muscles **1**: 237–240
– ligaments of interphalangeal joints of foot **1**: 213
– – – metatarsophalangeal joints **1**: 213
– metatarsal arteries **1**: 279–280
– tarsometatarsal ligaments **1**: 213
– tendinous sheath of fibularis longus muscle **1**: 238
Plantaris muscle **1**: 195, 200, 222, 224, 229, 233–234, 267–268
Platysma **2**: 28–30, 32–33, 45, 49, 74, 85, 91–93, 98–99
Pleura **2**: 111, 152, 209
Pleural borders → Borders of pleura
– cavity **2**: 153–154, 156–157, 159–160, 164
– cupula → Dome of pleura
Plica semilunaris conjunctivae **2**: 364–365
Pocket of pectoralis **1**: 110
Pons **1**: 22; **2**: 13, 303–306, 309, 311, 321, 324, 333, 341, 344, 352–353, 359, 361, 384, 408–409
Pontine arteries **2**: 292, 298–299
– nuclei **2**: 340
Pontocerebellar cistern **2**: 321, 341, 352–353, 359
Popliteal artery **1**: 245, 250, 255–256, 261, 264–265, 267–269, 272
– fascia **1**: 218, 230
– fossa **1**: 217, 222, 245, 254–256, 261, 266–268
– surface of femur **1**: 180, 195, 199, 224, 233–234
– vein **1**: 245, 247, 255–256, 261, 264–265, 267–268, 272
Popliteus muscle **1**: 195, 199–200, 229, 233–235, 265, 267–268, 272, 276–277

Porta hepatis **2**: 181
Portal triad **2**: 183, 185
– vein → Hepatic portal vein
Postcentral gyrus **2**: 314, 316, 348, 362
– sulcus **2**: 297, 314, 316
Postcommunicating part of anterior cerebral
    artery **2**: 292, 298, 300–302, 347, 351,
    356–357
– – – posterior cerebral artery **2**: 292, 298
Posterior **1**: 5
– abdominal wall **2**: 206–207, 228
– ampullary nerve **2**: 405
– antebrachial cutaneous nerve **1**: 133, 135,
    142–143, 150, 154
– arch of atlas **1**: 30, 36–37, 49–51, 55, 58–60;
    2: 284, 294, 302, 321
– articular facet of dens axis **1**: 30, 50
– atlanto-occipital membrane **1**: 49, 55, 60
– attachment of linea alba **1**: 77
– auricular artery **2**: 76–77, 85–86, 91–92,
    98–99
– – nerve **2**: 85–86, 91–92, 99
– – vein **2**: 80, 85
– axillary line **1**: 4
– – lymph nodes → Subscapular axillary lymph
    nodes
– basal segment of left lung [S X] **2**: 117
– – – – right lung [S X] **2**: 116
– – segmental bronchus of left lung [B X]
    2: 108–109, 114
– – – – – right lung [B X] **2**: 108–109, 114,
    120–121
– belly of digastric muscle **2**: 30, 34, 37, 44,
    49–51, 87, 98–100
– bony ampulla **2**: 401–402
– border of fibula **1**: 182–183
– – – radius **1**: 88
– – – testis **2**: 270
– – – ulna **1**: 89, 118
– brachial cutaneous nerve **1**: 61, 133, 135,
    142–143, 150–151
– branch(es) of great auricular nerve **2**: 82–83,
    91–92
– – – inferior pancreaticoduodenal artery
    2: 198
– – – medial antebrachial cutaneous nerve
    1: 132, 135–136, 150–151
– – – obturator artery **1**: 193
– – – – nerve **1**: 252
– – – ulnar recurrent artery **1**: 153
– calcaneal articular facet of talus **1**: 187, 207
– cerebellomedullary cistern **2**: 294–295, 305,
    321, 343
– cerebral artery **2**: 292, 298–302, 351, 358
– cervical intertransversarii muscles **1**: 55, 59
– – region **1**: 4
– chamber of eyeball **2**: 374, 384
– circumflex humeral artery **1**: 138–140, 143
– clinoid process **2**: 10, 19, 291, 301
– commissure of diencephalon **2**: 307, 310, 320,
    324, 340
– – – labia majora **2**: 269
– communicating artery **2**: 292, 298–301, 351,
    358
– cord of brachial plexus **1**: 134, 140–141;
    2: 93–95, 166
– cranial fossa **2**: 5, 10–11, 291, 394, 399, 407
– crico-arytenoid muscle **2**: 51, 66–68, 101
– cruciate ligament **1**: 196, 198–204, 272
– cusp of mitral valve **2**: 133, 135, 140
– – – tricuspid valve **2**: 132, 134–135

Posterior
– cutaneous nerve of arm → Posterior brachial
    cutaneous nerve
– – – – forearm → Posterior antebrachial
    cutaneous nerve
– – – – thigh → Posterior femoral cutaneous
    nerve
– deep temporal artery **2**: 76
– ethmoidal artery **2**: 77, 88, 90, 380–382
– – cells **2**: 13, 57, 60, 62–63, 359, 369, 385,
    387
– – foramen **2**: 21, 367–368
– – nerve **2**: 88, 381–382
– – vein **2**: 381
– extremity of spleen **2**: 189
– femoral cutaneous nerve **1**: 61, 243–244,
    254–257, 266; **2**: 226, 279–280
– fold of malleus **2**: 392, 398
– fontanelle **2**: 17
– fornix of vagina **1**: 17
– funiculus of spinal cord **2**: 288
– gastric artery **2**: 188, 199, 219
– – branches of posterior vagal trunk **2**: 167
– gluteal line of ilium **1**: 176
– horn of lateral meniscus **1**: 201
– – – – ventricle → Occipital horn of lateral
    ventricle
– – – medial meniscus **1**: 201
– – – spinal cord **1**: 23, 79; **2**: 288
– inferior cerebellar artery **2**: 292, 298–299,
    302
– – iliac spine **1**: 175–176
– – nasal nerves **2**: 88–89
– intercavernous sinus → Intercavernous
    sinus(es)
– intercondylar area **1**: 182
– intercostal arteries **1**: 14, 76; **2**: 96, 106,
    162–163, 167, 285–286
– – veins **1**: 14, 76; **2**: 162–163, 167, 285–286
– intermediate sulcus of spinal cord **2**: 284, 288,
    310–311
– internal vertebral venous plexus **2**: 285–287
– interosseous artery **1**: 138, 153–155, 157, 165
– – nerve **1**: 154
– interpositus nucleus **2**: 309
– interventricular branch of left coronary artery
    2: 144
– – – – right coronary artery **2**: 135, 143–144,
    146, 148
– – sulcus **2**: 125, 141, 145
– – vein → Middle cardiac vein
– labial branches of perineal artery **2**: 280
– – nerves **2**: 280–281
– lacrimal crest **2**: 368
– lateral choroidal branches of posterior
    cerebral artery **2**: 300
– – nasal arteries **2**: 77, 88–89
– – segment of liver [VII] **2**: 184
– layer of rectus sheath **1**: 65, 68, 75, 77
– – – thoracolumbar fascia **1**: 53–55
– left ventricular branch of left coronary artery
    2: 135, 143–144, 147–148
– ligament of fibular head **1**: 195
– – – incus **2**: 398
– limb of internal capsule **2**: 332–334, 348, 350,
    355–357
– – – stapes **2**: 397
– lobe of pituitary gland → Neurohypophysis
– – – prostate **2**: 237
– longitudinal ligament **1**: 37, 39, 47–48; **2**: 285
– medial choroidal branches of posterior
    cerebral artery **2**: 300

Posterior medial
– – segment of liver [VIII] **2**: 184
– median line **1**: 4
– – sulcus of medulla oblongata **2**: 310–311
– – – – spinal cord **2**: 284, 286, 288, 310–311
– mediastinum **2**: 104
– membranous ampulla **2**: 405
– meningeal artery **2**: 77, 100
– meniscofemoral ligament **1**: 199–200
– muscles of thigh **1**: 221–224; **2**: 253, 255
– nasal aperture(s) → Choana(e)
– – spine of palatine bone **2**: 8, 12, 23–24, 30,
    57
– nucleus of hypothalamus **2**: 328
– palpebral margin **2**: 364, 366
– papillary muscle of left ventricle of heart
    2: 133–134, 137, 140, 145
– – – – right ventricle of heart **2**: 132
– para-olfactory sulcus **2**: 317
– parietal artery **2**: 297
– part of dorsum of tongue → Posterior part
    of tongue
– – – medial palpebral ligament **2**: 365
– – – tongue **2**: 51, 101
– – – vaginal fornix **2**: 233
– perforated substance **2**: 306, 335
– petroclinoid fold **2**: 291, 293
– pillar of fauces → Palatopharyngeal arch
– pole of eyeball **2**: 374
– – – lens **2**: 377
– process of talus **1**: 184, 187
– quadrangular lobule of cerebellum **2**: 308
– ramus(-i) of cervical nerves **1**: 60; **2**: 32, 37,
    82–83, 284, 286
– – – lateral cerebral sulcus **2**: 316
– – – lumbar nerves **2**: 284
– – – sacral nerves **2**: 284
– – – spinal nerve **1**: 23, 61, 227; **2**: 284–286
– – – thoracic nerves **1**: 133
– recess of tympanic membrane **2**: 398
– region of elbow **1**: 142–143
– – – forearm **1**: 150
– – – thigh **1**: 4
– root of ansa cervicalis → Inferior root of ansa
    cervicalis
– – – cervical nerve **2**: 95, 166, 288–289
– – – sacral nerve **2**: 232
– – – spinal nerve **1**: 23; **2**: 95, 166, 284–286,
    288–289
– – – thoracic nerve **2**: 166, 284, 286
– rootlets of cervical nerve **2**: 284, 311
– – – spinal nerve **1**: 23; **2**: 284, 288, 311
– sacral foramina **1**: 34–35; **2**: 284
– sacro-iliac ligament **1**: 190–191
– scalene muscle **2**: 33–35, 37, 75, 92, 96
– scrotal branches of perineal artery **2**: 279
– – nerves **2**: 279
– segment of liver [I] **2**: 184
– – – right lung [S II] **2**: 116
– segmental bronchus of right lung [B II]
    2: 108–109, 114, 120–121
– semicircular canal **2**: 399–401, 407, 409
– – duct **2**: 399, 405, 407
– semilunar cusp of aortic valve **2**: 133–135,
    137, 141
– septal branches of sphenopalatine artery
    2: 77, 88, 90
– spinal artery **2**: 285–286, 289, 299
– – veins **2**: 285–286
– spinocerebellar tract **2**: 288
– superior alveolar artery **2**: 76, 86–87

Posterior superior alveolar
– – – branches of maxillary nerve **2**: 86–87
– – iliac spine **1**: 52, 55, 175–176, 191, 218, 222, 254–255, 257
– – lateral nasal branches of maxillary nerve **2**: 88–89
– – medial nasal branches of maxillary nerve **2**: 90
– – pancreaticoduodenal artery **2**: 188, 198, 203, 219
– surface of cornea **2**: 374
– – – eyelid **2**: 366
– – – fibula **1**: 182–183
– – – humerus **1**: 86
– – – kidney **2**: 208, 218
– – – lens **2**: 376–377
– – – petrous part of temporal bone **2**: 20, 405
– – – prostate **2**: 236–237
– – – radius **1**: 88
– – – scapula **1**: 84
– – – tibia **1**: 182–183, 234
– – – ulna **1**: 89
– talar articular surface of calcaneus **1**: 187, 207
– talocalcaneal ligament **1**: 212
– talofibular ligament **1**: 212, 214
– temporal branch(es) of lateral occipital artery **2**: 298, 302
– – – – middle cerebral artery **2**: 302
– tibial artery **1**: 250, 266–268, 273–275, 277, 279–281
– – vein(s) **1**: 246–247, 267, 273–275, 277
– tibiofibular ligament **1**: 206, 212
– tibiotalar part of medial ligament of ankle joint **1**: 212
– triangle → Lateral cervical region
– tubercle of atlas **1**: 30–31, 49–50, 55, 59–60; **2**: 302
– – – cervical vertebra **1**: 30–31; **2**: 33
– vagal trunk **1**: 25; **2**: 167, 248–249
– vein of left ventricle of heart **2**: 135, 143
– – – septum pellucidum **2**: 300
– wall of vagina **2**: 239–240
Posterolateral central arteries **2**: 300
– fissure of cerebellum **2**: 308
– fontanelle → Mastoid fontanelle
– nucleus of spinal cord **2**: 288
– sulcus of medulla oblongata **2**: 310–311
– – – spinal cord **1**: 23; **2**: 284, 286, 288, 310–311
Posteromedial frontal branch of callosomarginal artery **2**: 299
Postganglionic nerve fibers **1**: 23, 79
Postpyramidal fissure of cerebellum → Secondary fissure of cerebellum
Postsulcal part of dorsum of tongue → Posterior part of dorsum of tongue
Prebiventral fissure of cerebellum **2**: 308–309
Precaval lymph node(s) **2**: 198
Precentral gyrus **2**: 314, 316, 348, 362
– sulcus **2**: 297–298, 314, 316
Prechiasmatic sulcus **2**: 19, 291
Preclival fissure of cerebellum → Primary fissure of cerebellum
Precommunicating part of anterior cerebral artery **2**: 292, 298, 301
– – – posterior cerebral artery **2**: 292, 298
Precuneal branch(es) of pericallosal artery **2**: 297, 299
Precuneus **2**: 317
Pre-epiglottic fat body **2**: 66, 68
Pregnancy **2**: 242–243
Pregnant uterus **2**: 243

Pre-ileal position of vermiform appendix **2**: 178
Prelaryngidal lymph node(s) **2**: 81, 110
Premaxilla → Incisive bone
Premolar tooth/teeth **2**: 39–42
Prenatal descent of testis **2**: 272
Pre-occipital notch of cerebrum **2**: 315–316
Pre-optic nuclei of hypothalamus **2**: 328
Preprostatic sphincter muscle → Internal urethral sphincter muscle
Prepuce of clitoris **2**: 269, 281
– – penis **1**: 17; **2**: 232, 274–276
Preputial sac of penis **2**: 276
Prepyramidal fissure of cerebellum → Prebiventral fissure of cerebellum
Prerectal fibers of levator ani muscle **2**: 236, 266
Presacral nerve → Superior hypogastric nerve plexus
Presternal region **1**: 4
Presulcal part of dorsum of tongue → Anterior part of dorsum of tongue
Pretracheal layer of cervical fascia **1**: 64; **2**: 33, 36
– lymph nodes **2**: 81, 110, 163
Prevertebral layer of cervical fascia **2**: 33
– part of vertebral artery **1**: 60; **2**: 79, 118
Primary fissure of cerebellum **2**: 307–308
– ovarian follicles **2**: 241
Princeps pollicis artery **1**: 162–163, 166
Procerus muscle **2**: 28–30, 366
Processus cochleariformis **2**: 396
– vaginalis of peritoneum → Vaginal process of peritoneum
Profunda brachii artery → Deep artery of arm
– femoris artery → Deep artery of thigh
– – vein → Deep vein of thigh
Prolapse of intervertebral disc **1**: 48
Proliferative stage **2**: 242
Prominence of facial canal **2**: 396
– – lateral semicircular canal **2**: 396
Promontory of sacrum **1**: 14, 28, 35, 38–40, 69, 172, 178, 190; **2**: 202, 220–221, 228, 233–234, 238, 244–245, 248, 260–261, 264
– – tympanic cavity **2**: 391, 393, 396, 399, 402
Pronation **1**: 5
Pronator quadratus muscle **1**: 114–117, 122, 129, 153, 158, 162
– teres muscle **1**: 101, 106–107, 113–117, 140–141, 147, 152–154, 156
Proper hepatic artery → Hepatic artery proper
– palmar digital arteries **1**: 160–163, 165, 167
– – – nerves **1**: 132–133, 160–162, 164–165, 167
– – – – of median nerve **1**: 132–133
– – – – – ulnar nerve **1**: 132–133
– plantar digital arteries **1**: 279–280
– – – nerves **1**: 279–280
Prosencephalon → Forebrain
Prostate **1**: 17, 20–21, 260; **2**: 170, 232, 234–237, 244, 247, 250, 254, 258–259, 261, 266, 277
Prostatic ducts **2**: 235, 277
– sinus **2**: 235, 277
– urethra **2**: 235–237, 258, 277
– utricle **2**: 235, 237
– venous plexus **2**: 250, 254, 276
Proximal **1**: 5
– carpal sulcus **1**: 105
– interphalangeal joint(s) of hand **1**: 104, 124–125
– phalanx/phalanges of foot **1**: 184–186, 188

Proximal phalanx/phalanges of
– – – hand **1**: 8, 92–94, 104, 123, 129, 167
– – – middle finger **1**: 167
– – – thumb **1**: 92–93, 123
– radio-ulnar joint **1**: 82–83, 90–91, 99–101
Psoas major muscle **1**: 14, 54–55, 69, 194, 219, 228, 252–253; **2**: 171, 182, 209, 211, 213, 217–218, 220–221, 223–225, 227–228, 230, 233, 244–245, 248, 250–252, 254
– minor muscle **1**: 69, 219; **2**: 228
Pterygoid canal **2**: 19, 23, 88–89
– fossa of sphenoidal bone **2**: 19, 23, 368
– fovea of mandible **2**: 25
– hamulus **2**: 17, 19, 23–24, 27, 30, 48, 51, 56, 395
– notch of sphenoidal bone **2**: 19, 23
– process of sphenoidal bone **2**: 8, 12, 17, 19, 23–24, 27, 30, 48, 55–56, 63, 89, 368, 395
– venous plexus **2**: 80, 383
Pterygomandibular raphe **2**: 48
Pterygomaxillary fissure **2**: 368
Pterygopalatine fossa **2**: 88–89, 368
– ganglion **2**: 88–89
Pterygospinous ligament **2**: 27
Pubic arch **1**: 172
– branch of obturator artery **2**: 244
– – – – vein **2**: 244
– crest **1**: 174, 176
– region **1**: 4, 77
– symphysis **1**: 17, 170–175, 177–178, 190, 193; **2**: 232–233, 237, 243, 245, 247, 252, 256–261, 264–265, 268
– tubercle **1**: 66, 172, 174, 176, 219; **2**: 228, 245
Pubis **1**: 40, 77, 172, 174–177, 194, 221, 259; **2**: 234, 244, 252, 254, 256–261, 264, 267–268, 275–276, 278
Pubocervical ligament **2**: 246–247
Pubococcygeus muscle **2**: 261, 264–266
Pubofemoral ligament **1**: 192–193
Puborectalis muscle **2**: 179, 236, 264–266
Pubovesical ligament **2**: 246–247
Pubovesicalis muscle **2**: 246–247
Pudendal anesthesia **2**: 281
– canal **2**: 251, 255, 279–280
– nerve **1**: 61, 227, 243–244, 254–257; **2**: 226, 231, 244, 251, 256, 267, 279–281
Pudendum **2**: 163
Pulmonary ligament **2**: 111
– nerve plexus **1**: 25; **2**: 96, 167
– pleura → Visceral pleura
– trunk **1**: 12–13, 43; **2**: 107, 115, 119, 122, 124, 126–130, 132, 134–135, 139, 141–142, 144, 149, 154, 157–158, 164
– valve **2**: 132, 134–135, 137, 141
– veins **1**: 12–13; **2**: 96, 107, 111, 123, 140, 155, 157, 167
Pulp canal of tooth → Root canal of tooth
– cavity **2**: 40
Pulvinar nuclei **2**: 327
– of thalamus **2**: 310–311, 329–332, 335
Puncture of cervicothoracic ganglion **2**: 95
– – posterior cerebellomedullary cistern **2**: 321
Pupil **2**: 364, 371–372, 376, 384
Pupillary margin of iris **2**: 376
Putamen **2**: 300, 323, 329–335, 337–341, 344, 346–351, 355–357, 360–362
Pyknic person **1**: 6; **2**: 153
Pyloric antrum **2**: 173–176
– canal **2**: 173–176
– lymph nodes **2**: 198
– orifice **2**: 174–176, 194

Pyloric
– part of stomach **2**: 173–176, 191, 194, 200, 223
– sphincter muscle **2**: 174
Pylorus **2**: 154, 173
Pyramid of medulla oblongata **2**: 306, 309, 340
– – vermis **2**: 307–309
Pyramidal eminence **2**: 396, 398
– lobe of thyroid gland **2**: 70, 149
– process of palatine bone **2**: 24, 57, 368
– tract **2**: 340
Pyramidalis muscle **1**: 64–65, 227–228; **2**: 276
Pyramis → Pyramid of vermis

Q

Quadrangular membrane **2**: 67
– space **1**: 110–111, 143
Quadrants of tympanic membrane **2**: 392
Quadrate ligament of elbow joint **1**: 99
– lobe of liver **2**: 181, 183–184, 191, 200, 223, 248
Quadratus femoris muscle **1**: 220, 223–224, 226–229, 256; **2**: 253, 255–256
– lumborum muscle **1**: 54–55, 58–59, 69, 219, 223, 227–228; **2**: 171, 209, 211, 218, 223–224, 227–228
– plantae muscle **1**: 208, 211, 214, 238, 240, 279–280
Quadriceps femoris muscle **1**: 10, 195–196, 202, 219–220, 226, 231, 235, 252–253, 258–264; **2**: 252, 254–255
Quadrigeminal plate → Tectal plate

R

Radial artery **1**: 123, 138–141, 152–153, 155, 157–163, 165
– collateral artery of deep artery of arm **1**: 138–139, 142–143, 152–154
– – ligament of elbow joint **1**: 98–99
– – – – wrist joint **1**: 102, 104
– fossa of humerus **1**: 86
– groove of humerus → Groove for radial nerve
– head of flexor digitorum superficialis muscle **1**: 115, 117
– nerve **1**: 61, 112–113, 117, 128, 132–134, 140–143, 145–147, 150–154, 157, 160–161, 164–165; **2**: 93–94
– notch of ulna **1**: 89, 99–100
– recurrent artery of radial artery **1**: 138–139, 141, 152–153
– styloid process **1**: 88, 92–94, 99, 102, 105, 116, 159
– tuberosity → Tuberosity of radius
– veins **1**: 140, 164
Radialis indicis artery **1**: 162–163
Radiate carpal ligament **1**: 102
– ligament of head of rib **1**: 46–47
– sternocostal ligaments **1**: 45
Radiated pain **1**: 79
Radiation of corpus callosum **2**: 337, 342, 345–346, 348
Radii of lens **2**: 377
Radiocarpal joint → Wrist joint
Radio-ulnar joints → Distal/proximal radio-ulnar joint
Radius **1**: 8, 82–83, 88, 90–94, 98–104, 116–119, 122, 125, 129–130, 139, 154–158
Ramus(-i) communicantes of spinal nerve **1**: 23, 25, 79; **2**: 95–96, 166–167, 248, 285

Ramus(-i)
– of ischium **1**: 172, 176, 220–221; **2**: 268, 275, 279
– – mandible **2**: 4–7, 25–26, 41, 49, 51, 58, 73, 100
Raphe of penis **2**: 274–275
– – scrotum **2**: 274, 276
Rectal ampulla **1**: 17; **2**: 170, 179, 230–232, 243, 253, 255, 260–261
– retinaculum **2**: 246
– venous plexus **2**: 251
Recto-uterine fold **2**: 239
– ligament **2**: 239, 246–247
– pouch **1**: 17; **2**: 233, 238–239, 241–243, 247, 256–257, 260
Rectovesical ligament **2**: 246–247
– pouch **2**: 170, 193, 206, 232, 247, 258
Rectovesicalis muscle **2**: 247
Rectum **1**: 16–21, 194, 261; **2**: 170, 179, 202, 204–206, 218, 220, 230–234, 238, 243, 245–248, 251, 253, 256–261, 272, 276
Rectus abdominis muscle **1**: 62–65, 67–69, 75–77, 194, 227–228; **2**: 193, 202, 225, 245, 256–261, 276
– capitis anterior muscle **2**: 37, 73
– – lateralis muscle **1**: 55; **2**: 37
– – posterior major muscle **1**: 55, 58–60; **2**: 32, 37, 73
– – – minor muscle **1**: 55, 58; **2**: 32, 37, 73
– femoris muscle **1**: 193–194, 216, 219–220, 226–228, 252–253, 258–259, 262–264; **2**: 228, 257–259
– sheath **1**: 63–65, 68, 75, 77
Recurrent branch of spinal nerve → Meningeal ramus of spinal nerve
– interosseous artery **1**: 138, 154–155
– laryngeal nerve **1**: 25; **2**: 96–97, 101, 149, 167
Red bone marrow **1**: 10
– nucleus **2**: 309, 315, 328, 331, 334–335, 340–341, 350, 357
Reflected inguinal ligament **1**: 66
Reflexion lines of peritoneum **2**: 207
Regions of human body **1**: 4
Renal artery **1**: 12, 14; **2**: 162, 167, 199, 203, 208, 210–215, 218–219
– calyx/calices **1**: 17; **2**: 212, 216–217
– columns **2**: 212
– cortex **2**: 208, 210, 212, 218
– ganglia **2**: 248
– impression on liver **2**: 181
– – – spleen **2**: 189
– medulla **2**: 208, 210, 212
– nerve plexus **1**: 25; **2**: 248–249
– papilla **2**: 212
– pelvis **1**: 17; **2**: 208, 211–212, 214, 216–217, 287
– pyramids **2**: 212
– segmental arteries **2**: 212, 214–215
– sinus **2**: 208, 210, 212–213, 218, 223
– vein(s) **1**: 14; **2**: 162, 199, 203, 208, 210–214, 218, 223
Respiratory region of nasal mucosa **2**: 90
– system **1**: 16; **2**: 52–53
Rete testis **2**: 270
Reticular membrane of spiral organ **2**: 404
– nucleus of thalamus **2**: 326–327, 330–331, 340, 344
– part of substantia nigra **2**: 328
Retina **2**: 373–377, 384–385
Retinacula of skin **1**: 11
Retro-articular process of temporal bone **2**: 20

Retrobulbar fat **2**: 58–59, 61, 336, 353, 358, 360, 378, 384–387
Retrocardial space **2**: 107, 127
Retrocecal position of vermiform appendix **2**: 178
Retrocolic position of vermiform appendix **2**: 178
Retro-ileal position of vermiform appendix **2**: 178
Retrolenticular limb of internal capsule → Retrolentiform limb of internal capsule
Retrolentiform limb of internal capsule **2**: 332–333
Retromandibular vein **2**: 80, 98–99, 383
Retromolar triangle of mandible **2**: 25
Retroperitoneal organs **2**: 171
– – of upper abdomen **2**: 199, 203
– position **2**: 171
– space **2**: 248–249
– viscera **2**: 171
– – of upper abdomen **2**: 199, 203
Retropubic space **2**: 232–233, 237, 246, 252, 260–261
Retropyloric lymph node(s) **2**: 198
Retrosternal space **2**: 127
Rhinal sulcus **2**: 304, 315, 317, 333–334
Rhombencephalon → Hindbrain
Rhomboid fossa **2**: 284, 289, 309–311, 342, 409
– major muscle **1**: 53–54, 60, 110–112, 142
– minor muscle **1**: 54, 110–112, 142
Ribs [I–XII] **1**: 18–21, 29, 38, 40–47, 55, 68–69, 73–74, 82–83, 85, 87, 148, 219; **2**: 35, 37, 75, 93, 105, 107, 118, 126, 153, 156–157, 161–162, 164, 167, 172, 209, 211, 213–215, 217, 222, 226, 287
Right atrioventricular orifice **2**: 135, 139, 141
– – valve → Tricuspid valve
– atrium of heart **1**: 12–13; **2**: 104, 122, 124–126, 128–132, 137, 139–143, 154, 158–161, 167
– auricle of heart **2**: 124, 128–129, 132, 139–142, 158, 166
– branch of hepatic artery proper **2**: 183–184, 197
– – – – portal vein **1**: 12–13
– bundle of atrioventricular bundle **2**: 140
– colic artery **2**: 200–203
– – flexure **2**: 154–155, 172, 191–192, 194, 205, 223
– – lymph nodes **2**: 203
– – vein **2**: 201–202
– coronary artery **2**: 104, 124, 129, 132–135, 140–144, 146, 148, 162, 167
– – cusp of aortic valve → Right semilunar cusp of aortic valve
– – vein → Small cardiac vein
– crus of lumbar part of diaphragm **1**: 69; **2**: 105–106, 155, 182, 196, 208, 220–223
– cupula of diaphragm **2**: 150–151, 172
– fibrous ring of heart **2**: 135
– – trigone of heart **2**: 135, 141
– gastric artery **2**: 196, 198
– – lymph nodes **2**: 198
– – vein **2**: 188, 196, 203
– gastro-epiploic artery → Right gastro-omental artery
– – vein → Right gastro-omental vein
– gastro-omental artery **2**: 196–198, 200, 202–203
– – lymph nodes **2**: 198
– – vein **2**: 196, 200
– hepatic duct **2**: 181, 183

Right hepatic
– – vein **2**: 167, 185
– inferior lobar bronchus **2**: 108–110, 114, 120–121
– – pulmonary vein **2**: 113, 123, 125, 132–133, 139, 141, 143, 158, 164–165, 167
– infracolic space **2**: 170–171
– lamina of thyroid cartilage → Lamina of thyroid cartilage
– lobe of liver **2**: 154–155, 172, 180–183, 191, 204, 220–224
– – – prostate **2**: 237
– – – thyroid gland **2**: 35, 47, 50, 68, 70–71, 75, 97–98, 101, 149, 164–165, 167
– lumbar lymph nodes → Lumbar lymph nodes
– lung **1**: 16, 20; **2**: 96, 108–109, 111–114, 116–117, 119–121, 126, 128–131, 149–152, 154–161, 165, 172, 191, 220, 222
– lymphatic duct **1**: 15, 76; **2**: 81
– main bronchus **1**: 16; **2**: 105–106, 108–111, 113–114, 119–121, 155, 157, 161
– marginal branch of right coronary artery **2**: 124, 135, 142, 144, 146, 148
– – vein of heart **2**: 135, 142
– parietocolic space **2**: 171
– part of diaphragmatic surface of liver **2**: 180
– posterolateral branch of right coronary artery **2**: 135, 143, 146
– pulmonary artery **1**: 13; **2**: 104, 110–111, 113, 119, 123–125, 131, 139, 142–143, 157, 161, 165
– – veins **2**: 111, 123
– semilunar cusp of aortic valve **2**: 133–135, 137
– – – – pulmonary valve **2**: 132, 135
– superior lobar bronchus **2**: 108–110, 114, 120–121
– – pulmonary vein **2**: 123, 125, 131–133, 139, 141, 143, 164–165, 167
– thoracic duct → Right lymphatic duct
– triangular ligament of liver **2**: 180, 207
– venous angle **1**: 15
– ventricle of heart **1**: 12–13; **2**: 104, 119, 124–125, 128–129, 132, 134–137, 139–143, 145, 154, 158–160, 166–167
Rima glottidis **2**: 68–69
Ring finger **1**: 105
Risorius muscle **2**: 28–29, 99
Roof of acetabulum **1**: 177
– – orbit **2**: 58–59, 336, 357, 360, 386–387
Root(s) apex of tooth **2**: 40
– canal of tooth **2**: 40
– of cervical nerves **1**: 51; **2**: 294
– – first cervical nerve **1**: 51
– – median nerve **2**: 149
– – mesentery **2**: 171, 199, 202, 204, 206
– – nail → Lunule of nail
– – penis **2**: 276, 278
– – sacral nerves **2**: 232
– – sigmoid mesocolon **2**: 206–207
– – spinal nerve **2**: 285
– – tongue **2**: 46
– – tooth **2**: 40–41
– – transverse mesocolon **2**: 200, 206
Rootlets of spinal nerve **2**: 284–285, 288, 311
Rostrum of corpus callosum **2**: 299, 307, 317, 325, 337
Rotatores thoracis breves muscles **1**: 56, 59
– – longi muscles **1**: 56, 59
Round ligament of liver **1**: 12; **2**: 180–181, 185, 190–191, 196, 200, 204, 248
– – – uterus **1**: 17; **2**: 163, 172, 233, 238–240, 245–246, 250–251

Round
– window **2**: 391, 393, 396, 398, 401–402, 405
Rubrospinal tract **2**: 288
Rupture of dorsal digital expansion of hand **1**: 125
Ruptured ovarian follicle **2**: 245

S

Sacciform recess of distal radio-ulnar joint **1**: 102, 104
Saccular nerve **2**: 405
– recess → Spherical recess
Saccule **2**: 405
Sacral canal **1**: 22, 34–35, 40, 174, 194; **2**: 225, 244
– cornu **1**: 34–35
– crests **1**: 34–35
– flexure of rectum **2**: 232
– ganglia **1**: 25
– hiatus **1**: 34–35, 175; **2**: 265
– horn → Sacral cornu
– kyphosis **1**: 28
– lymph nodes **2**: 163
– nerves **1**: 22; **2**: 232, 284
– plexus **1**: 227–229, 244; **2**: 226–227, 231, 234, 244–245, 248
– spine **2**: 288
– splanchnic nerves **1**: 25; **2**: 231
– tuberosity **1**: 34–35
– venous plexus **2**: 287
– vertebra(e) **1**: 191, 194; **2**: 225, 232, 243–244, 260–261, 264
Sacro-iliac joint **1**: 38, 170–175, 178, 194; **2**: 220, 225, 253, 255
Sacropelvic surface of ilium **1**: 176
Sacrospinous ligament **1**: 190–193, 225–226, 257; **2**: 230, 265, 279, 281
Sacrotuberous ligament **1**: 190–193, 223–226, 256–257; **2**: 230, 265, 279–281
Sacrum [sacral vertebrae I–V] **1**: 9, 14, 28–29, 34–35, 38–39, 170–175, 177–178, 190–191, 194, 225; **2**: 202, 225, 232–234, 243–245, 253, 255, 258–261, 264–265, 281, 284
Sagittal axes **1**: 5
– border of parietal bone **2**: 22
– connective tissue strands of lesser pelvis **2**: 246–247
– planes **1**: 5
– suture **2**: 3, 5, 17, 295
Salpingopharyngeal fold **2**: 45, 50, 90
Salpingopharyngeus muscle **2**: 51
Saphenous branch of descending genicular artery **1**: 252, 269
– nerve **1**: 242–243, 248, 252, 263, 266, 270, 278
– opening **1**: 63–65, 218, 248–249
Sartorius muscle **1**: 194, 199–200, 204, 216, 219, 221–222, 224, 226–228, 231, 233, 235, 252–253, 255, 258–265, 267, 272, 277; **2**: 228, 256–259
Scala tympani **2**: 391, 402–405
– vestibuli **2**: 391, 402–405
Scalene gap **2**: 34–35, 37
– tubercle **1**: 44
Scalenus anterior muscle → Anterior scalene muscle
– medius muscle → Middle scalene muscle
– posterior muscle → Posterior scalene muscle
Scan of bones **1**: 3
– – thyroid gland **2**: 71
Scapha **2**: 390

Scaphoid **1**: 8, 92–94, 102, 104, 123, 129–130, 159
– fossa of sphenoidal bone **2**: 19
Scapula **1**: 20, 43, 53, 73, 82–85, 87, 95–97, 105, 107–109, 111–112, 136–137, 140–144, 148–149; **2**: 92, 156, 161
Scapular line **1**: 4
– region **1**: 4
Sciatic nerve **1**: 223, 227, 229, 235, 240, 244, 256–257, 261–262; **2**: 226, 230, 253, 256–259, 279–280
Sclera **2**: 372–376, 384
Scleral venous sinus **2**: 372–375
Sclerocorneal boundary **2**: 372–373
Scrotal cavity **2**: 170, 232, 271–273
Scrotum **1**: 17, 67; **2**: 170, 232, 234, 261, 271–274, 276
Sebaceous glands of external acoustic meatus **2**: 392
– – – eyelid **2**: 366
Second cervical vertebra → Axis [C II]
– functional areas of cerebral cortex **2**: 319
– toe [II] **1**: 184–185, 188
Secondary fissure of cerebellum **2**: 307–308
– retroperitoneal position → Retroperitoneal position
– somato-afferent nerve fibers **1**: 23, 79
– spiral lamina **2**: 402–403
– tympanic membrane **2**: 391, 398, 405
Secretory stage **2**: 242
Segment I of liver → Posterior segment of liver [I]
– II of liver → Left posterior lateral segment of liver [II]
– III of liver → Left anterior lateral segment of liver [III]
– IV of liver → Left medial segment of liver [IV]
– IVa of liver → Left posterior medial segment of liver [IVa]
– IVb of liver → Left anterior medial segment of liver [IVb]
– V of liver → Anterior medial segment of liver [V]
– VI of liver → Anterior lateral segment of liver [VI]
– VII of liver → Posterior lateral segment of liver [VII]
– VIII of liver → Posterior medial segment of liver [VIII]
Segmental arteries of kidney **2**: 212, 214–215
– – – lung **2**: 115
– bronchus(-i) **2**: 115
– innervation of body wall **1**: 61, 78
– – – dorsal body wall **1**: 61
– – – head **2**: 82–83
– – – human body **1**: 134, 244
– – – lower limb **1**: 134, 242–244
– – – neck **2**: 82–83
– – – trunk **1**: 61, 78, 134, 244
– – – upper limb **1**: 132–134, 244
– – – ventral body wall **1**: 78
– ramifications of portal triad **2**: 183
Segmentation of bronchi **2**: 114, 120–121
– – liver **2**: 184–185
– – lungs **2**: 116–117
Sella turcica **2**: 23, 57
Sellar diaphragm → Diaphragma sellae
Semicircular canals **2**: 396, 398–402, 406–407, 409
– ducts **2**: 399, 405–407
Semilunar cusps of aortic valve **2**: 129–130, 133–135, 138

Semilunar cusps of
– – – pulmonary valve **2**: 134–135, 137
– folds of colon **2**: 177–178
– gyrus **2**: 317, 324, 334, 338
– hiatus **2**: 55–57
– line → Linea semilunaris
Semimembranosus muscle **1**: 195, 199–200, 217, 221–222, 224, 226–227, 232–235, 255–256, 258, 261–265, 267–268, 272
Seminal colliculus **2**: 235, 237, 277
– gland **1**: 17, 77, 260; **2**: 234, 236–237, 244, 247, 255, 258–259, 261
– vesicle → Seminal gland
Semispinalis capitis muscle **1**: 53–54, 56–60; **2**: 32–33, 37, 73–75
– cervicis muscle **1**: 56, 58–59; **2**: 33, 74
– thoracis muscle **1**: 56–59
Semitendinosus muscle **1**: 200, 219, 221–224, 227, 231, 233, 235, 255–256, 258, 261–265, 267, 272
Sensory root of cervical/sacral/spinal/thoracic nerve → Posterior root of cervical/sacral/spinal/thoracic nerve
– – – ciliary ganglion **2**: 381–382
– – – trigeminal nerve **2**: 84, 89, 306, 380
– speech area of cerebral cortex **2**: 319
Septa testis **2**: 270–271
Septal cusp of tricuspid valve **2**: 132, 135, 140
– nasal cartilage **2**: 13, 54
– olfactory region of nasal mucosa **2**: 90
– papillary muscle of right ventricle of heart **2**: 132, 140
Septum of frontal sinuses **2**: 59, 61
– – glans penis **2**: 275
– – musculotubal canal **2**: 393, 396, 398
– – scrotum **2**: 232, 271, 274
– – sphenoidal sinuses **2**: 61, 293
– pellucidum **2**: 300, 304–305, 307, 317, 322–324, 332, 337–340, 347–350, 354–355, 360
– penis **2**: 275
Sequence of eruption of deciduous teeth **2**: 42
– – – – permanent teeth **2**: 39
Serosa → Serous coat
Serous coat **2**: 171
– – of bladder **2**: 235, 245
– – – jejunum **2**: 176
– – – small intestine **2**: 176
– – – stomach **2**: 173
– – – urinary bladder **2**: 235, 245
– – – uterus → Perimetrium
– pericardium **2**: 104, 123–125, 132–134, 142–143, 154–155
Serratus anterior muscle **1**: 63–65, 68, 72, 110, 112, 144, 148; **2**: 35
– posterior inferior muscle **1**: 54–55, 57
– – superior muscle **1**: 54, 57, 60
Sesamoid bones of foot **1**: 184–186, 188
– – – hand **1**: 92–94, 102
Shaft of clavicle/femur/fibula/humerus/phalanx/radius/rib/tibia/ulna → Body of clavicle/femur/fibula/humerus/phalanx/radius/rib/tibia/ulna
Shape differences of skull **2**: 2
Sheath(s) of optic nerve → Inner/outer sheath of optic nerve
– – styloid process of temporal bone **2**: 20
Shenton's line **1**: 177
Shin bone → Tibia
Short ciliary nerves **2**: 381–382
– gastric arteries **2**: 198
– gyri of insula **2**: 323, 344–345

Short
– head of biceps brachii muscle **1**: 64, 106–107, 110, 112, 141
– – – – femoris muscle **1**: 199, 221–222, 224, 226, 229, 232–234, 255–256, 261, 263, 267–268, 271
– limb of incus **2**: 397–398
– posterior ciliary arteries **2**: 371–373, 381–382
– saphenous vein → Small saphenous vein
Shoulder **1**: 106–111, 135–137, 140, 142–144
– girdle → Pectoral girdle
– joint → Glenohumeral joint
Sigmoid arteries **2**: 202, 219, 229–230
– colon **1**: 16, 18–19, 21, 194; **2**: 172, 193, 196, 202, 204–205, 220–221, 225, 230, 232, 238, 248, 251–255, 257, 260–261, 276
– mesocolon **2**: 193, 196, 206–207, 230
– sinus **2**: 49, 100, 291, 294, 352–353, 395, 400, 409
– veins **2**: 202
Silhouette of heart **2**: 122, 153
Simple bony limb of lateral semicircular canal **2**: 401–402
– membranous limb of lateral semicircular duct **2**: 405
Sinu-atrial nodal branch of right coronary artery **2**: 144
– node **2**: 140
Sinus of epididymis **2**: 270–271
– – pulmonary trunk **2**: 139
– tympani **2**: 396
Skeletal system → Skeleton of human body
Skeleton of foot → Bones of foot
– – hand → Bones of hand
– – human body **1**: 2–3
– – larynx **1**: 65–66
– – nose **2**: 23, 54
– – trunk **1**: 40
Skin **1**: 11, 65, 67, 74; **2**: 271
Skull **2**: 2–17, 32, 58–59, 61, 76–77, 290, 336, 394–395, 400
– cap **2**: 2–3, 17
– of newborn child **2**: 17
Small cardiac vein **2**: 129, 135, 140, 143
– intestine **1**: 16; **2**: 170–171, 174, 176, 188, 192–196, 200, 203, 225, 232
– saphenous vein **1**: 245, 247, 254–256, 266–268, 272, 274–275, 277–278
Socket of glenohumeral joint **1**: 96
– – hip joint **1**: 193
Soft palate **2**: 7, 38–39, 45, 50, 52, 55, 57, 90, 395
Sole of foot **1**: 217, 237–238, 279–281
Soleal line of tibia **1**: 182
Soleus muscle **1**: 211, 217, 221, 231–235, 241, 255, 267–268, 271, 273–274, 276–277
Somatic afferent nerve fiber(s) **1**: 23, 79
– efferent nerve fiber(s) **1**: 23
– nerve fiber(s) **1**: 23, 79
Somatosensory areas of cerebral cortex **2**: 319
Spaces of iridocorneal angle **2**: 375
Spatial orientations **1**: 5
Spermatic cord **1**: 63–66, 216; **2**: 234, 261, 273–274, 276
Spheno-ethmoidal recess **2**: 9, 11, 55, 62, 359
– suture **2**: 10
Sphenofrontal suture **2**: 4, 6, 10, 12, 368
Sphenoid → Sphenoidal bone
Sphenoidal angle of parietal bone **2**: 22
– bone **1**: 51; **2**: 4–6, 8, 10, 12, 14–17, 19, 23–24, 30–31, 48, 55–56, 58, 60, 63, 89, 359, 367–368, 380, 395

Sphenoidal
– concha **2**: 19
– fontanelle **2**: 17
– lingula **2**: 10,19
– margin of temporal bone **2**: 20
– part of middle cerebral artery **2**: 298
– process of palatine bone **2**: 57
– rostrum **2**: 19
– sinus **2**: 7, 9, 11–13, 23, 27, 52, 55–57, 60–62, 88–90, 293–294, 302, 305, 352–353, 359–360, 369, 378, 385, 406–407, 409
– yoke → Jugum sphenoidale
Sphenomandibular ligament **2**: 27, 86
Spheno-occipital synchondrosis **2**: 10, 17
Sphenopalatine artery **2**: 76–77, 88–90
– foramen **2**: 55–56, 368
– notch of palatine bone **2**: 57
Sphenoparietal sinus **2**: 291, 294
– suture **2**: 4, 6, 10, 12
Sphenosquamous suture **2**: 6, 8, 10, 12
Sphenozygomatic suture **2**: 4, 6, 368
Spherical recess **2**: 401–402
Spheroidal joint **1**: 10
Sphincter pupillae muscle **2**: 375
– urethrovaginalis muscle **2**: 247, 250–251
Spinal arachnoid mater **2**: 73, 285–286, 295, 321
– branch(es) of dorsal branch of posterior intercostal artery **1**: 76; **2**: 285–286
– – – – – – – – vein **2**: 285–286
– – – lateral sacral artery **2**: 244
– – – vertebral artery **2**: 286
– – – – vein **2**: 286
– cord **1**: 22–23, 37, 39, 60, 79; **2**: 73–75, 95, 158, 160–161, 166, 284–286, 288, 292, 294, 303–304, 307, 310–311, 320–321, 324, 340
– dura mater **2**: 73, 75, 284–286, 289, 321
– ganglion **1**: 23, 48, 79; **2**: 95, 166, 284–287, 289
– nerve(s) **1**: 22–23, 48, 60–61, 79; **2**: 95–96, 166–167, 248, 284–286, 288–289, 311
– part of accessory nerve → Spinal root of accessory nerve
– – – deltoid muscle **1**: 108
– pia mater **2**: 285–286, 295
– reticular formation **2**: 288
– root of accessory nerve **1**: 22; **2**: 292, 294–295, 306, 311
Spinalis muscle **1**: 56–58
Spine of helix **2**: 390
– – scapula **1**: 53, 84–85, 87, 95–96, 105, 108–109, 111, 142, 148; **2**: 92
– – sphenoidal bone **2**: 19
Spinoreticular tract **2**: 288
Spinotectal tract **2**: 288
Spinous process of axis **1**: 30–31, 36–37, 40, 49–51, 55; **2**: 294
– – – vertebra **1**: 29–33, 36–40, 42, 46–48, 50–51, 55, 60, 190; **2**: 75, 287, 289
– – – – prominens **1**: 31
Spiral arteries of uterus **2**: 243
– canal of cochlea **2**: 403
– – – modiolus cochleae **2**: 402–404
– crest of cochlear duct **2**: 404
– ganglion → Cochlear ganglion
– ligament of cochlear duct **2**: 404
– membrane → Tympanic surface of cochlear duct
– organ **2**: 404
– prominence of cochlear duct **2**: 404
Spleen **1**: 15–16, 18–19, 21; **2**: 155, 171–172, 182, 186, 189, 191, 198–199, 204, 208, 220–222, 248

Splenic artery **2**: 167, 188–189, 196–200, 203, 207, 219, 221
– branches of splenic artery **2**: 197, 219
– hilum **2**: 189
– lymph nodes **2**: 198, 203
– nerve plexus **2**: 248–249
– vein **2**: 188–189, 198–200, 203, 207, 221
Splenium of corpus callosum **2**: 307, 315, 317, 322, 324–325, 335, 342–343, 345–347, 349, 354–356, 361
Splenius capitis muscle **1**: 53–54, 56–57, 60; **2**: 30, 32–35, 37, 73–75, 92–93
– cervicis muscle **1**: 54, 56–57, 60; **2**: 33, 74
Splenography **2**: 197
Splenorenal ligament **2**: 206–207
Spongy bone **1**: 7, 10
– urethra **2**: 170, 232, 237, 266–267, 275, 277–278
Squamosal border of parietal bone **2**: 22
– margin of greater wing of sphenoidal bone **2**: 19
Squamous part of frontal bone **1**: 87; **2**: 3–4, 6–7, 10, 12, 21, 23, 368
– – – occipital bone **1**: 37, 51, 87; **2**: 3, 6–7, 10, 12, 17–18, 290, 294, 321, 352
– – – temporal bone **2**: 4, 6, 10, 12, 17, 20, 26, 368, 391–392, 399
– suture **2**: 6, 12
Stalk of epiglottis **2**: 64–65
Stapedial membrane **2**: 398
Stapedius muscle **2**: 398
Stapes **2**: 391, 397–399, 405
Stellate ganglion → Cervicothoracic ganglion
Sternal angle **1**: 45; **2**: 161
– branches of internal thoracic artery **1**: 76
– end of clavicle **1**: 84
– facet of clavicle **1**: 84, 110; **2**: 96
– line **1**: 4
– part of diaphragm **1**: 68–69
Sternoclavicular joint **1**: 45, 62, 82
Sternocleidomastoid artery **2**: 97, 99
– branches of occipital artery **2**: 76
– muscle **1**: 53–54, 60, 62–64, 68, 112; **2**: 30, 32–37, 44, 68, 71–75, 81, 85, 92–93, 95, 98–99
– region **1**: 4
– vein **2**: 99
Sternocostal head of pectoralis major muscle **1**: 63–65
– joints **1**: 45
– triangle **1**: 68–69
Sternohyoid muscle **1**: 68, 112; **2**: 33–36, 44–45, 68, 71, 75, 93, 97–99
Sternopericardial ligaments **2**: 122
Sternothyroid muscle **1**: 68; **2**: 33–36, 68, 71, 75, 93, 97, 99, 149
Sternum **1**: 40–41, 45, 68, 76, 82, 87; **2**: 104, 107, 118, 127, 150, 154, 156–159, 161, 172
Stomach **1**: 16, 18–19, 21, 43; **2**: 106–107, 128, 130, 154–155, 167, 170–176, 182, 186, 189–191, 194, 196, 198, 200, 208, 222–223, 248
Straight gyrus **2**: 317, 335, 337
– part of cricothyroid muscle **2**: 66, 70
– sinus **2**: 52, 289, 291, 294, 321, 354–359
Stratum corneum of epidermis **1**: 11
– germinativum of epidermis **1**: 11
Stress trajectories of bone **1**: 7
Stria medullaris of thalamus **2**: 300, 307, 324–326, 340
– terminalis **2**: 300, 322, 325–326, 331, 340, 344, 346

Stria
– vascularis of cochlear duct **2**: 404
Striate area of cerebral cortex **2**: 322, 346
– body → Corpus striatum
Striatum **2**: 300, 329, 332
Stroma of iris **2**: 375
Styloglossus muscle **2**: 32, 34–35, 37, 46–49, 51, 87, 97, 99
Stylohyoid ligament **2**: 27, 35, 51
– muscle **2**: 32, 34, 36–37, 44, 47, 49, 51, 86–87, 97–98, 100
Styloid process of radius → Radial styloid process
– – – temporal bone **2**: 6, 8, 12, 20, 27, 34–35, 47–49, 51, 100, 290, 395, 399, 402
– – – third metacarpal bone **1**: 92, 94
– – – ulna → Ulnar styloid process
Stylomandibular ligament **2**: 26–27
Stylomastoid artery **2**: 76, 100
– foramen **2**: 8, 20, 84
Stylopharyngeus muscle **2**: 35, 37, 46–51, 100
Subacromial bursa **1**: 96
Subarachnoid cisterns **2**: 321
– space **2**: 73, 75, 232, 285–287, 289, 294–295, 321, 326, 352–353, 405
– – of optic nerve **2**: 374, 378
Subarcuate fossa of temporal bone **2**: 20
Subcallosal area **2**: 304, 317, 357
– gyrus → Subcallosal area
Subclavian artery **1**: 12, 14, 60, 64, 72, 75, 138–139; **2**: 35, 72, 78–79, 81, 92–93, 96–97, 100, 105–107, 118, 122–125, 130, 139, 142–143, 156, 162–163, 165, 167
– lymphatic trunk **1**: 15, 76; **2**: 149, 163
– nerve **1**: 112, 134; **2**: 93–94, 98, 149
– triangle → Omoclavicular triangle
– trunk → Subclavian lymphatic trunk
– vein **1**: 12, 14, 64, 72–73, 75, 137; **2**: 93, 97, 122, 149, 162–164
Subclavius muscle **1**: 64, 68, 106–107, 112, 140; **2**: 93, 149
Subcostal nerve **2**: 209, 226–227, 248
Subcutaneous nerves of anterior region of elbow **1**: 151
– – – – – forearm **1**: 151
– – – arm **1**: 135–136
– – – dorsum of foot **1**: 278
– – – – hand **1**: 164
– – – foot **1**: 270, 278
– – – forearm **1**: 150
– – – gluteal region **1**: 254
– – – hand **1**: 164
– – – leg **1**: 266, 270
– – – neck **2**: 91–92
– – – popliteal fossa **1**: 254, 266
– – – posterior region of forearm **1**: 150
– – – shoulder **1**: 135–136
– – – thigh **1**: 248, 254
– prepatellar bursa **1**: 218, 230, 232
– tissue **1**: 11
– veins of anterior region of elbow **1**: 151
– – – – – forearm **1**: 151
– – – arm **1**: 135–137
– – – dorsum of foot **1**: 270, 278
– – – – hand **1**: 164
– – – foot **1**: 270, 278
– – – forearm **1**: 137, 150
– – – gluteal region **1**: 254
– – – hand **1**: 164
– – – leg **1**: 266, 270
– – – lower limb **1**: 246
– – – neck **2**: 91–92

Subcutaneous veins of
– – – popliteal fossa **1**: 254, 266
– – – posterior region of forearm **1**: 150
– – – shoulder **1**: 135–137
– – – thigh **1**: 248, 254
Subdeltoid bursa **1**: 96, 109
Subdivision of bronchial tree **2**: 114
– – mediastinum **2**: 104
Subdural space **2**: 285–286, 289, 295
Subependymal stratum **2**: 338
Subepicardial fat **2**: 133–135
Subfascial prepatellar bursa **1**: 200
Subhepatic space **2**: 170–171
Subiculum of hippocampus **2**: 326
– – promontory of tympanic cavity **2**: 396
Sublenticular limb of internal capsule → Sublentiform limb of internal capsule
Sublentiform limb of internal capsule **2**: 332–333, 344
Sublingual artery **2**: 47, 97–99
– caruncle **2**: 38, 45
– fold **2**: 38
– fossa of mandible **2**: 25
– gland **2**: 38, 45, 47, 87, 99
– vein **2**: 47, 99
Submandibular duct **2**: 45, 47, 87, 99
– fossa of mandible **2**: 25
– ganglion **2**: 87
– gland **2**: 33–34, 36, 44–45, 49–50, 85, 87, 98–99
– lymph nodes **2**: 44, 81
Submental artery **2**: 44, 76–77, 98–99
– lymph nodes **2**: 44, 81
– vein **2**: 80, 383
Suboccipital nerve **1**: 60; **2**: 289
– puncture **2**: 321
Subparietal sulcus **2**: 304, 317
Subperitoneal space **2**: 250–251
Subphrenic space of peritoneal cavity **2**: 154, 170, 190
Subpleural lymphatic vessels **2**: 113
Subpopliteal recess **1**: 10, 200
Subpubic angle **1**: 172, 175
Subpyloric lymph nodes **2**: 198
Subscapular artery **1**: 140–141
– axillary lymph nodes **1**: 72
– fossa **1**: 85
– lymph nodes → Subscapular axillary lymph nodes
– nerves **1**: 112–113, 134, 140; **2**: 94
Subscapularis muscle **1**: 64, 95, 97, 106–107, 110, 112–113, 140–141, 144, 149
Subserosa of parietal/visceral peritoneum **2**: 171, 230, 232
Subserous layer → Subserosa
Substantia nigra **2**: 309, 315, 328, 330–331, 335, 340, 344, 350–351
– propria of cornea **2**: 375
– – – sclera **2**: 375
Subtalar joint **1**: 188, 206–215
Subtendinous bursa of subscapularis muscle **1**: 96
Subthalamic nucleus **2**: 330, 340, 344, 350
Sulcomarginal fasciculus **2**: 288
Sulcus limitans **2**: 310–311
– of auditory tube **2**: 8, 19
– – corpus callosum **2**: 304, 317, 319, 337
– sclerae **2**: 374
– tali **1**: 187
– terminalis cordis **2**: 125
Superciliary arch **2**: 21

Superficial arteries of brain **2**: 297
– – – face **2**: 85
– – – head **2**: 85
– – – neck **2**: 92
– branch of lateral plantar nerve **1**: 279–280
– – – medial circumflex femoral artery
    1: 252–253
– – – – plantar artery **1**: 279–281
– – – radial nerve **1**: 132–133, 140, 150–154,
    157, 160–161, 164
– – – ulnar nerve **1**: 152–153, 161–162
– cervical artery **2**: 91–92, 98, 100, 149
– – vein **2**: 98
– circumflex iliac artery **1**: 75, 248, 251, 253;
    2: 228
– – – vein **1**: 75, 248
– dorsal veins of penis **2**: 275–277
– epigastric artery **1**: 75, 248, 252–253; **2**: 228
– – vein **1**: 75, 245, 248, 252; **2**: 276
– external pudendal artery(-ies) **1**: 248,
    252–253; **2**: 228
– facial region **2**: 84–85
– – veins **2**: 80
– fascia of penis **2**: 275–276
– fibular nerve **1**: 235, 240, 242, 270–271, 278
– head of flexor pollicis brevis muscle **1**: 103,
    121, 123–124, 166–167
– inguinal lymph nodes **1**: 248; **2**: 163
– – ring **1**: 66–67, 218; **2**: 273–274
– investing fascia of perineum → Perineal fascia
– lateral cervical lymph nodes **2**: 81, 91
– layer of cervical fascia → Investing layer of
    cervical fascia
– – – temporal fascia **2**: 30
– middle cerebral vein **2**: 291, 295–297, 300
– nuchal fascia **2**: 91
– palmar arch **1**: 138, 161, 163
– – branch of radial artery **1**: 152–153, 155,
    160–163
– – fascia **1**: 160
– parotid lymph nodes **2**: 81
– part of masseter muscle **2**: 30, 98–99
– perineal compartment → Superficial perineal
    pouch
– – pouch **2**: 250–251
– – space → Superficial perineal pouch
– peroneal nerve → Superficial fibular nerve
– popliteal lymph nodes **1**: 245
– posterior sacrococcygeal ligament **1**: 190
– temporal artery **2**: 76–77, 81, 85–89, 98–99
– – branches of auriculotemporal nerve
    2: 86–87
– – vein(s) **2**: 80–81, 85, 98–99, 383
– transverse metacarpal ligament **1**: 160
– – perineal muscle **1**: 227; **2**: 265–267,
    279–280
– veins of anterior region of elbow **1**: 151
– – – arm **1**: 135–137
– – – brain **2**: 297
– – – dorsum of foot **1**: 270, 278
– – – – hand **1**: 164
– – – face **2**: 85
– – – foot **1**: 270, 278
– – – forearm **1**: 137, 150–151
– – – hand **1**: 164
– – – head **2**: 85
– – – leg **1**: 266, 270
– – – lower limb **1**: 246, 248, 254, 266, 270,
    278
– – – thigh **1**: 248, 254
– – – upper limb **1**: 135–137, 150–151, 164

Superior **1**: 5
– aberrant ductule of epididymis **2**: 270
– alveolar nerves **2**: 84, 86
– anastomotic vein **2**: 296–297
– angle of scapula **1**: 84–85, 108
– articular facet of vertebra → Articular facet
    of superior articular process of vertebra
– – process of axis **2**: 72
– – – – sacrum **1**: 34–35, 38, 172
– – – – vertebra **1**: 29–33, 36, 38, 42, 46–48,
    55; **2**: 72, 286
– – surface of atlas **1**: 30–31, 50
– – – – tibia **1**: 182
– belly of omohyoid muscle **2**: 34, 36, 81, 97–99
– border of petrous part of temporal bone
    2: 20
– – – scapula **1**: 84–85
– – – spleen **2**: 189
– branch(es) of oculomotor nerve **2**: 379, 381
– – – transverse cervical nerve **2**: 91–92
– bulb of jugular vein **2**: 49, 100
– cerebellar artery **2**: 292, 298–299, 302
– – peduncle **2**: 308–311, 334, 343
– cerebral veins **2**: 294, 296–297
– cervical cardiac branches of vagus nerve **1**: 25;
    2: 100, 149
– – – nerve **2**: 95–96, 100, 166
– – ganglion **1**: 25; **2**: 88, 95–96, 100, 166
– choroid vein **2**: 300
– clunial nerves **1**: 61, 243, 254–255
– colliculus **2**: 310–311, 324, 328, 335, 350, 357
– conjunctival fornix **2**: 365, 384
– constrictor muscle **2**: 46–49, 100
– costal facet of thoracic vertebra **1**: 32, 46–47
– costotransverse ligament **1**: 46
– dental nerve plexus **2**: 84, 86
– diaphragmatic lymph nodes **1**: 76; **2**: 113
– duodenal flexure **2**: 191
– – fold **2**: 206
– – fossa **2**: 193
– epigastric artery **1**: 75–76
– – vein **1**: 75
– extensor retinaculum of foot **1**: 230–232, 236,
    241
– extremity of kidney **2**: 208, 215, 218, 222
– – – thyroid gland → Superior pole of thyroid
    gland
– eyelid **2**: 362, 364, 379, 384
– facet of talus **1**: 187–188
– fascia of pelvic diaphragm **2**: 250–251
– fibular retinaculum **1**: 232–234, 241, 268
– fovea of fourth ventricle **2**: 310
– frontal gyrus **2**: 314, 316–317, 337–338, 348
– – sulcus **2**: 314, 316
– ganglion of vagus nerve **2**: 100
– gemellus muscle → Gemellus superior muscle
– genial spine of mandible → Superior mental
    spine of mandible
– glenohumeral ligament **1**: 95–96
– gluteal artery **1**: 256–257; **2**: 230, 234,
    244–245
– – nerve **1**: 227, 229, 244, 257; **2**: 226, 228
– – vein(s) **1**: 257
– horn of falciform margin of saphenous
    opening **1**: 218
– – – thyroid cartilage **2**: 51, 64–67, 70, 101
– hypogastric nerve plexus **1**: 25; **2**: 231,
    248–249
– hypophysial artery **2**: 301
– ileocecal recess **2**: 177
– labial branch(es) of facial artery **2**: 76, 85–87
– – – – infra-orbital nerve **2**: 85, 87

Superior labial
– – vein **2**: 80, 383
– lacrimal canaliculus **2**: 365
– – – papilla **2**: 364–365
– laryngeal artery **2**: 97–99, 101
– – nerve **2**: 50, 96–101, 167
– lateral brachial cutaneous nerve **1**: 61, 78,
    132–133, 135, 142–143
– – cutaneous nerve of arm → Superior lateral
    brachial cutaneous nerve
– – genicular artery **1**: 250, 255–256, 267, 269,
    271
– ligament of epididymis **2**: 270
– – – incus **2**: 391, 398
– – – malleus **2**: 391, 398
– lingular bronchus of left lung [B IV]
    2: 108–109, 114
– – segment of left lung [S IV] **2**: 117
– lobar arteries of left lung **2**: 119
– – – – right lung **2**: 113, 119
– lobe of left lung **2**: 111–112, 114, 117,
    149–150, 154–156, 160
– – – right lung **2**: 111–114, 116, 150, 154–155,
    165
– longitudinal fasciculus **2**: 333
– – muscle of tongue **2**: 46–47
– macular arteriole **2**: 377
– – venule **2**: 377
– margin of cerebral hemisphere **2**: 314,
    316–317, 337–338
– medial genicular artery **1**: 250, 256, 267–269
– mediastinum **2**: 104, 153
– medullary velum **2**: 304, 307–311
– mental spine of mandible **2**: 25
– mesenteric artery **1**: 12, 14; **2**: 105, 162, 167,
    188, 198–203, 207, 211, 213–214, 218–219,
    223–224
– – ganglion **1**: 24–25; **2**: 167, 248
– – lymph nodes **2**: 203
– – nerve plexus **1**: 25; **2**: 248–249
– – vein **2**: 188, 199–203, 207, 223–224
– nasal concha **2**: 22, 50, 52, 55–56, 58, 88–89,
    336
– – meatus **2**: 55–56, 365
– – retinal arteriole **2**: 377
– – – venule **2**: 377
– nuchal line **1**: 55; **2**: 8, 18
– oblique muscle **2**: 58, 360, 370–371, 379–383,
    386–387
– ophthalmic vein **2**: 58, 80, 379, 382–384
– orbital fissure **2**: 4, 9–10, 19, 23, 58–59,
    367–369, 379
– palpebral groove **2**: 364
– pancreatic lymph nodes **2**: 198, 203
– pancreaticoduodenal artery **2**: 197
– – lymph nodes **2**: 203
– parathyroid gland **1**: 15; **2**: 49, 100–101
– parietal lobule **2**: 314, 316–317
– part of diaphragmatic surface of liver **2**: 180
– – – duodenum **2**: 171, 173–176, 188, 194,
    199, 204, 206, 223
– – – vestibular nerve **2**: 405
– peroneal retinaculum → Superior fibular
    retinaculum
– petrosal sinus **2**: 80, 291
– pole of kidney → Superior extremity of
    kidney
– – – testis → Upper pole of testis
– – – thyroid gland **2**: 71
– pubic ligament **1**: 190, 193
– – ramus **1**: 172–176, 221; **2**: 268
– recess of omental bursa **2**: 170, 206–207

Superior
– rectal artery **2**: 202, 229–231, 234
– – nerve plexus **2**: 248
– rectus muscle **2**: 58, 360, 362, 370–371, 379–382, 384, 386–387
– root of ansa cervicalis **2**: 87, 93–94, 97–100
– sagittal sinus **2**: 289–291, 294–295, 297, 300, 321, 336, 339, 341–343, 347, 349, 354–361, 408
– segment of left lung [S VI] **2**: 117
– – – right lung [S VI] **2**: 116
– segmental artery of kidney **2**: 212, 214
– – bronchus of left lung [B VI] **2**: 109, 114
– – – – right lung [B VI] **2**: 109, 114, 120–121
– semilunar lobule of cerebellum **2**: 308
– suprarenal artery(-ies) **2**: 162
– tarsal muscle **2**: 366
– tarsus **2**: 365–366, 383–384
– temporal gyrus **2**: 316, 323, 337–338, 348
– – line of parietal bone **2**: 6, 22, 31
– – retinal arteriole **2**: 377
– – – venule **2**: 377
– – sulcus **2**: 316
– thalamostriate vein **2**: 300, 322, 326, 344, 346, 348
– thoracic aperture **1**: 41
– thyroid artery **2**: 74, 76–77, 79, 93, 97–101, 149
– – notch **2**: 64–65, 70
– – tubercle **2**: 64
– – vein **2**: 80, 98–99, 149
– tibiofibular joint → Tibiofibular joint
– tracheobronchial lymph nodes **2**: 110, 113
– transverse scapular ligament **1**: 95, 140, 143
– trunk of brachial plexus **1**: 134; **2**: 94–95, 166
– tympanic artery **2**: 380
– ulnar collateral artery **1**: 138–143, 152–153
– veins of cerebellar hemisphere **2**: 295
– vena cava **1**: 12–15; **2**: 97, 107, 122–125, 129–130, 132–133, 139–143, 157, 161–165, 167, 172
– vertebral notch **1**: 32–33, 35
– vesical artery(-ies) **2**: 234, 244–245
– vestibular area of internal acoustic meatus **2**: 401–403
Superolateral superficial inguinal lymph nodes **1**: 245
Superomedial superficial inguinal lymph nodes **1**: 245
Supination **1**: 5
Supinator crest **1**: 89
– muscle **1**: 101, 113, 116–117, 119, 140, 152–154, 156
Suprachiasmatic nucleus **2**: 328
Supraclavicular lymph nodes **2**: 81
– nerves **1**: 61, 78, 132–133; **2**: 82–83, 91–92, 94, 98
– part of brachial plexus **1**: 134
Supracollicular sphincter muscle → Internal urethral sphincter muscle
Supracondylar process of humerus **1**: 86
Supraglenoid tubercle **1**: 85
Suprahyoid branch of lingual artery **2**: 98
– muscles **2**: 36
Supramarginal gyrus **2**: 314, 316
Supra-optic nucleus **2**: 328
– recess **2**: 301, 307, 320, 351
Supra-orbital artery **2**: 76–77, 85–87, 380–381, 383
– foramen **2**: 21, 367
– margin of frontal bone **2**: 4–5, 21, 367
– nerve **2**: 82–83, 85–87, 380–381, 383

Supra-orbital
– notch **2**: 4, 21
– vein **2**: 80
Suprapatellar bursa **1**: 10, 195
Suprapineal recess **2**: 307, 310–311, 320
Suprapiriform foramen **1**: 223–225, 257; **2**: 281
Suprapyloric lymph node **2**: 198
Suprarenal gland **1**: 14–15, 19; **2**: 171, 182, 199, 210, 215–216, 218, 220–222, 248
– nerve plexus **2**: 248
– vein(s) **1**: 14; **2**: 162
Suprascapular artery **1**: 140; **2**: 78–79, 92–93, 98, 100, 149
– nerve **1**: 112–113, 134, 140, 143; **2**: 93–94, 149
– notch **1**: 84–85, 95
– region **1**: 4
– vein **2**: 122
Supraspinatus muscle **1**: 95, 97, 106, 108–113, 142–143, 148–149
Supraspinous fossa **1**: 84–85, 87, 95
– ligament **1**: 39, 46–48, 190
Suprasternal notch → Jugular notch of sternum
– space **2**: 33
Supratarsal part of superior eyelid **2**: 364
Supratragic tubercle **2**: 390
Supratrochlear artery **2**: 76, 85–87, 381, 383
– foramen of humerus **1**: 86
– nerve **2**: 82–83, 85–87, 380–381, 383
– vein(s) **2**: 80, 85, 383
Supravaginal part of cervix of uterus **2**: 233, 239–240
Supraventricular crest **2**: 132
Supravesical fossa **1**: 67, 77; **2**: 238
Supreme intercostal artery **2**: 79, 118
Sural arteries **1**: 250, 255–256, 266–267, 269
– communicating branch of common fibular nerve **1**: 266
– nerve **1**: 242–243, 266–267, 278
Surface anatomy of abdomen **1**: 62
– – – back **1**: 52
– – – lower limb **1**: 216–217
– – – thorax **1**: 62
– – – upper limb **1**: 105
– projections of viscera **1**: 18–21
Surfaces of permanent teeth **2**: 40
Surgical neck of humerus **1**: 86
Suspensory ligament(s) of breast **1**: 70–71, 74
– – – ovary **2**: 233, 238–241, 251
– – – penis **1**: 63–64, 66
– retinacula of breast → Suspensory ligaments of breast
Sustentaculum tali of calcaneus **1**: 184, 186–188, 210
Sutural bone(s) **2**: 3
Sympathetic ganglion(-ia) **1**: 25
– innervation of eyeball **2**: 382
– nervous system **1**: 24–25
– – – in lesser pelvis **2**: 231
– – – – neck **2**: 95–96, 166
– – – – retroperitoneal space **2**: 248–249
– – – – upper thorax **2**: 95–96, 166
– part of autonomic division of peripheral nervous system → Sympathetic nervous system
– pathways **1**: 24
– root of ciliary ganglion **2**: 382
– – – pterygopalatine ganglion → Deep petrosal nerve
– trunk **1**: 23, 25; **2**: 33, 95–96, 100, 166–167, 231, 248–249, 285

Symphysial surface **1**: 40, 176, 191, 221; **2**: 264, 276
Synchondrosis → Cartilaginous joint
– of first rib **1**: 45
Syndesmosis → Fibrous joint
Synostosis → Bony union
Synovial bursa **1**: 51
– fold(s) **1**: 10–11
– joint **1**: 10
– layer of articular capsule **1**: 10–11, 198, 200
– membrane → Synovial layer of articular capsule
– sheath(s) **1**: 10
– – of digits of hand **1**: 121–122, 130–131
– – – toes **1**: 238
Systole **2**: 136–138

T

Taenia → Tenia
Tail of caudate nucleus **2**: 322, 326, 329–332, 340, 344, 346, 348, 350–351, 355–356, 361
– – epididymis **2**: 270, 272
– – helix **2**: 390
– – pancreas **2**: 188, 199–200, 203, 206–207, 248
Talar articular surface of navicular **1**: 207
– shelf → Sustentaculum tali of calcaneus
Talocalcaneal interosseous ligament **1**: 188, 206–208, 210–211, 214–215
– joint → Subtalar joint
Talocalcaneonavicular joint **1**: 188, 206–207, 209–215
Talocrural joint → Ankle joint
Talonavicular ligament **1**: 212
– portion of talocalcaneonavicular joint **1**: 209, 215
Talus **1**: 184–188, 207–211, 214–215, 277
Tapetum **2**: 333–334
Tarsal bones **1**: 170–171, 184–185, 188
– glands **2**: 366, 384
– interosseous ligaments **1**: 215
– part of superior eyelid **2**: 364
– sinus **1**: 184, 188, 209–211, 215
– tendinous sheaths **1**: 241
Tarsometatarsal joints **1**: 207, 215
Tectal part of column of fornix **2**: 324, 328, 334
– plate **2**: 304–305, 315, 348
Tectorial membrane of cochlear duct **2**: 404
– – – median atlanto-axial joint **1**: 49, 51
Tectum of midbrain **2**: 289, 328, 334–335, 350–351, 357–358, 361
Teeth → Tooth/Teeth
Tegmental nuclei **2**: 328
– roof of tympanic cavity → Tegmental wall of tympanic cavity
– wall of tympanic cavity **2**: 391, 396
Tegmentum of midbrain **2**: 304, 309–310, 324, 328, 350–353, 358–359
Tela choroidea of fourth ventricle **2**: 304, 307, 309, 324
– – – third ventricle **2**: 299–300, 307, 322, 326, 344, 346, 348
Telencephalon → Cerebrum
Temporal bone **2**: 4–6, 8, 10–12, 14–17, 20, 26, 48, 51, 58, 100, 290, 302, 352–353, 359, 361–362, 368, 391–396, 399–400, 402, 405–409
– branches of facial nerve **2**: 84–85, 98
– fascia **2**: 30, 58
– fossa **2**: 9, 11
– genu of optic radiation **2**: 335

Temporal
– gyri **2**: 331
– horn of lateral ventricle **2**: 300, 320, 322–323, 326, 333–334, 340–341, 344, 350, 357–358, 361–362, 385, 408
– line of frontal bone **2**: 20–21
– lobe **2**: 61–63, 312–313, 329, 339, 341–343, 345, 349, 352–353, 356–362, 385, 400, 408–409
– operculum of superior temporal gyrus **2**: 323, 338
– plane of parietal bone **2**: 6, 22
– pole **2**: 306, 315–316, 323
– surface of frontal bone **2**: 21
– – – greater wing of sphenoidal bone **2**: 19, 58
Temporalis muscle **2**: 31–32, 37, 58, 62–63, 73, 86–87, 352–353, 358–360, 362, 380, 387, 391
Temporomandibular joint **2**: 11, 26–27, 31
Temporoparietalis muscle **2**: 28–29
Temporopontine fibers **2**: 328, 332
Temporozygomatic suture **2**: 6, 8
Tendinous arch of levator ani muscle **2**: 244, 250–251, 255, 264
– – – soleus muscle **1**: 268
– chiasm of digits of hand **1**: 124
– cords of heart → Chordae tendineae of heart
– fossae of radius **1**: 88
– intersection(s) of rectus abdominis muscle **1**: 62–65
– sheath(s) of abductor longus and extensor pollicis brevis muscles **1**: 130
– – – extensor carpi ulnaris muscle **1**: 130
– – – – digiti minimi muscle **1**: 130
– – – – digitorum and extensor indicis muscles **1**: 130
– – – – – longus muscle **1**: 241
– – – – hallucis longus muscle **1**: 241
– – – – pollicis longus muscle **1**: 130
– – – extensores carpi radiales muscles **1**: 130
– – – flexor carpi radialis muscle **1**: 130
– – – – digitorum longus muscle **1**: 214–215, 241
– – – – hallucis longus muscle **1**: 214–215, 241
– – – – pollicis longus muscle **1**: 121, 130–131
– – – foot **1**: 241
– – – hand **1**: 130–131
– – – superior oblique muscle **2**: 370–371
– – – tibialis anterior muscle **1**: 241
– – – – posterior muscle **1**: 214–215, 241
– – on ankle **1**: 241
– – – fingers **1**: 130–131
– – – wrist **1**: 130–131
Tendon **1**: 10
– of infundibulum of right ventricle of heart **2**: 135
– sheath **1**: 10
Tenia fimbriae **2**: 326
– habenulae **2**: 326
– of fornix **2**: 300, 322, 324, 326
– thalami **2**: 310–311, 324, 326
Tensile stress trajectories **1**: 7
Tensor fasciae latae muscle **1**: 194, 216, 219, 226–227, 253, 259; **2**: 228, 256–259
– tympani muscle **2**: 391, 398–399
– veli palatini muscle **2**: 37, 48, 51, 73, 89, 395
Tentorial nerve of ophthalmic nerve **2**: 293, 380
– notch **2**: 291
Tentorium cerebelli **2**: 289, 291–294, 343, 353, 356–359, 361–362
Teres major muscle **1**: 52–54, 97, 105–113, 140–144, 148–149

Teres
– minor muscle **1**: 95, 97, 109–113, 142–144, 148
Terminal filum → Filum terminale
– ileum **2**: 177–178, 190, 194–195, 200, 202, 204, 225, 238
– notch of auricle **2**: 390
– sulcus of tongue **2**: 46, 101
Testicular artery **1**: 67, 77; **2**: 162, 211, 215, 218, 228, 230, 270–272, 274
– nerve plexus **2**: 248–249
– vein **1**: 77; **2**: 162, 218, 228, 270–272, 274, 278
Testis **1**: 15, 17, 67; **2**: 170, 232, 258, 261, 270–274, 278
Thalamic fasciculus **2**: 340
Thalamoparietal fibers **2**: 332
Thalamus **2**: 300, 304–305, 307, 310–311, 317, 324–332, 335, 340–341, 344, 346–349, 354–356, 360–361, 408
Thenar eminence **1**: 105, 114–115, 120, 160
Thigh **1**: 2, 216–224, 226, 248, 251–256, 258–265; **2**: 228
– bone → Femur
Third molar tooth/teeth **2**: 40–41
– occipital nerve **1**: 60; **2**: 82–83
– trochanter **1**: 180
– ventricle **2**: 299–301, 304, 307, 310, 320–322, 326–327, 329, 332, 338–341, 344, 346, 348–351, 355–357, 361, 408
Thoracic aorta **1**: 14, 76; **2**: 78–79, 104–107, 126, 157–163, 165, 167
– aortic nerve plexus **2**: 167
– cardiac branches of thoracic ganglia **2**: 166–167
– – – – vagus nerve **2**: 149
– cavity **2**: 153
– constriction of esophagus **2**: 106
– duct **1**: 15; **2**: 149, 155, 163, 167
– ganglia **1**: 25; **2**: 96, 166–167
– intertransversarii muscles **1**: 59
– kyphosis **1**: 28
– lymph nodes **1**: 15; **2**: 113
– nerves [T 1–T 12] **1**: 22–23, 133; **2**: 166, 284, 286
– organs **2**: 126–127, 150–151, 154–161, 172
– part of esophagus **2**: 105–106
– – – iliocostalis lumborum muscle **1**: 56–58
– – – sympathetic trunk **2**: 96, 166
– – – thoracic duct **1**: 15
– – – vertebral column → Thoracic spine
– spine **1**: 28, 42, 46–47; **2**: 288
– vertebra(e) [T I–T XII] **1**: 28–29, 32, 36, 38, 42–43, 47, 60; **2**: 37, 72, 75, 104, 107, 127, 156–161, 182, 186, 209, 214–215, 217, 222, 284
– viscera **1**: 18–21; **2**: 126–127, 150–151, 154–161, 172
Thoraco-acromial artery **1**: 135, 142; **2**: 91–93, 98, 149
– vein(s) **1**: 73, 137
Thoracodorsal artery **1**: 72; **2**: 93, 149
– nerve **1**: 72, 112–113, 134, 140–141, 227; **2**: 93–94, 149
Thoraco-epigastric lymph nodes **1**: 72
– vein(s) **1**: 75; **2**: 149
Thoracolumbar fascia **1**: 53–55, 222, 226
Thorax **1**: 2, 40–43, 62, 68, 75–76, 82–83; **2**: 93, 96, 118, 126–131, 149–151, 153–167, 172
Thumb **1**: 92–93, 104–105, 123
Thymus **1**: 15; **2**: 104, 151
Thyro-arytenoid muscle **2**: 67–68

Thyrocervical trunk **1**: 139; **2**: 78–79, 93, 100, 118
Thyro-epiglottic ligament **2**: 66
Thyrohyoid branch of ansa cervicalis **2**: 94, 98–99
– foramen **2**: 46–48, 65–67, 70
– membrane **2**: 44, 46–48, 65–68, 70, 74, 97, 101
– muscle **2**: 34–35, 44–48, 66, 93, 97, 99, 149
Thyroid articular surface on cricoid cartilage **2**: 64, 67
– cartilage **1**: 18, 20–21; **2**: 35–36, 44, 47–48, 51–52, 64–68, 70, 97, 99, 101, 106, 110, 149, 164
– gland **1**: 15, 18, 20–21; **2**: 35–36, 47, 49–50, 52, 68, 70–71, 75, 96–98, 100–101, 149–151, 164–165, 167, 172
Thyropharyngeal part of inferior constrictor muscle **2**: 46–47, 68
Tibia **1**: 10, 170–171, 182–183, 188, 195–203, 205, 208–212, 214, 216, 220–221, 226, 230–232, 234–235, 241, 247, 268–270, 272–277
Tibial collateral ligament **1**: 195–196, 199–200, 220–221, 272
– division of sciatic nerve **1**: 227, 229, 235, 240
– nerve **1**: 227, 229, 235, 240, 242–243, 245, 255–256, 263–268, 270, 272–275, 277, 279
– nutrient artery **1**: 268
– tuberosity **1**: 10, 181–183, 195–197, 205, 216, 218–219, 230–232, 252, 270–271
Tibialis anterior muscle **1**: 198, 207, 211–213, 216, 231–232, 235, 240–241, 271, 273–278
– posterior muscle **1**: 208, 212–215, 231, 233–235, 238, 240–241, 267–268, 273–277
Tibiocalcaneal part of medial ligament of ankle joint **1**: 212–214
Tibiofibular joint **1**: 170–171, 205, 272
– syndesmosis **1**: 205–206, 208–209, 212, 214, 275
– trunk **1**: 269
Tibionavicular part of medial ligament of ankle joint **1**: 206, 212
Tip of nose → Apex of nose
– – tongue → Apex of tongue
Toes → Digits of foot
Tongue **2**: 13, 38–39, 46–47, 50–52, 58, 68, 87, 97, 101, 336
Tonsil of cerebellum **2**: 294, 307–309
Tonsillar branch of facial artery **2**: 76
Tooth/Teeth **2**: 41, 61
– of lower jaw **2**: 25, 39–43, 86
– – upper jaw **2**: 24, 39–43, 86
Torus tubarius **2**: 45, 50, 52, 57
Trabeculae carneae of left ventricle of heart **2**: 133, 140
– – – right ventricle of heart **2**: 132, 134, 140
Trabecular architecture of bone **1**: 7
– tissue of sclera **2**: 375
Trachea **1**: 14–16, 18, 43; **2**: 36, 47, 49–50, 52–53, 65–66, 68, 70–71, 75, 100, 104–110, 113–115, 119–121, 126–127, 130–131, 150–151, 155–156, 161, 165, 172
Tracheal bifurcation **2**: 104, 106, 108, 110, 155
– branches of inferior thyroid artery **2**: 100
– cartilages **2**: 47–48, 50, 65–66, 68, 70, 105–106, 108–109
– glands **2**: 67, 109
Trachealis muscle **2**: 66
Tracheobronchial lymph nodes **2**: 104, 110, 157
Tracts of extrapyramidal system **2**: 288
– – spinal cord **2**: 288

Tractus spiralis foraminosus **2**: 401–403
Tragal lamina **2**: 390
Tragus **2**: 390
Trajectories of bone **1**: 7
Transversalis fascia **1**: 65–67
Transverse acetabular ligament **1**: 190, 193
– arch of foot **1**: 189
– arytenoid muscle **2**: 51–52, 67–68
– axes **1**: 5
– branch of lateral circumflex femoral artery
  1: 251
– cervical artery **1**: 60; **2**: 81, 92–93, 118, 149,
  162
– – ligament → Cardinal ligament
– – nerve **1**: 78; **2**: 82–83, 91–94, 98–99
– – vein(s) **2**: 149, 164
– colon **1**: 16, 18, 20–21; **2**: 154, 170, 172, 179,
  186, 190–194, 196, 200, 202–205, 208,
  223–224
– costal facet **1**: 32, 46
– crest of internal acoustic meatus **2**: 401, 403
– diameter of pelvis **1**: 178
– facial artery **2**: 76, 85–86, 98
– fascicles of palmar aponeurosis **1**: 120, 160
– – – plantar aponeurosis **1**: 237
– folds of rectum **2**: 179, 232, 243
– head of adductor hallucis muscle **1**: 238, 240
– – – – pollicis muscle **1**: 121–122, 124
– ligament of atlas **1**: 50–51; **2**: 294
– – – knee **1**: 196
– mesocolon **2**: 154, 170, 179, 191–193, 200,
  204, 206
– muscle of tongue **2**: 46–47
– occipital sulcus **2**: 314–315
– palatine folds **2**: 38–39, 45
– – suture **2**: 8, 24
– part of duodenum → Inferior part of
  duodenum
– – – nasalis muscle **2**: 28–30
– pericardial sinus **2**: 104, 123, 130, 143
– perineal ligament **2**: 266–267
– planes **1**: 5
– pontine fibers **2**: 340
– process of atlas **1**: 30–31, 49, 55, 59–60;
  2: 37, 72, 289
– – – axis **1**: 30
– – – coccyx **1**: 35
– – – first thoracic vertebra **2**: 37
– – – vertebra **1**: 29–32, 35–37, 42, 47, 51;
  2: 33, 37, 72, 74–75, 284
– ridges of sacrum **1**: 9, 34
– sinus **2**: 289, 291, 294, 359, 362, 409
– temporal gyri **2**: 323, 338, 345
– vesical fold **1**: 77
Transversus abdominis muscle **1**: 54, 58, 65–69,
  76–77, 194, 227–228; **2**: 196, 211, 220–221,
  225, 228
– thoracis muscle **1**: 68, 76
– vaginae muscle **2**: 250–251, 265
Trapezium **1**: 8, 92–94, 102–104, 123, 129
Trapezius muscle **1**: 52–54, 60, 62–64, 97, 105,
  111–112, 148–149; **2**: 30, 32–37, 73–75, 81,
  92–93, 98
Trapezoid **1**: 8, 92–94, 102–104, 129
– ligament **1**: 95–96, 107
– line of clavicle **1**: 84
Triangular fossa of auricle **2**: 390
– fovea of arytenoid cartilage **2**: 64
– part of inferior frontal gyrus **2**: 316
– recess **2**: 307, 320
– space **1**: 106, 110–111, 140, 143

Triceps brachii muscle **1**: 52, 62, 95, 101,
  105–119, 141–149, 152–154
– surae muscle **1**: 203, 207, 211–213, 215–216,
  221, 230, 232–234, 240–241, 255, 267–268,
  276–277, 279
Tricuspid valve **2**: 104, 132, 134–135, 140,
  159–160
Trigeminal cave **2**: 294
– cavity → Trigeminal cave
– cistern **2**: 295
– ganglion **1**: 22; **2**: 84, 86, 89, 293, 295, 301,
  306, 380
– impression **2**: 20, 399–400
– nerve [V] **1**: 22; **2**: 32, 34, 37, 82–84, 86–89,
  284, 289, 291–295, 306, 309, 311, 341, 344,
  352, 359, 380, 382
– tubercle **2**: 310–311
Trigone of bladder **2**: 235, 237
– – hypoglossal nerve → Hypoglossal trigone
– – lateral lemniscus **2**: 311
– – vagus nerve → Vagal trigone
Triquetrum **1**: 8, 92–94, 102, 104, 123, 129, 159
Triticeal cartilage **2**: 65–67
Trochanter tertius → Third trochanter
Trochanteric bursa of gluteus maximus muscle
  1: 223–224, 256
– – – – medius muscle **1**: 224
– fossa **1**: 180, 194
Trochlea of humerus **1**: 86, 90–91, 98, 100–101,
  149
– – superior oblique muscle **2**: 370–371,
  381–383
– – talus **1**: 184, 187–188, 210–211
Trochlear fovea **2**: 367–368
– nerve [IV] **1**: 22; **2**: 88, 284, 289, 291–295,
  306, 310–311, 379–382
– notch of ulna **1**: 89–91, 99
True conjugate **1**: 178
– pelvis → Lesser pelvis
Trunk **1**: 14, 40, 61–65, 68, 78, 134, 154–155,
  244
– of accessory nerve **2**: 100
– – atrioventricular bundle **2**: 140
– – corpus callosum **2**: 300, 307, 317, 325,
  337–341, 344–345, 360
– – spinal nerve **1**: 23, 48; **2**: 95, 166, 285–286
Tubal branch(es) of ovarian artery **2**: 241
– – – uterine artery **2**: 241, 245
– extremity of ovary **2**: 239–240
Tuber cinereum **2**: 301, 306–307, 315, 330–331,
  334–335
– of vermis of cerebellum **2**: 307
Tuberal nuclei of hypothalamus **2**: 328
Tubercle of fifth metacarpal bone **1**: 94
– – rib **1**: 41, 44; **2**: 75
– – scaphoid **1**: 94, 102, 123, 130
– – trapezium **1**: 94, 102–103
– – upper lip **2**: 44
Tuberculum of iliac crest **1**: 256
– sellae **2**: 10
Tuberosity for coracoclavicular ligament **1**: 84
– – serratus anterior muscle **1**: 44
– of cuboid **1**: 186
– – distal phalanx of foot **1**: 186
– – – – – hand **1**: 94
– – fifth metatarsal bone **1**: 186, 188, 232
– – navicular **1**: 186, 188, 279
– – radius **1**: 88, 90–91, 100
– – ulna **1**: 89, 99
Tunica albuginea of corpora cavernosa **2**: 275,
  278
– – – corpus spongiosum **2**: 275

Tunica albuginea of
– – – testis **2**: 270–271
– – vaginalis testis **1**: 67; **2**: 170, 270–274
Tympanic canaliculus **2**: 20, 393, 402
– cavity **2**: 11, 361, 391, 393–394, 396, 398–400,
  402, 405–407
– cells **2**: 396
– membrane **2**: 17, 89, 391–392, 398–400, 405
– nerve **2**: 89, 393
– opening of pharyngotympanic tube **2**: 398
– part of temporal bone **2**: 20, 391–392
– plexus **2**: 89, 398
– ring **2**: 17
– sulcus **2**: 396
– surface of cochlear duct **2**: 404
Tympanomastoid fissure **2**: 20

U

Ulna **1**: 8, 82–83, 89–94, 98–105, 116–119, 122,
  125, 129–130, 135, 139, 142, 149–150,
  154–158
Ulnar artery **1**: 123, 138–139, 152–153, 155,
  157–163, 165
– collateral ligament of elbow joint **1**: 98–99
– – – – wrist joint **1**: 102, 104
– head of flexor carpi ulnaris muscle **1**: 117
– – – pronator teres muscle **1**: 115–117
– nerve **1**: 113, 117, 123, 128, 132–134,
  140–143, 145–147, 150–154, 156–162,
  164–165; **2**: 93–94, 149
– notch of radius **1**: 88, 92
– recurrent artery **1**: 138–139, 143, 153
– styloid process **1**: 89, 92, 94, 99, 102, 105
– tuberosity → Tuberosity of ulna
– veins **1**: 164
Umbilical artery(-ies) **1**: 12–13; **2**: 230, 234,
  243–246
– cord **1**: 13; **2**: 242–243
– hernia **1**: 63
– region **1**: 4, 65, 75, 77
– ring **1**: 63
– vein **1**: 13; **2**: 243
Umbilicus **1**: 12–13, 63–65, 75; **2**: 172, 196, 202,
  209, 243
Umbo of tympanic membrane **2**: 392, 398
Uncinate fasciculus **2**: 333
– gyrus **2**: 317, 325
– process of cervical vertebra → Uncus of body
  of cervical vertebra
– – – ethmoidal bone **2**: 22, 55–56
– – – head of pancreas **2**: 188, 199, 202
– – – vertebral body → Uncus of body of
  cervical vertebra
Uncus **2**: 315, 324–325, 333–334
– of body of cervical vertebra **1**: 30–31
Unpaired thyroid venous plexus **1**: 14; **2**: 149
Upper abdomen **2**: 171, 182, 191, 198–199, 203,
  208, 222–223
– accessory renal artery **2**: 162, 214
– arm → Arm
– eyelid → Superior eyelid
– limb **1**: 74, 82–83, 105, 132–134, 138–139,
  244
– lip **2**: 44–45, 52, 55
– lobe of left/right lung → Superior lobe of
  left/right lung
– part of trunk **2**: 154–155
– pleura-free triangle **2**: 150
– pole of testis **2**: 270
– trunk of brachial plexus → Superior trunk of
  brachial plexus

Urachus **1**: 13; **2**: 246
Ureter **1**: 14, 17–20, 77; **2**: 162, 199, 208–214, 216–218, 223, 230, 234–236, 238–239, 241, 244–246, 248, 251, 261, 276
Ureteric nerve plexus **2**: 248–249
– orifice **1**: 17; **2**: 232–233, 235, 237, 246, 250
Urethra **1**: 17, 20–21; **2**: 170, 232–233, 235–237, 243, 250, 257–260, 266–267, 275–278
Urethral artery **2**: 267
– crest **2**: 235, 277
– hiatus **2**: 266
– lacunae **2**: 277
Urinary bladder **1**: 12–13, 16–18, 20–21, 77, 194; **2**: 163, 170, 172, 193, 202, 204, 206, 211, 217–218, 220–221, 232–238, 242–247, 250, 252, 254, 256–261, 276–278
– system **1**: 17; **2**: 218, 232–233
Urogenital diaphragm → Deep perineal pouch
– hiatus of pelvic diaphragm **2**: 264–265
– system **1**: 17; **2**: 232–233
Uterine artery **2**: 241, 245–247, 251
– cavity **1**: 17; **2**: 233, 240, 242, 252, 256–257
– extremity of ovary **2**: 239–240
– horn **2**: 240
– ostium of tube **2**: 240
– part of tube **2**: 240
– tube **1**: 17; **2**: 163, 172, 233, 238–241, 245, 250–252
– vein(s) **2**: 251
Uterosacral ligament → Recto-uterine ligament
Uterus **1**: 17; **2**: 163, 172, 233, 238–243, 245–247, 250–252, 256–257, 260, 268
Utricle **2**: 405
Utricular nerve **2**: 405
– recess of bony labyrinth → Elliptical recess of bony labyrinth
Utriculo-ampullary nerve **2**: 405
Utriculosaccular duct **2**: 405
Uvula of bladder **2**: 235
– – palate **2**: 13, 38–39, 45, 50–52
– – vermis of cerebellum **2**: 307–309

V

Vagal part of accessory nerve → Cranial root of accessory nerve
– trigone **2**: 310–311
Vagina **1**: 17; **2**: 233, 239–240, 243, 245, 251, 256–257, 260, 268–269
Vaginal artery **2**: 245
– branch of uterine artery **2**: 241
– fornix **2**: 233, 240, 256–257
– orifice **2**: 265, 268–269, 280
– part of cervix of uterus **1**: 17; **2**: 233, 239–240, 251, 268
– process of peritoneum **2**: 272–273
– – – sphenoidal bone **2**: 19, 23
– rugae **2**: 233, 240, 269
– venous plexus **2**: 251
Vagus nerve [X] **1**: 22, 25, 51; **2**: 33–35, 37, 75, 82, 93, 96–97, 100, 149, 167, 248–249, 284, 289, 291–292, 294–295, 306, 311, 340
Vallate papillae **2**: 39, 46, 101
Vallecula of cerebellum **2**: 308
Valve of coronary sinus **2**: 132, 140
– – foramen ovale **2**: 133
– – inferior vena cava **2**: 132, 140
Variations in form of stomach **2**: 173
– – position of vermiform appendix **2**: 178
– of coronary arteries of heart **2**: 144–145
– – orifices of bile and pancreatic ducts **2**: 187
– – renal artery **2**: 214

Vas deferens → Ductus deferens
– spirale **2**: 404
Vascular circle of optic nerve **2**: 372–373
– lamina of choroid **2**: 373
– space **1**: 219
Vasto-adductor membrane **1**: 219, 252–253
Vastus intermedius muscle **1**: 220, 229, 253, 258–264
– lateralis muscle **1**: 216–217, 219, 223–224, 226, 229, 231–232, 252–253, 255–256, 259–264; **2**: 228
– medialis muscle **1**: 216, 219, 221, 229, 231, 252–253, 258–260, 262–264; **2**: 228
Vein(s) of abdomen **2**: 218
– – anterior abdominal wall **1**: 77
– – – region of elbow **1**: 140
– – arm **1**: 137, 140
– – axilla **1**: 73; **2**: 93, 149
– – brain **2**: 300
– – caudate nucleus **2**: 300
– – dorsal body wall **2**: 162
– – dorsum of foot **1**: 278
– – eyeball **2**: 372–373
– – face **2**: 80
– – gluteal region **1**: 255–257
– – head **2**: 80
– – heart **2**: 142–143
– – leg **1**: 267–268
– – lower limb **1**: 246–247
– – male pelvis **2**: 234, 244
– – mediastinum **2**: 149, 164
– – neck **2**: 93, 97–99, 149, 164
– – orbit **2**: 383
– – perineum **2**: 279–280
– – peripharyngeal space **2**: 100
– – popliteal fossa **1**: 255–256, 267–268
– – posterior abdominal wall **2**: 228
– – retroperitoneal organs of upper abdomen **2**: 203
– – sheath of optic nerve **2**: 373
– – shoulder **1**: 140
– – spinal cord **2**: 286–287
– – thigh **1**: 252, 255–256; **2**: 228
– – thorax **1**: 76; **2**: 93, 97
– – tongue **2**: 97
– – trunk **1**: 14
– – upper limb **1**: 137
– – ventral body wall **1**: 75
– – vertebral column **2**: 286–287
Vena comitans of hypoglossal nerve **2**: 99
Venous angle **1**: 15
– sinuses of cranial dura mater → Dural venous sinuses
– valve(s) **1**: 73, 246–247
Ventral **1**: 5
– anterior nucleus of thalamus **2**: 327
– body wall **1**: 75–76
– corticospinal tract → Anterior corticospinal tract
– funiculus of spinal cord → Anterior funiculus of spinal cord
– horn of spinal cord → Anterior horn of spinal cord
– intermediate nucleus of thalamus **2**: 327
– median fissure of medulla oblongata → Anterior median fissure of medulla oblongata
– median fissure of spinal cord → Anterior median fissure of spinal cord
– muscles of trunk **1**: 62–65, 68
– nuclei of thalamus **2**: 326–327, 331, 344
– paraflocculus → Tonsil of cerebellum

Ventral
– posterior nuclei of thalamus **2**: 340
– posterolateral nucleus of thalamus **2**: 327
– posteromedial nucleus of thalamus **2**: 327
– ramus(-i) of cervical nerves → Anterior rami of cervical nerves
– – – lumbar nerves → Anterior rami of lumbar nerves
– – – sacral nerves → Anterior rami of sacral nerves
– – – spinal nerve → Anterior ramus of spinal nerve
– – – thoracic nerves → Intercostal nerves
– root of spinal nerve → Anterior root of spinal nerve
– rootlets of spinal nerve → Anterior rootlets of spinal nerve
– spinocerebellar tract → Anterior spinocerebellar tract
– spinothalamic tract → Anterior spinothalamic tract
– white commissure of spinal cord → Anterior white commissure of spinal cord
Ventricles of brain **2**: 320
Ventricular system of brain **2**: 320
Ventrolateral sulcus of medulla oblongata → Anterolateral sulcus of medulla oblongata
– – – spinal cord → Anterolateral sulcus of spinal cord
Ventromedial nucleus of hypothalamus **2**: 328
– – – spinal cord → Anteromedial nucleus of spinal cord
Vermiform appendix **1**: 16, 18–19; **2**: 172, 177–178, 193, 195, 202–204, 238
Vermis of cerebellum **2**: 306–309, 322, 334, 342–343, 345, 348, 350–353, 356–359, 409
Vertebra(e) **1**: 28–33, 36–39, 42–43, 47–48, 50–51, 55; **2**: 284, 286–287, 289
– prominens [C VII] **1**: 28, 31, 37, 40, 60
Vertebral arch **1**: 29–30, 33, 47, 60; **2**: 284–286
– artery **1**: 14, 51, 60; **2**: 33, 68, 72–75, 77–79, 96–97, 100, 118, 162, 286, 289, 291–292, 294–295, 298–299, 301–302
– body **1**: 7, 29–33, 35–40, 43, 46–48, 51, 55; **2**: 71–72, 158–161, 287, 294
– – of axis **1**: 30, 36, 51; **2**: 72, 294
– canal **1**: 22, 39–40, 46–47, 50, 60; **2**: 74, 158, 160–161, 243, 253, 284–285, 289
– column **1**: 28, 30–39, 42–43, 46–51; **2**: 161
– foramen **1**: 30–33, 47
– ganglion **2**: 96, 167
– region **1**: 4
– vein **2**: 68, 73, 75, 165, 286
Vertex **2**: 6
Vertical axes **1**: 5
– muscle of tongue **2**: 47
Vesical retinaculum **2**: 246
– surface of uterus **2**: 242
– venous plexus **2**: 250, 254, 276
Vesico-uterine pouch **1**: 17; **2**: 233, 238, 243, 247, 260
Vesicular appendix of epoöphoron **2**: 239
– ovarian follicle(s) **2**: 245
Vestibular aqueduct **2**: 405
– area **2**: 310
– canaliculus **2**: 20, 400–402
– fold **2**: 52, 68
– fossa of vagina **2**: 269
– ganglion **2**: 405
– labyrinth **2**: 400
– ligament **2**: 66, 68

Vestibular
– lip of limbus of osseous spiral lamina **2**: 404
– membrane → Vestibular surface of cochlear duct
– nerve **2**: 399, 405
– surface of cochlear duct **2**: 404
– – – tooth **2**: 39–40
Vestibule **2**: 400–402, 406
– of vagina **2**: 233, 250–251, 268–269
Vestibulocochlear nerve [VIII] **1**: 22, 51; **2**: 284, 289, 291–292, 294–295, 306, 308–309, 311, 340, 399, 405, 408–409
Vincula tendinum of digits of hand **1**: 124
Virgin **2**: 269
Visceral afferent nerve fiber(s) **1**: 23, 79
– efferent nerve fiber(s) **1**: 23, 79
– layer of serous pericardium **2**: 104, 123–125, 132–134, 142–143, 154
– – – synovial sheath **1**: 10
– – – tunica vaginalis testis **2**: 270–271, 274
– peritoneum **2**: 171, 176, 232
– pleura **2**: 115, 151, 154–157
– surface of liver **2**: 181, 184, 191, 204
– – – spleen **2**: 189
Viscerocranium **2**: 369
Visual area(s) of cerebral cortex **2**: 319, 322, 335, 346
– pathway **2**: 335
Vitreous body **2**: 374, 384–385
Vocal fold **2**: 52, 68
– ligament **2**: 66
– process of arytenoid cartilage **2**: 64, 68
Vocalis muscle **2**: 68
Vomer **2**: 8, 12–17, 23, 58, 395
Vomerovaginal groove **2**: 19
Vorticose vein(s) **2**: 372–373, 381
V-phlegmona **1**: 131
Vulva → Pudendum

W

Waldeyer's ring **2**: 45
Wall of pharynx **2**: 45–51
Ward's triangle **1**: 7
White laminae of cerebellum **2**: 309
– matter/substance of cerebellum **2**: 309, 334
– – – cerebrum **2**: 289, 338
– – – spinal cord **2**: 285
– ramus communicans of spinal nerve **1**: 23, 79; **2**: 96, 166–167, 285
Wing of central lobule of cerebellum **2**: 308
– – ilium → Ala of ilium
– – sacrum → Ala of sacrum
Wisdom tooth/teeth → Third molar tooth/teeth
Wrist **1**: 92–94, 103–105, 123, 129–131
– joint **1**: 82–83, 102, 104, 159

X

Xiphisternal joint **1**: 45
Xiphoid process **1**: 40–41, 45, 62, 64, 68; **2**: 150

Y

Yellow bone marrow **1**: 10

Z

Zenker's diverticulum → Pharyngo-esophageal diverticulum
Zona fasciculata of cortex of suprarenal gland **2**: 216
– glomerulosa of cortex of suprarenal gland **2**: 216
– incerta **2**: 340
– orbicularis of hip joint **1**: 192

Zona
– reticularis of cortex of suprarenal gland **2**: 216
Zone(s) of hyperalgesia of inner organs **1**: 79
– – – kidney **2**: 209
Zonular fibers **2**: 374–375, 377
– spaces **2**: 374–375, 377
Zygapophysial joint **1**: 36, 48, 51, 55; **2**: 75, 289
Zygomatic arch **2**: 6, 8, 31, 48, 58, 368
– bone **2**: 4, 6, 14–17, 26, 48, 58–59, 62–63, 367–368
– branches of facial nerve **2**: 84–85, 98–99, 383
– margin of greater wing of sphenoidal bone **2**: 19
– nerve **2**: 82–86, 88, 379–380
– process of frontal bone **2**: 4, 21, 58, 367
– – – maxilla **2**: 8, 24
– – – temporal bone **2**: 20, 26, 399
Zygomaticofacial branch of zygomatic nerve **2**: 82–83, 85–86, 379
– foramen **2**: 4, 6, 26, 367–368
Zygomaticomaxillary suture **2**: 4, 6, 8, 367–368
Zygomatico-orbital artery **2**: 76, 85, 98
Zygomaticotemporal branch of zygomatic nerve **2**: 82–83, 85, 379
Zygomaticus major muscle **2**: 28–30, 32, 48, 85, 98, 366
– minor muscle **2**: 28–30, 32, 366